The Health Professional's Guide to
Gastrointestinal Nutrition

Laura E. Matarese, PhD, RDN, LDN, CNSC, FADA, FAND, FASPEN,
Gerard E. Mullin, MD, CNSP, FACN, AGAF, and
Janice L. Raymond, MS, RDN, CD, CSG

Editors

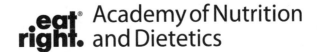

eat right. Academy of Nutrition and Dietetics

Cathy Iammartino, Publisher

Elizabeth Nishiura, Manager of Production and Digital Content Development

The Health Professional's Guide to Gastrointestinal Nutrition

Laura E. Matarese, Gerard E. Mullin, and Janice L. Raymond, Editors

ISBN 978-0-88091-450-5

10 9 8 7 6 5 4 3 2

For more information on the Academy of Nutrition and Dietetics, visit: www.eatright.org

Contents

PART VI: THERAPEUTIC INTERVENTIONS FOR GASTROINTESTINAL DISORDERS

About the Editors

Laura E. Matarese, PhD, RDN, LDN, CNSC, FADA, FAND, FASPEN

Laura Matarese is an associate professor of Medicine in the Division of Gastroenterology, Hepatology, and Nutrition, Department of Internal Medicine, the Brody School of Medicine at East Carolina University in Greenville, NC. She is the author of numerous books, chapters, articles, abstracts, and videos and currently serves on the editorial boards of several journals. She has lectured extensively, both nationally and internationally, and has held numerous positions within the Academy of Nutrition and Dietetics and the American Society for Parenteral and Enteral Nutrition.

Dr. Matarese is the past president of the National Board of Nutrition Support Certification. She currently serves on the Board of Trustees of the Oley Foundation and as a commissioner for the Commission on Dietetic Registration. She is the recipient of numerous honors and awards, including the American Dietetic Association Medallion Award; the American Dietetic Association Foundation Award for Excellence in the Practice of Clinical Nutrition; the American Society for Parenteral and Enteral Nutrition (A.S.P.E.N.) Awards for Distinguished Achievement in Nutrition Support Dietetics, Excellence in Nutrition Support Education, and Advanced Clinical Practice (first recipient); and the Dietitians in Nutrition Support Distinguished Service Award.

Gerard E. Mullin, MD, CNSP, FACN, AGAF

Gerard Mullin is an associate professor in the Department of Medicine at the Johns Hopkins Hospital. He is an internist, gastroenterologist, and nutritionist. Dr. Mullin is nationally and internationally renowned for his work in integrative gastroenterology and nutrition. He has accumulated over 20 years of clinical experience in the field of integrative gastroenterology and earned his master's degree in nutrition while in practice.

In 2009 Dr. Mullin was named an honorary member of the American Dietetic Association (now the Academy of Nutrition and Dietetics). He is an associate editor of multiple nutrition and integrative medicine journals and serves on several certification exam committees and boards. Dr. Mullin has authored and edited a number of books in nutrition and integrative medicine (http://thefoodmd.com/books). He has been interviewed on radio and television and has contributed to many stories in the print media. Dr. Mullin's biography has been included in Marquis and Covington's *Who's Who* numerous times, and he has been selected as one of America's Top Physicians since 2004.

Janice L. Raymond, MS, RDN, CD, CSG

Janice Raymond has a diverse background in dietetics practice. She has worked in research, critical care, foodservice management, outpatient services, long-term care, and home infusion. Ms. Raymond has held appointed and elected positions with the Academy of Nutrition and Dietetics at both the state and national levels. She has authored numerous peer-reviewed publications and contributed chapters to several books. She currently works for Thomas Cuisine Management as director of Clinical Nutrition Services at Providence Health Care in Seattle, WA, and has an affiliate faculty appointment at Bastyr University. Janice is the coeditor of *Krause's Food and the Nutrition Care Process*, 13th and 14th editions.

Contributors

Mary Jo Alberino, RD, CNSC
Registered Dietitian
Center for Gut Rehabilitation
    and Transplant Center
Cleveland Clinic
Cleveland, OH

Therese L. Austin, MS, RD, LD, CNSC
Infusion Dietitian
Coram Specialty Infusion Services
Cleveland, OH

Kathy T. Barco, RD, CNSC
Outpatient Clinical Dietitian
Cleveland Clinic
Cleveland, OH

Nora Rahn Baumgart, MS, RD, CNSC
Physician Assistant Student
Northwestern University
Feinberg School of Medicine
Chicago, IL

Amy C. Brown, PhD, RD
Associate Professor, Complementary and
    Alternative Medicine
John A. Burns School of Medicine
University of Hawaii
Honolulu, HI

Karen M. Buzby, RD, LDN
Clinical Dietitian Specialist
Metabolic and Bariatric Surgery Program
Penn Medicine
Philadelphia, PA

Annette M. Carpenter, RD, CNSC
Senior Clinical Nutrition Specialist
Medstar Washington Hospital Center
Washington, DC

Jennifer R. Carter, RD, CNSC
Clinical Nutrition Manager
Valley Health Systems
Winchester Medical Center
Winchester, VA

Yolanda Cartwright, PhD, RD
Medical Writer/Independent Consultant
Flossmoor, IL

Bani Chander Roland, MD
Assistant Professor of Medicine
Division of Gastroenterology and Hepatology
The Johns Hopkins School of Medicine
Baltimore, MD

Gail A. Cresci, PhD, RD, CNSC
Associate Staff, Department of Gastroenterology
    and Pathobiology
Assistant Professor of Medicine, Cleveland Clinic
    Lerner College of Medicine
Cleveland Clinic
Cleveland, OH

Sheila E. Crowe, MD, FRCPC, FACP, FACG, AGAF
Director of Research
Division of Gastroenterology, Department
    of Medicine
University of California, San Diego
San Diego, CA

Amy K. Fischer, MS, RD
Registered Dietitian
New York, NY

Barbara J. Goodin, MS, RD, CDE
Pediatric Nutrition Specialist
Department of Pediatrics, Division of Genetics
University of Virginia Health Sciences Center
Charlottesville, VA

James H. Grendell, MD
Professor of Medicine, State University of New York
    at Stony Brook School of Medicine
Chief, Division of Gastroenterology, Hepatology,
    and Nutrition, Winchester University Hospital
Mineola, NY

Tiffani Lynn Hays, MS, RD, LDN
Director of Pediatric Nutrition
Johns Hopkins Children's Center
Baltimore, MD

Mary E. Hise, PhD, RD, CNSC
Director, Global Medical Affairs
Baxter Healthcare
Deerfield, IL

Mary Margaret Huizinga, MD, MPH
Assistant Professor of Medicine
Vanderbilt University School of Medicine
Nashville, TN

Hossam M. Kandil, MD, PhD
Associate Professor and Chief
Division of Gastroenterology, Hepatology,
    and Nutrition
Brody School of Medicine
East Carolina University
Greenville, NC

Jennifer C. Lefton, MS, RD, CNSC, FAND
Clinical Nutrition Specialist
Medstar Washington Hospital Center
Washington, DC

John Leung, MD
Director of Food Allergy Center at Tufts Medical
    Center and Floating Hospital for Children
Department of Gastroenterology, Department of
    Pediatric Gastroenterology, Department of Allergy
    and Immunology, Tufts Medical Center
Boston, MA

Suzanne M. Lugerner, MS, RN, LDN, CNSC, CNS
Director, Clinical Nutrition
Medstar Washington Hospital Center
Washington, DC

Angela A. MacDonald, DCN, RD, CNSC
Consultant Dietitian
Sombra, ON

Mary J. Marian, MS, RD, CSO
Clinical Dietitian and Instructor, University
    of Arizona
Consultant for Arizona Oncology
Tucson, AZ

Neha R. Parekh, MS, RD, LD, CNSC
Intestinal Transplant Coordinator
Cleveland Clinic Center for Gut Rehabilitation
    and Transplant
Cleveland, OH

Carol Rees Parrish, MS, RD
Nutrition Support Specialist
University of Virginia Health System, Digestive Health
    Center
Charlottesville, VA

S. Devi Rampertab, MD, FACG, AGAF
Assistant Professor of Medicine
Rutgers—Robert Wood Johnson Medical School
New Brunswick, NJ

Monica L. Riegert, MSN, DNP, CRNP
Nurse Practitioner
The Johns Hopkins University
Baltimore, MD

Kristen M. Roberts, MS, RD, LD
GI Nutrition Specialist
ThriveRX
Cincinnati, OH

Carol J. Rollins, MS, PharmD, RD, BCNSP, FASPEN
Coordinator, Nutrition Support Team, University of Arizona Medical Center
Associate Professor, College of Pharmacy, University of Arizona
Tucson, AZ

Carolyn Coker Ross, MD, MPH
Clinical Assistant Professor of Medicine
University of Arizona Medical Center
Center for Integrative Medicine
Denver, CO

Denise Baird Schwartz, MS, RD, CNSC, FADA, FAND, FASPEN
Nutrition Support Coordinator
Providence Saint Joseph Medical Center
Burbank, CA

Karen M. Sexton-Hamilton, MS, RD, LD, CNSC
Director, Nutrition Services and Programs
Coram Healthcare
Moscow, PA

Sunita Sidhu-Buonocore, MD

Arlene Stein, MS, RD, CDN, CNSD
Nutrition Support Dietitian
Department of Gastroenterology, Hepatology, and Nutrition
Winchester University Hospital
Mineola, NY

Jenifer L. Thompson, MS, RD, LDN, CSP
Advance Practice Dietitian
Johns Hopkins Children's Center
Baltimore, MD

Dawn McDowell Torres, MD
Transplant Hepatologist/Chief of Hepatology
Walter Reed National Military Medical Center
Bethesda, MD

Jodi Wolff, MS, RD, LD, CNSC
Pediatric Clinical Dietitian
Rainbow Babies and Children's Hospital
UH Case Medical Center
Cleveland, OH

Acknowledgments

Success is rarely achieved in isolation, and this book is no exception. I would like to offer my sincerest thanks to my coeditors, Dr. Gerry Mullin and Janice Raymond, for their vision, efforts, and perseverance during the production of this book. It has been an honor and privilege to work with them. This book would not have been possible without the extraordinary assistance and guidance we received from Elizabeth Nishiura from the Academy of Nutrition and Dietetics. She worked tirelessly to see this book through production and provided us with superb publishing and editorial guidance. I would like to thank Cathy Iammartino and Barbara J. Visocan, also from the Academy, for their ability to make things happen. Thank you as well to Dr. Marion Winkler for writing the Foreword.

Rarely do people have the opportunity to publicly acknowledge the individuals in their life who have provided inspiration, support, and guidance to them. First, to my family and friends who tolerated my many absences while I finished this book, I thank you. I am grateful to my many multidisciplinary colleagues who over the years have become dear friends, many of whom contributed chapters. The best part of volunteerism is the lasting friendships that are cultivated. I would also like to acknowledge a number of physicians who have influenced and mentored me over the course of my career. In particular, I acknowledge and appreciate the opportunities and insights afforded to me by Drs. Richard E. Miller, Josef E. Fischer, Ezra Steiger, and Kareem Abu-Elmagd. I consider myself to be fortunate and privileged to have an exceptional Chief, Dr. Hossam Kandil, and appreciate the continued encouragement, support, and wisdom that I receive from him daily.

Finally, a very special, sincere, and heartfelt thanks goes to the patients who have allowed me to care for them. I have learned a great deal from them over the course of my career. They were and remain an inspiration to me, professionally and personally.

Laura E. Matarese, PhD, RDN, LDN, CNSC, FADA, FAND, FASPEN

My sincere thanks to my coeditors, Dr. Laura Matarese and Janice Raymond, for their support and outstanding editorial management. My deepest appreciation to Elizabeth Nishiura from the Academy of Nutrition and Dietetics publishing team for her tireless efforts to make this book possible. Thank you to the Academy of Nutrition and Dietetics for conferring upon me honorary membership as well as for providing collaboration and support. I also express my gratitude to the many experts whose exceptional contributions made this book possible and to Dr. Marion Winkler who contributed the Foreword.

There are many individuals I would like to recognize for shaping my career and sparking my interest in gastroenterology and nutrition. Thank you to my mentors who have guided my career over the years—in particular, Drs. Anthony Kalloo, Andrew Weil, Victoria Maizes, and Ben Caballero. Thank you as well to the nutritionists whose collaborations have fostered my career development and friendships over the years: Drs. Laura Matarese, Carol Ireton-Jones, Mark DeLegge, Steve McClave, Kelly Tappenden, Jeanette Hassee, Deborah Rubin, Alan Buchmann, Tim Lipman, Ron Koretz, and Amy Brown, and

Ms. Kathy Swift. A special thank you to those who have supported my clinical practice at Johns Hopkins: my medical office assistant, Julie McKenna-Thorpe; Ms. Erin O'Keefe and Ms. Abena Carr-Walker; nurse clinician Kimberly Kidd-Watkins; administrators Lisa Bach-Burdsall and Nathan Smith; administrative director Tiffany Boldin; Dr. Myron L. Weisfeldt, chairman of medicine at Johns Hopkins; and Dr. Linda A. Lee, clinical director of the Johns Hopkins Division of Gastroenterology and Hepatology.

Gerard E. Mullin, MD, CNSP, FACN, AGAF

Thanks go first to Laura Matarese and Gerard Mullin for inviting me to participate as an editor of this book. To be associated with two such renowned individuals is truly an honor. I would like to express my gratitude to the editorial staff at the Academy of Nutrition and Dietetics; their expertise and support was invaluable. I sincerely appreciate the many chapter contributors, who spent countless hours writing and editing so that others may benefit by their expertise.

Many people have shared their knowledge and wisdom with me over the years. I would like to particularly thank James Becker, MD, who was my real mentor in the area of gastroenterology. Kathleen Mahan, RDN, and Sylvia Escott-Stump, RDN, who invited me to become an editor of *Krause's* nutrition textbook, changed my life forever, and without them I would not be a part of this endeavor. Finally, I cannot forget to thank my always supportive family.

Janice L. Raymond, MS, RDN, CD, CSG

Thank you to the following manuscript reviewers: Alan P. Agins, PhD; Tracy Burch, RD, CNSC; Anne Cox, MS, RD, CSO; Tracie M. Dalessandro, MS, RD, CDN; Erin Fennelley, RD, LD, CNSC; Trisha Fuhrman, MS, RD, LD, CNSC, FADA; Michelle L. Henry, MPH, RD; Laura A. Jeffers, MEd, RD, LD; Patti Landers, PhD, RD, LD; Julie O'Sullivan Maillet, PhD, RD, FADA; Ainsley M. Malone, MS, RD, LD, CNSC; Marcia Nahikian-Nelms, PhD, RD, LD; Patti H. Perks, MS, RD, CNSC; Brandis Roman, RD, CNSC; Karen Schmidt, RD, CSP; Rebecca A. Weseman, RD, LMNT, CNSC; and Marion F. Winkler, PhD, RD, LDN, CNSC, FASPEN.

Foreword

The intestine is an amazing organ and is central to the study of nutrition. With a length that is often compared to a football field and an absorptive capacity nearly the size of a tennis court, this dynamic and elaborate organ is essential in nutrient digestion and absorption and vital for the regulation of the immune system. Home to thousands of bacterial species, the intestine is a physiologic biome shedding new light on our understanding of health, disease, inflammation, and obesity. Dysregulation or a subtle imbalance in this delicate system can wreak havoc in the body, and intestinal dysfunction and disease can significantly affect the ability to eat and enjoy food, and ultimately influence quality of life. The intense focus on the intestinal microflora and the environmental milieu in the intestine is expected to increase our understanding of disease and set the stage for the future development of innovative therapeutic strategies.

The practice of clinical nutrition goes hand-in-hand with the anatomy and physiology of the gastrointestinal (GI) system. Understanding the relationship between food and health requires comprehensive knowledge of the science of nutrient digestion, absorption, metabolism, and elimination. The interrelationship between the two fields, nutrition and gastroenterology, has led to the development of textbooks targeting clinical nutrition education to gastroenterologists. Yet, the converse, publications that educate dietetics professionals about gastroenterology, is less common. *The Health Professional's Guide to Gastrointestinal Nutrition,* edited by esteemed colleagues Laura Matarese, Gerard Mullin, and Janice Raymond, fills this unique niche. These distinguished professionals combine their expertise in nutrition, gastroenterology, hepatology, internal medicine, intestinal failure, complementary and alternative care, and the Nutrition Care Process and sustainable food delivery systems to produce a scholarly and practical text. Their humanism and patient-centered approach to care is evident while delivering a well-referenced and research-based guide for practitioners. The profound wisdom of Hippocrates (420 BC), "Our medicine should be food, and food should be our medicine," is evident throughout.

The content of this book is central to everything I do on a daily basis in the nutrition care and management of patients and clients. For years, I have lugged a heavy satchel across the hospital campus from the office to the clinic and to the classroom, filled with needed resources, patient educational materials, food lists, and references. As I read *The Health Professional's Guide to Gastrointestinal Nutrition,* it was increasingly clear that this book contains everything I need, and more, in one comprehensive volume. The editors, in collaboration with 40 distinguished practitioners and authors, have created a superb guide to relevant GI pathophysiology, current research, diagnostic criteria, treatment plans, practice points, and evidence-based guidelines for GI disorders, liver and exocrine disorders, GI oncology and surgery, and systemic disorders. From assessment to therapeutic interventions, this easy-to-read book provides brief narratives, key facts, anatomic illustrations and figures, tables, algorithms, charts, and references. Interesting contributions include obesity, eating disorders, food allergy and intolerances, drug-nutrient interactions with GI drugs, nutraceutical supplements, probiotics, and ethical and legal issues. Enteral and parenteral nutrition for adults and pediatrics in the hospital and home are included; in addition, there is extensive coverage of food-related topics, strategies for management of treatment-related symptoms, food choices to manage diarrhea, and food source tables for phytochemicals and cancer prevention, fat, dietary fiber, and FODMAPs.

Dietetics practitioners and other health care professionals must be cognizant of and address nutrition and quality-of-life issues. In my research, the definition of *quality of life* includes "being able to eat what you want to eat, when you want to eat it." Frequently, patients and clients suffer from life-altering GI symptoms and distress, and many experience enormous challenges around eating and enjoyment of food. Often left to trial-and–error interventions, severe dietary restrictions, or avoidance of food altogether, these patients comprise a group of individuals who greatly benefit from collaborative practice by dietetics professionals and gastroenterologists. As recommended in one of the chapters, "a careful dietary history to discern whether food intolerances are provoking symptoms" is an essential component of care. This book combines the knowledge-, evidence-, and practice-based wisdom of expert clinicians and educators in the disciplines of nutrition and gastroenterology. If the GI tract excites you, this book is great reading. I plan to use the material for patient counseling, for dietetics training, and as a core for our fellows in Gastroenterology. *The Health Professional's Guide to Gastrointestinal Nutrition* will not sit on my bookshelf; rather, it will accompany me on my daily rounds.

Marion F. Winkler, PhD, RD, LDN, CNSC, FASPEN
Associate Professor of Surgery
Surgical Nutrition Specialist
Alpert Medical School of Brown University
Rhode Island Hospital
Providence, RI

Preface

At the opening of Chapter 5: Small Intestine Malabsorptive Disorders, our colleagues Parrish, Baumgart, and Goodin observe, "The process of digestion and absorption is a complex cascade of events. As with most other physiologic processes, it is not appreciated until it goes awry." In this concise statement, these authors identify two of the primary concerns of *The Health Professional's Guide to Gastrointestinal Nutrition*. This book is intended to help registered dietitian nutritionists (RDNs) and other health care providers understand both the "complex cascade of events" involved in digestion and absorption and the many ways that this process can "go awry." At the same time, the book is also a practice-oriented guide to what RDNs, physicians, and allied health professionals can do to help identify, alleviate, and/or resolve the nutritional problems that affect the quality of life of our patients.

Part I: Gastrointestinal Anatomy, Diagnostics, and Assessment comprises four chapters that introduce basic and essential concepts in gastrointestinal (GI) nutrition and foreground the discussion in the subsequent parts of the book. The descriptions and illustrations in Chapter 1 can serve an "atlas" of the anatomy of the GI tract and the accessory digestive organs. Chapter 2 surveys many tests and procedures used to diagnose and evaluate GI problems, explaining clearly and succinctly how these tools are used and what they can and cannot tell us about a patient's health status. Chapters 3 and 4 address the important topic of nutrition assessment—the first step in the Nutrition Care Process—as it relates to the care of individuals with GI disorders and those who are critically ill.

Part II: Nutrition and Gastrointestinal Tract Disorders includes six chapters. The first two provide broader reviews of malabsorptive disorders (Chapter 5) and GI symptoms (Chapter 6), whereas the latter four examine specific GI tract diseases: inflammatory bowel disease (Chapter 7), short bowel syndrome (Chapter 8), irritable bowel syndrome (Chapter 9), and celiac disease (Chapter 10). Part III: Nutrition and Liver and Exocrine Disorders has separate chapters covering diseases of the liver and pancreas (Chapters 11 and 12, respectively). In both Part II and Part III, readers will find a wealth of information on disease etiologies, symptoms, diagnostic techniques, and nutritional implications. These chapters also offer practical suggestions about selecting nutrition interventions that are appropriate for specific patients.

Part IV: Gastrointestinal Oncology and Surgery has three chapters, on oncology (Chapter 13), GI tract surgeries (Chapter 14), and bariatric procedures (Chapter 15). In each chapter, the contributors explore how these medical interventions are used to address serious health problems but can also have significant consequences (sometimes lifelong ones) for the nutritional well-being of patients. As in Parts III and IV, the chapters in Part IV feature research- and evidence-based insights into nutrition assessment and intervention strategies. Additionally, the illustrations in Chapter 14: Gastrointestinal Tract Surgery and Chapter 15: Bariatric Surgery can help readers understand how surgical procedures alter digestion and absorption.

Part V: Systemic Disorders and Specific Populations covers obesity, eating disorders, and food allergy and food intolerance. Chapter 16 identifies what we know (and don't know) about several weight loss strategies, including energy- and macronutrient-restricted diets. Given the impact that excess weight can have on health outcomes for our patients, this information is of considerable relevance. The chapter on eating disorders (Chapter 17) presents the latest DSM-V diagnostic criteria (2013) and discusses the role of the RDN on the interdisciplinary team caring for the patient with anorexia nervosa, bulimia nervosa, binge eating disorder, or another type of eating disorder. The final chapter in this part (Chapter 18) emphasizes the crucial distinctions between food allergy and food intolerance and explains the diagnosis and management of various adverse reactions to foods.

Part VI: Therapeutic Interventions for Gastrointestinal Disorders includes eight chapters. The first four (Chapters 19–22) focus on nutrition support, including the uses of enteral and parenteral nutrition in adult and pediatric patients as well as the special challenges of administering nutrition support in the home care setting. The information in these chapters complements and expands upon the coverage of nutrition support interventions for specific GI disorders found in many of the earlier chapters of this book. Chapter 23 is a quick guide to drug-nutrient interactions that may occur with the medications used to treat GI disorders. The next two chapters examine the uses of nutraceutical supplements (Chapter 24) and probiotics (Chapter 25) to treat GI and liver disorders. Although further scientific investigation of these therapies is needed, these chapters can help readers separate the more promising options from those that have not demonstrated efficacy. Finally, Chapter 26 frames the ethical and legal issues that health care professionals may face when providing GI nutrition interventions, particularly when a patient or authorized caregiver chooses to refuse artificial nutrition and hydration. The Appendix to this book lists more information on ethical and legal topics.

There are many ways to use this book. You may wish to start at the beginning and read this book from cover to cover. Alternatively, we encourage you to turn first to the chapters that are most relevant to the types of care you provide or begin with the topics that are least familiar to you. Whatever your strategy, we hope that you find *The Health Professional's Guide to Gastrointestinal Nutrition* to be an essential and helpful professional resource.

Laura E. Matarese, PhD, RDN, LDN, CNSC, FADA, FAND, FASPEN
Gerard E. Mullin, MD, CNSP, FACN, AGAF
Janice L. Raymond, MS, RDN, CD, CSG

PART I

Gastrointestinal Anatomy, Diagnostics, and Assessment

CHAPTER 1

The Gastrointestinal System

Gerard E. Mullin, MD, CNSP, FACN, AGAF,
and Monica L. Riegert, MSN, DNP, CRNP

The gastrointestinal (GI) system extends from the mouth to the anus. It digests and absorbs food, provides a physical and immunologic barrier, and participates in many regulatory, metabolic, and immunologic functions. It is generally categorized as follows:

- The upper GI tract: mouth, esophagus, stomach, and duodenum
- The lower GI tract: jejunum, ileum, colon, rectum, and anus
- Accessory digestive organs: salivary glands, liver, pancreas, and gallbladder

The Mouth and Oral Phase of Digestion

The mouth—containing teeth, tongue, and salivary glands that facilitate digestion in the oral phase—is where the digestion process initiates. The oral phase of digestion involves the following:

- Teeth mechanically break down food.
- Salivary glands produce and release saliva to moisten food; amylase in saliva breaks down starch.
- The tongue begins the pharyngeal phase of swallowing.

Swallowing

The act of swallowing includes a series of three phases:

1. In the *oral phase,* food is placed in the mouth and combined with saliva, chewed if necessary, and formed into a bolus by the tongue.
2. In the *pharyngeal phase,* the bolus of food is moved involuntarily to the back of the mouth. The soft palate then elevates to close off the nasopharynx to prevent the bolus from entering the respiratory tract.

3. The *esophageal phase* is the final stage, during which peristaltic waves continue to move the bolus through the esophagus into the stomach. The lower esophageal sphincter must relax to allow the bolus to pass into the stomach.

Stomach and the Gastric Phase of Digestion

The term *gastric* refers to the stomach, which is a pouch-like structure that receives food from the esophagus. In normal-weight individuals, the stomach is approximately the size of a clenched fist. Once a bolus of food enters the stomach, the bolus is broken down both mechanically and chemically into a thick liquid known as *chyme*. Gastric acids, hormones, and digestive enzymes are secreted by glands in the stomach walls to aid digestion:

- *Hydrochloric acid (HCl)* is produced by the parietal cells in the lining of the stomach. The acidic pH inhibits bacteria. Mucous is secreted by the goblet cells in the stomach. This mucous protects the stomach lining that could otherwise be damaged by the gastric acids, bile, ingested chemicals, and enzymes.
- *Pepsin* is a protease or proteolytic enzyme that is produced and released by the chief cells of the stomach.
- *Intrinsic factor,* a glycoprotein secreted by the epithelial cells in the stomach, is necessary for absorption of vitamin B-12.
- *Gastrin* is a gastric hormone that stimulates secretion of HCl and pepsinogen (the precursor of pepsin) and increases gastric motility.

Four major anatomical sections comprise the stomach:

- The first portion of the stomach, the *cardiac region,* is situated directly below the lower esophageal sphincter (LES) and receives contents from the esophagus as it empties into the stomach.
- The *fundus* comprises the stomach's upper curvature and body (ie, the central region of the stomach).
- The *antrum* is located below the body of the stomach and is distinguishable from the other regions of the stomach by the absence of rugae (gastric folds).
- The most distal section of the stomach, the *pylorus,* has two parts: the *pyloric antrum,* which is situated directly below the body of the stomach, and the *pyloric canal*—the narrowest section of the stomach—which connects to the small intestine at the duodenum and serves as the control mechanism in the process of gastric emptying. Chyme remains in the pyloric canal until it is broken down to the appropriate consistency that allows it to pass into the small intestine via the pyloric sphincter.

After food is processed in the stomach, it passes into the small intestine, where most digestion and absorption occurs (see Figure 1.1).

The Small Intestine

The small intestine is the longest portion of the digestive tract, measuring approximately 6 meters (20 feet) in the average adult. Millions of finger-like projections, called *villi,* that are critical for absorption are

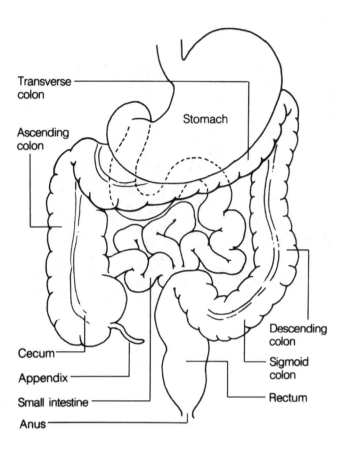

FIGURE 1.1 Stomach and intestines. Source: National Cancer Institute. NCI Visuals Online. http://visualsonline .cancer.gov/details.cfm?imageid=1768. Accessed October 28, 2013.

found throughout the entire lining of the small intestine (see Figure 1.2 on page 6). *Microvilli* and *capillary beds* are found on each of the villi. The microvilli are microscopic projections that house brush-border cells containing many digestive enzymes. Before the bloodstream transports absorbed nutrients to the liver via the hepatic portal vein, those nutrients pass through the capillary beds for filtering, processing, and distribution to the rest of the body.

Myriad microscopic folds populate the entire small intestine to maximize absorption. Two types of folds found in the intestinal wall are *rugae* and *plicae circulares*. The small intestine can extend and contract as necessary because the rugae provide extra tissue, where plicae circulares are fixed ridges on the intestinal wall. Along with the villi and microvilli, these intestinal folds maximize the digestion and nutrient absorption processes by markedly increasing the available surface area of the small intestine. The small intestine comprises three sections: the duodenum, jejunum, and ileum. Each section performs distinct functions in the digestion process.

- The *duodenum* is the first segment of the small intestine, connected to the stomach at the pylorus. The duodenum is approximately 26 cm (9.8 in) long and is the site of cholecystokinin release. *Cholecystokinin* stimulates pancreatic secretion of enzymes and causes the contraction of the gallbladder. *Secretin,* which is also released in the duodenum, increases the pancreatic output

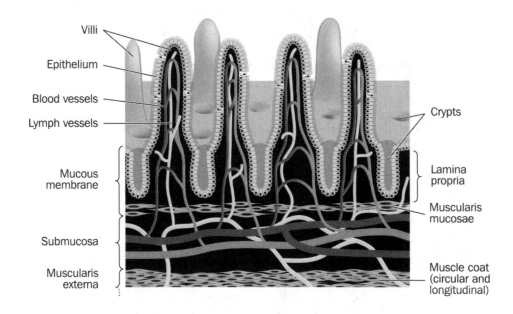

FIGURE 1.2   Small intestinal villi. Source: © Can Stock Photo Inc. www.canstockphoto.com.

of water and bicarbonate. In the duodenum, carbohydrates, proteins, and fats are broken down into monosaccharides, amino acids, glycerol, and fatty acid chains. Bile is released from the gallbladder, which emulsifies fats to allow for absorption.

- The next segment of the small intestine, the *jejunum,* is where most of the absorption process occurs. It is 2.5 meters (8.2 feet) in length. Absorption is complex, combining the intricate process of active transport with the simple process of passive diffusion. *Active transport* moves ions or other substances, in combination with a transport protein, across a membrane against an energy gradient. *Passive diffusion* is the random movement through openings in or between the membranes of the mucosal cell walls. *Facilitated diffusion* is movement that requires a carrier protein, and *pinocytosis* occurs when an epithelial cell membrane engulfs a small drop of intestinal contents. It allows large particles such as whole proteins to be absorbed in small quantities.

- The final segment of the small intestine, the *ileum,* is where residual absorption occurs. The ileum is approximately 3.5 meters (11.5 feet) in length. It absorbs vitamins, electrolytes, and other nutrients that passed unabsorbed through the jejunum while selectively absorbing vitamin B-12 and bile salts.

Large Intestine

Three main parts—the cecum, the colon, and the rectum—comprise the large intestine, which is approximately 1.5 meters (5 feet) long (see Figure 1.1, earlier in this chapter).

- Food from the small intestine is transported first to the *cecum,* a small pouch at the end of the large intestine, via the terminal ileum.
- The two main functions of the *colon* are to absorb water and electrolytes that remain in the material passing through it and to compress the remaining contents into a bolus to facilitate

excretion from the body. The colon is divided into the ascending colon, the transverse colon, and the descending colon. The *ascending colon* extends straight to the liver's lower border from the cecum. The *transverse colon* spans from the border of the liver to the border of the spleen. The *descending colon* is routed downward and connects to the S-shaped sigmoid colon, which is connected to the rectum.

- The *rectum* is the final portion of the large intestine, which serves as a reservoir for stool until it is excreted though the anus. This excretion is regulated by the anal sphincter. When pressure is detected in the rectum, involuntary smooth muscle relaxation of the internal anal sphincter and voluntary skeletal muscle contraction and relaxation of the external anal sphincter allow for the passage of stool out of the body.

Accessory Digestive Organs

Accessory organs—specifically, the pancreas, liver, and gallbladder—are not direct components of the digestive tract but have important functions in the GI system by aiding the digestion process (Figure 1.3).

Pancreas

The *pancreas* is an elongated gland located behind the stomach. It connects to the duodenum via the pancreatic duct. The pancreas has both endocrine and exocrine functions. The endocrine pancreatic function does not play a direct role in digestion; rather, it assists in regulating blood glucose levels through

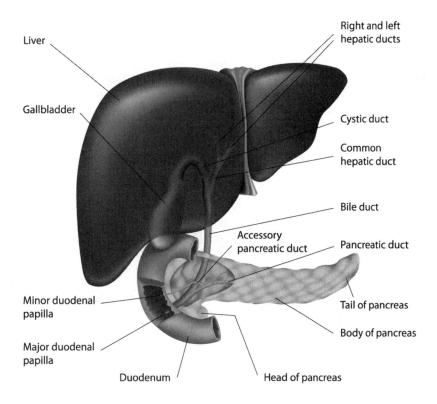

FIGURE 1.3 Liver, gallbladder, pancreas, and bile passage. Source: © Can Stock Photo Inc. www.canstockphoto.com.

insulin production. The exocrine pancreatic function includes the synthesis of digestive juices—containing sodium bicarbonate; amylase; lipase; and trypsin and chymotrypsin, which are major proteases—that are secreted into the small intestine via the pancreatic duct.

- *Sodium bicarbonate* keeps the intestinal system at a neutral pH by neutralizing acidic material from the stomach.
- *Amylase* breaks down carbohydrates into monosaccharides.
- *Lipase* breaks down fats into glycerol and fatty acid chains.
- *Proteases* break down proteins into amino acids.

Liver

The largest gland in the human body, the *liver* is located just below the diaphragm in the right upper quadrant of the abdomen. Among its numerous vital functions in the body, the liver's most direct role in the digestion and detoxification processes involves its secretory and excretory functions, particularly in the synthesis and secretion of bile. Once the liver has synthesized bile, that bile is transported to and stored in the gallbladder.

Gallbladder

The liver transports bile, which enables enzymatic breakdown of fats via emulsification, to the *gallbladder*, a pear-shaped sac located under the liver. Until bile is released to the small intestine by way of the common bile duct, it is concentrated and stored in the gallbladder.

Conclusion

The anatomy and physiology of the digestive tract and accessory organs are essential to the understanding of disorders of maldigestion and malabsorption of nutrients. The pathophysiology of many disease processes is best understood in context of the anatomy and physiology of the GI system.

Sources

Berkow R, Beers MH, eds. *The Merck Manual of Medical Information.* 2nd ed. Whitehouse Station, NJ: Merck; 2003.

Copstead-Kirkhorn LC, Banasik JL. *Pathophysiology,* 4th ed. St. Louis, MO: Saunders; 2009.

Mahan LK, Escott-Stump S, Raymond JL. *Krause's Food and the Nutrition Care Process.* 13th ed. St. Louis, MO: Elsevier; 2013

Porth CM, Matfin G. *Pathophysiology: Concepts of Altered Health States,* 8th ed. Philadelphia, PA: Wolters Kluwer Health: Lippincott Williams & Wilkins; 2008.

CHAPTER 2

Gastrointestinal Tests and Procedures

Gerard E. Mullin, MD, CNSP, FACN, AGAF,
and Amy K. Fischer, MS, RD

This chapter reviews the relevance and importance of gastrointestinal (GI) tests to the diagnosis and treatment of GI nutritional disorders. Disorders relating to the GI tract are considered digestive disorders (see Chapter 1). "Good" digestive health is described as an ability to process nutrients through properly functioning GI organs, including the stomach, intestine, liver, pancreas, and gallbladder. When these organs do not function properly, patients may need to consult a gastroenterologist for further testing and diagnosis (1).

Many different types of disorders can affect the digestive system and require GI testing. These disorders may include (1):

- Colorectal cancer (see Chapter 13)
- Irritable bowel syndrome (IBS; see Chapter 9)
- Inflammatory bowel disease (IBD), including Crohn's disease and ulcerative colitis (see Chapter 7)
- Diverticulitis
- Diverticulosis
- Ischemic bowel disease
- Celiac disease (see Chapter 10)
- Heartburn and gastroesophageal reflux disease (GERD)
- Gastroparesis
- Functional illnesses, such as constipation, diarrhea, vomiting, belching, and flatulence (see Chapter 6)
- Peptic ulcer disease
- Gallbladder disease
- Nutritional deficiencies
- GI infections from viruses, bacteria, fungi, and protozoa
- Obesity (see Chapter 16)

Finally, if the patient is unable to be sustained on an oral diet but is able to absorb nutrients, a feeding tube can be placed by the gastroenterologist. For more information on enteral nutrition, refer to Chapters 19, 21, and 22.

Upper Endoscopy

An upper endoscopy (also known as *endoscopy, gastroscopy,* or *esophagogastroduodenoscopy* [EGD]) is a procedure that allows a physician to examine the lining of the upper GI tract, including the esophagus, stomach, and duodenum (first portion of the small intestine) (2,3). The procedure is used to visually examine the upper digestive system by passing a flexible tube (with a light and tiny camera on the distal end) into the esophagus. This tube, known as an *endoscope,* can view, photograph, and biopsy and can identify inflammation, erosions, ulcerations, changes in blood vessels, and destruction of surface cells (2,3).

Upper endoscopy procedures are used for many different indications, including the following (1,2):

- Removal of stuck objects, including food
- Detection of ulcers, abnormal growths, precancerous conditions, bowel obstruction or inflammation, and hiatal hernias
- Treatment of bleeding ulcers
- Tissue biopsy
- Determination of the cause of abdominal pain, nausea, vomiting, swallowing difficulties, gastric reflux, unexplained weight loss, or bleeding in the upper GI tract

Preparation and Procedure

The upper GI tract must be empty before the procedure; the patient should not eat or drink anything during the 8 hours before the test. Before the procedure, patients should discuss all health conditions, medications, and vitamins they are taking. Prior to the procedure, patients are sedated. Physicians may numb the patient's throat with a local anesthetic spray before the procedure.

During the procedure, the patient lies on his or her back or side on an examining table. The endoscope is carefully passed through the mouth and down the esophagus into the stomach and duodenum. The camera on the endoscope transfers images of the intestinal lining to a monitor. Air pumped through the endoscope inflates the stomach and duodenum to make it easier to see. During this procedure, the physician can perform biopsies, stop bleeding, and remove abnormal growths (1).

Risks

Risks associated with upper endoscopy include adverse reactions to sedatives, bleeding from the biopsy site, and accidental puncture of the GI tract (1,2).

Colonoscopy

Colonoscopy is used to see inside the rectum and detect inflamed tissue, abnormal growths, and early signs of colorectal cancer. It also used to investigate potential causes of changes in bowel habits, abnormal pain, bleeding from the anus, and weight loss. Colonoscopy is considered the criterion standard for detecting colorectal cancers and adenoma (4–6).

Preparation and Procedure

To prepare for the colonoscopy, patients typically follow a clear liquid diet for 1 day, unless there is a history of constipation and/or known slow gut transit, in which case the recommended duration of bowel preparation is 2 days. After preparation, all solids must be emptied from the GI tract before the procedure. Acceptable liquids include fat-free bouillon, strained fruit juice, water, plain coffee, plain tea, sport drinks, and gelatin. The day prior to the procedure, the patient must have consumed only clear liquids and then consume some form of purgative (low-volume sodium phosphate purge or high-volume polyethylene glycol purge). A laxative or enema may be required the night before a colonoscopy. Because sedation is administered, patients cannot drive after the procedure and should be accompanied by another individual to escort them home. Recovery time for the patient is approximately 2 to 3 hours (1,7).

During a colonoscopy, the patient is placed on his or her left side. A long flexible lighted tube known as a *colonoscope* is inserted into the anus and slowly guided through the rectum into the colon. The scope inflates the large intestine with carbon gas and a camera is mounted on the scope. Once the camera reaches the small intestine, it is slowly withdrawn and the large intestine is examined again. During the procedure, the physician can remove growths and polyps to detect signs of colorectal cancer. Routine colonoscopy should typically begin at age 50 years; starting earlier may be recommended for people with a history of colorectal cancer or inflammatory bowel disease (5,6).

Risks

Colonoscopy risks include severe abdominal pain, bowel perforation, fever, bloody bowel movements, dizziness, and weakness. The removal of polypoid growths increases the aforementioned risks, as does the presence of widespread colonic diverticulosis or severe colitis. Rare complications include splenic or hepatic trauma and splenic rupture.

Flexible Sigmoidoscopy

A flexible sigmoidoscopy is an internal examination of the lower large bowel/colon and rectum using a flexible sigmoid scope. The test can help diagnose the causes of a bowel obstruction; diarrhea; colon polyps; diverticulitis; inflammatory bowel disease; blood, mucus, or pus in stool; and colorectal cancer. Normal findings show that the lining of the sigmoid colon, rectal mucosa rectum, and anus are normal in color, texture, and size. Abnormal results may indicate anal fissures, anal rectal abscesses, bowel construction, cancer, colorectal polyps, diverticulitis, hemorrhoids, inflammatory bowel disease, inflammation, and proctitis.

Preparation and Procedure

The morning of the procedure, the patient should consume a light breakfast. One hour before the procedure, one to two saline enemas are required. The examination can be done in a physician's office or in the hospital. Sedation is not administered, and the patient usually experiences some tolerable abdominal pain (6,7).

During sigmoidoscopy, the patient lies on his or her left side with his or her knees drawn toward the chest. First, the physician performs a digital rectal exam to enlarge the anus for the sigmoidscope. Next, a 60-cm flexible sigmoidscope is inserted into the rectum; air is introduced into the colon to expand the area and may cause the urge to have a bowel movement. The sigmoidscope is usually inserted to the sigmoid colon or descending colon. The scope is used to observe the lining of the bowel, and a hollow channel in the center of the scope allows the physician to take biopsies. The procedure usually takes 7 to 15 minutes. The patient may return to ordinary daily activities immediately after the procedure (6,7).

Risks

The risk of complications is very low. Rare side effects include bowel perforation and bleeding at biopsy site (6,7).

Capsule Endoscopy Procedures

Capsule endoscopy is used to see regions of the small intestine that cannot be reached in an endoscopy. The use of capsule endoscopy procedures is indicated in the diagnosis of obscure GI bleeding, iron-deficiency anemia, and intestinal malabsorption of unclear significance. Capsule endoscopy is also used for screening and surveillance of polyps in familial polyposis syndromes, to assess suspected Crohn's disease without intestinal obstruction, and to stage celiac disease (8).

Wireless Capsule Endoscopy

A wireless capsule endoscopy is a wireless miniature camera that is swallowed by the patient. As it makes its way through the digestive tract, the endoscopy captures pictures of the GI mucosa. Wireless capsule endoscopy is used for the following (8,9):

- To investigate potential cause(s) of obscure GI bleeding following a negative upper and lower endoscopy. Capsule endoscopy has a diagnostic yield of 65% of detecting the cause of occult GI bleeding.
- To diagnose small bowel Crohn's disease (see Chapter 7).
- Assessment of celiac disease extent and activity throughout the small intestine (see Chapter 10).
- Screening and surveillance for polyps in familial polyposis syndromes.

PREPARATION AND PROCEDURE

The patient prepares for the endoscopy in the same manner as for a colonoscopy. The procedure is done using an 11 × 26 capsule endoscope, a device that consists of an optical dome, four light-emitting electrodes, a sensor, two batteries, and a microtransmitter.

The capsule acquires and transmits digital images at the rate of two per second to a sensor array attached to the patient's abdomen. It is able to capture video images of the mucosal surface of the entire length of the small intestine directly. The procedure is virtually pain-free because the capsule is propelled forward through the GI tract by peristalsis (9,10).

The patient can engage in normal daily activities after the procedure. Also, the patient can eat a normal diet 4 hours after ingesting the capsule; however, if the patient has delayed gastric emptying, that can interfere with the test (8,11).

RISKS

There is a risk of capsule retention or entrapment in strictures or diverticula. Presence of intestinal obstruction, fistulas, or strictures may impede the excretion of the capsule and can cause a bowel obstruction. Capsule endoscopy is contraindicated in patients with known strictures or swallowing disorders. Patients with extensive small bowel Crohn's, those who chronically use nonsteroidal anti-inflammatory drugs, and those with abdominal radiation injury are at higher risk of capsule retention (8,11).

Small bowel series have been used by clinicians to look for strictures and determine whether the capsule will safely pass through the small intestine and into the colon. However, a negative small bowel series does not exclude a stricture and has been associated with a number of capsule retentions. The history of obstructive symptoms or a prior history of intestinal surgery is more predictive of a capsule retention than a negative small bowel series.

SmartPill Capsule

The SmartPill is a wireless, ingestible capsule that measures pressure, pH, and temperature data at regular intervals as it travels through the GI tract. Gastric emptying and whole GI tract transit can be assessed. The information gathered also helps diagnose gastroparesis and other GI motility disorders such as slow transit constipation (11,12).

PREPARATION AND PROCEDURE
The preparation for the SmartPill is a standard overnight fast. On the day of the study, all patients are given a standardized SmartBar bar (255 kcal, 75% carbohydrate, 21% protein, 3% fat, and 3% fiber) just before they ingest the SmartPill. They are then expected to fast for 6 hours, with the exception of small quantities of water (up to ½ cup).

RISKS
The only potential risk is capsule retention in the setting of a stricture in the GI tract.

BRAVO pH Capsule

The Bravo pH monitoring system is a catheter-free pH test used to measure and monitor acid reflux in the setting of GERD. The Bravo pH monitoring system uses a small pH capsule that is attached to the esophageal wall during a standard upper endoscopy and transmits pH data every 12 seconds to a small receiver unit via radiofrequency telemetry for 48 hours (11,13). The BRAVO is used to either diagnose GERD or determine whether medical therapy is working to prevent acid reflux.

PREPARATION AND PROCEDURE
Preparation for a BRAVO procedure is the same as for a standard upper endoscopy—ie, overnight fast. For the procedure, the patient either sits or lies down while the physician places the capsule into the esophagus. After the capsule is in place, suction is applied, drawing a small amount of tissue into the capsule and locking it into place. The pH recording starts immediately after the application of the capsule and continues for 48 hours, transmitting pH measurements wirelessly to a small receiver worn by the patient on a waistband or belt. Patients are instructed to keep a diary and record mealtimes, position changes, and the time and type of their symptoms. They are encouraged to pursue their daily activities and diet. On completion of the procedure, the patient returns the recording device to the physician, who uploads the data. The capsule is disposable and passes naturally through a bowel movement within a few days after the test (11,13).

RISKS
Risks of this procedure include the following (13):

- Premature detachment of the pH capsule
- Failure of the capsule to detach from the esophagus within a few days after placement
- Tears in the mucosal and submucosal layers of the esophagus, causing bleeding
- Perforation

Enteroscopy

The small bowel can be a difficult area to examine due to its anatomy, location, and relative tortuosity. Because the small intestine is 18 to 22 feet in length, conventional endoscopy cannot provide adequate visualization. Enteroscopy is the use of scopes to examine the small intestine (14–16). There are several different types of enteroscopes.

Push Enteroscopy

Push enteroscopy is one of the most frequently used endoscopic methods for small bowel examination. It is usually considered the next diagnostic step in the evaluation of a patient with obscure GI bleeding after a negative endoscopy and colonoscopy (3,8). Indications for push enteroscopy include the following:

- Determining the cause of malabsorption
- Determining the cause of unexplained diarrhea
- Diagnosing refractory celiac disease
- Determining the cause of unexplained GI bleeding

PREPARATION AND PROCEDURE
Patients should not take products containing aspirin for 1 week before the procedure. They should also tell doctors if they are taking blood thinners such as warfarin (Coumadin) or clopidogrel (Plavix), because these medications can interfere with the test. Patients should follow a liquid diet the day before the procedure, and they may consume clear liquids up to 4 hours before the exam. A numbing medication is usually administered to reduce a gagging feeling that patients may experience when the tube is inserted into the mouth.

A thin, flexible tube (endoscope) is inserted through the mouth and is advanced into the proximal jejunum. The patient must remain alert to swallow and turn during the procedure, so only a mild sedative can be administered. Push enteroscopy is an outpatient procedure, done under conscious sedation, and lasts between 15 and 45 minutes. The patient may experience mild cramping (1,8).

RISKS
Risks are rare and include the following (8):

- Excessive bleeding at the biopsy site
- Bowel perforation
- Infection of the biopsy site
- Vomiting

Double-Balloon and Single-Balloon Enteroscopy

The main uses for balloon enteroscopy are to visualize the small bowel and perform diagnostic and therapeutic procedures. The double-balloon enteroscopy, also known as the *push-and-pull enteroscopy*, allows for visualization of the entire small intestine, tissue sampling, and therapeutic intervention (14,15). Single-balloon enteroscopy was designed to mimic the functions of double-balloon enteroscopy. The single balloon system looks just like double-balloon enteroscopy except that it lacks a balloon at the tip of the endoscope (14,15).

Patients prepare for this procedure in the same way as for capsule endoscopy and colonoscopy. During a double-balloon enteroscopy, balloons are attached to the endoscope and are inflated to allow the physician to view the large part of the small intestine (1).

The main risks for balloon enteroscopy procedures are related to the administration of anesthesia, possible perforation of the intestine, and bleeding.

Endoscopic Retrograde Cholangiopancreatography

Endoscopic retrograde cholangiopancreatography (ERCP) is used to diagnose and treat problems in the liver, gallbladder, bile ducts, and pancreas, including gallstones, inflammatory strictures (scars), leaks (from trauma and surgery), and cancer (1).

Preparation and Procedure

The stomach and duodenum must be empty to obtain accurate results. Patients should not consume any food or beverages after midnight the night before the procedure or 6 to 8 hours beforehand.

X-rays and an endoscope are used in the procedure. The patient lies on his or her left side on an examining table in an X-ray room. Medication is administered to numb the back of the throat, and a sedative is given before the exam. The patient swallows the endoscope, and the physician guides the scope through the esophagus, stomach, and duodenum until it reaches the location where the ducts of the biliary tree and pancreas open into the duodenum. At this time, the patient will be turned to lie flat on his or her stomach and the physician will pass a small plastic tube through the scope. Dye is injected into the ducts to allow visualization by X-ray. X-rays are taken immediately after the dye injection. In the case of a gallstone obstructing the ducts, instruments can be inserted into the scope to remove or relieve the obstruction. A biopsy can be done for further testing.

ECRP requires 30 minutes to 2 hours to complete. Patients may experience discomfort when air is blown into the duodenum and dye is injected into the ducts. This discomfort can generally be managed with sedation and mild pain medication. Tenderness or lump at the site of sedative injection usually subsides within in a few days.

Risks

Risks of ERCP include pancreatitis and, less commonly, infection, bleeding, and perforation of the duodenum (1).

Motility Procedures

Disorders of gastric motor function include impaired accommodation, gastroparesis, and dumping syndrome (17–19). The symptoms that occur in patients with gastric motor disorders are nonspecific, and they consist of poor appetite, postprandial fullness, and bloating, nausea, vomiting, epigastric pain, and early satiety (inability to finish a normal-size meal).

GI motility and functional bowel diseases include achalasia, scleroderma, GERD, gastroparesis, functional dyspepsia, irritable bowel syndrome, colonic inertia, pelvic floor dyssynergia, and fecal incontinence (19,20).

Esophageal Motility Study

Esophageal motility study or esophageal manometry is a procedure used to evaluate lower- and upper-esophageal sphincter pressure, esophageal body contraction amplitude, and peristaltic sequence. The procedure is useful in evaluating patients with dysphagia, unexplained or noncardiac chest pain, or symptoms suggestive of GERD. It is also used to assess patients prior to antireflux surgery. The two manometric methods used are the low-compliance water-perfused catheter system and the solid-state pressure system (12,21). The preparation for this procedure involves an overnight fast, and the main risk is discomfort to the patient during the procedure.

Anorectal Motility Study

Anorectal manometry is a test to evaluate patients with fecal incontinence and constipation. The test measures the pressure of the anal sphincter muscles together with an assessment of rectal sensation, recto-anal reflexes, and rectal compliance (21,22).

PREPARATION AND PROCEDURE

The patient should use one or two enemas 2 hours before the procedure. No food or liquids should be consumed during the 2 hours prior to the procedure. Regular medications and water are allowed up to 2 hours prior to the exam. Patients who are allergic to latex should inform the physician of this allergy before the test so that a latex-free balloon can be used.

The procedure lasts approximately 30 minutes. The patient lies on his or her left side. A small flexible tube with a balloon on the end is inserted into the rectum. The small balloon is attached to a catheter that may be inflated in the rectum to assess the normal reflex pathways. The physician or nurse may request that the patient squeeze, relax, and push at various times throughout the exam to measure the anal sphincter muscle pressures (21,22).

Two other tests may be done: (*a*) an anal sphincter electromyography (EMG) to evaluate the nerve supply to the anal muscles and (*b*) a balloon expulsion test to measure the time it takes to expel a balloon from the rectum (21,22). Anal sphincter EMG is recorded with a small plug electrode placed in the anal canal. The patient is asked to relax, squeeze, and push at different times. The anal sphincter muscle electrical activity is recorded and displayed on a computer screen. Anal sphincter EMG confirms the proper muscle contractions during squeezing and muscle relaxation during pushing. Normal anal EMG activity with low anal squeeze pressures on manometry may indicate a torn sphincter muscle that can be repaired (21,22). The test is used to look for defects in anal sphincter smooth muscle dysfunction.

In a balloon expulsion test, a small balloon is inserted into the rectum and inflated with water. The patient then tries to defecate (expel) the small balloon from the rectum. The amount of time it takes to expel the balloon is recorded. Prolonged balloon expulsion suggests a dysfunction in the anorectum area (22). The patient can drive after the procedure and resume normal activities.

RISKS

Anorectal manometry is a safe procedure with minimal risks and is unlikely to cause any pain. The main risk is discomfort to the patient during the procedure. Rare complications include a perforation (tearing) or bleeding of the rectum (23).

Gastric Emptying

Gastroparesis is impaired gastric motility that results in delayed or irregular contractions of the stomach, leading to various GI symptoms, such as early satiety, bloating, nausea, vomiting, diarrhea, or constipation. Tests used to evaluate a patient with impaired gastric emptying include upper endoscopy, barium X-ray, and ultrasound to rule out obstructions or mucosal or structural disorders. Once other causes are ruled out, SmartPill tests, gastric emptying scintigraphy, and breath tests can be done to diagnose gastroparesis (24).

As described earlier in this chapter, the SmartPill is a small wireless device in capsule form that can be swallowed. For a gastric emptying scintigraphy, the patient eats a meal consisting of eggs that contain a small amount of radioisotope, a radioactive substance that shows up on scans. The scan measures the rate of gastric emptying at 1, 2, 3, and 4 hours. When more than 10% of the meal is still in the stomach at 4 hours, the diagnosis of gastroparesis is confirmed.

For a breath test, the patient ingests a meal containing a small amount of isotope; then breath samples are taken to measure the presence of the isotope in exhaled carbon dioxide. The results reveal how fast the stomach is emptying.

Feeding Tubes

Feeding tubes provide nutrition support to patients who cannot take food by mouth or who cannot eat enough to support their nutritional needs (see Chapter 19 for more information on enteral nutrition). Percutaneous endoscopic gastrostomy (PEG), jejunal extension through a PEG (gastrojejunostomy), or direct endoscopic jejunostomy is appropriate when nutrition support will be required for more than 3 weeks. Short-term tube feeding is generally managed by placing a nasoenteric tube (25,26).

Percutaneous Endoscopic Gastrostomy (PEG)

PEG is a nonsurgical procedure that places a feeding tube through the skin and abdominal wall, directly into the stomach, with an endoscope. Appropriate indications for PEG placement include esophageal obstruction, head and neck cancer, dysphagia, and supplemental nutrition during chemotherapy or radiation (27).

PREPARATION AND PROCEDURE

A patient prepares for this procedure by fasting overnight, as for an upper endoscopy, and receives a dose of intravenous antibiotics according to physician preference.

During an upper endoscopy, the endoscopist must first demonstrate the transillumination of light across the abdominal wall to ensure that no overlying bowel is present. After successful transillumination, an incision is made on the abdominal wall under sterile conditions after local anesthesia. A thin wire is introduced though the incision and into the stomach under visualization and then delivered externally though the oral cavity. The gastrostostomy tube is delivered over the wire placed via a push-and-pull technique. Successful placement is confirmed via visualization with the endoscopy. The gastrostostomy tube is secured to the abdominal wall externally with a fastener then dressed with gauze at the conclusion of the procedure. The procedure takes 15 to 20 minutes.

The gastrostomy tube can be used once the patient is discharged from the endoscopy unit. Use of a PEG feeding tube can be temporary or permanent, depending on the medical condition. The lifespan of the tube is about 1 year. Replacement gastrostomy tubes that use a balloon inflation system can be used when the original tube has to be replaced (25,26).

Protocols for immediate postplacement care of the tube should be implemented to ensure that the feeding tube site is kept clean and the feeding tube is kept patent. If the tube is accidentally dislodged, the physician should be contacted immediately and the tube should be replaced within 24 hours to prevent the incision from closing (25).

RISKS

Minor complications include leakage of food or fluid around the tube. Mild bleeding or infection may occur at the incision site.

Percutaneous Endoscopic Jejunostomy (PEJ)

A percutaneous endoscopic jejunostomy (PEJ) tube, also known as a jejunostomy tube, is surgically implanted in the upper section of the small intestine (jejunum) just below the stomach. The PEJ bypasses the stomach and the patient is fed directly into the intestinal tract. The placement of a PEJ tube is indicated in patients with the following (25,28):

- Unsuitable stomach access
- High risk for aspiration
- Gastric resection (partial or total)
- Gastric pull-up, gastric outlet obstruction, or obstructed or nonfunctioning gastrojejunostomy
- Gastric dysmotility
- Gastroparesis
- Stenosis
- Previous esophageal surgery

PREPARATION AND PROCEDURE

Preparation is the same as for an upper endoscopy (an overnight fast). Although it is similar to PEG placement, direct endoscopic jejunostomy placement is considerably more difficult. If necessary, the tube can be secured in place with sutures by a physician. The skin surrounding the tube should be kept clean, dry, and covered with gauze dressing (26).

Conclusion

Digestive disorders are one of the most common reasons people seek medical advice, and many digestive problems are multifactorial. Diagnosis and treatment generally involves GI tests and procedures.

References

1. National Digestive Diseases Information Clearinghouse (NDDIC). Diagnostic Tests for Digestive Diseases. http://digestive.niddk.nih.gov/ddiseases/topics/diagnostic.aspx. Accessed December 5, 2013.
2. Fefferman DS, Farrell RJ. Endoscopy in inflammatory bowel disease: indications, surveillance, and use in clinical practice. *Clin Gastroenterol Hepatol.* 2005;3(1):11–24.

3. Concha R, Amaro R, Barkin JS. Obscure gastrointestinal bleeding: diagnostic and therapeutic approach. *J Clin Gastroenterol.* 2007;41(3):242–251.

4. Rao VS, Ahmad N, Al-Mukhtar A, Stojkovic S, Moore PJ, Ahmad SM. Comparison of rigid vs flexible sigmoidoscopy in detection of significant anorectal lesions: colorectal disease. *J Clin Gastroenterol.* 2007;41(3):242–251.

5. Walsh JM, Terdiamn JP. Colorectal cancer screening: clinical applications. *JAMA.* 2003;289(10):1297–1302.

6. Walsh JM, Terdiamn JP. Colorectal cancer screening: scientific review. *JAMA.* 2003;289(10):1288–1296.

7. Torpy JM, Lynm C, Glass RM. Colon cancer screening. *JAMA.* 2003;289(10):1334.

8. Sidhu R, Sanders DS, Morris AJ, McAlindon ME. Guidelines on small bowel enteroscopy and capsule endoscopy in adults. *Gut.* 2008;57:125–136.

9. Urbain D, Van Laer W, Mana F. Capsule endoscopy for detection of small bowel malignancies. *Surg Technol Int.* 2008;17:126–30.

10. Zuckerman GR, Prakash C, Askin MP, Lewis BS. AGA technical review on the evaluation and management of occult and obscure gastrointestinal bleeding. *Gastroenterology.* 2000;118(1):201–221.

11. Ang D, Teo EK, Ang TL, Ong J, Poh CH, Tan J, Fock KM. To Bravo or not? A comparison of wireless esophageal pH monitoring and conventional pH catheter to evaluate non-erosive gastroesophageal reflux disease in a multiracial Asian cohort. *Singapore J Dig Dis.* 2010;11:19–27.

12. Katz P. Utility and standards in esophageal manometry. *J Clin Gastroenterol.* 2008;42(5):62.

13. Kwiatek MA, Pandolfino JE. The Bravo pH capsule system. *Dig Liver Dis.* 2008;40(3):156–160.

14. Kawamura T, Yasuda K, Tanaka K, Uno K, Ueda M, Sanada K, Nakajima M. Clinical evaluation of a newly developed single-balloon enteroscope. *Gastrointest Endosc.* 2008;68(6):1112–1116.

15. Lo SK. Techniques, tricks, and complications of enteroscopy. *Gastrointest Endosc Clin N Am.* 2009;19(3): 381–388.

16. Tennyson CA, Lewis BA. Enteroscopy: an overview. *Gastrointest Endosc Clin N Am.* 2009;19:315–324.

17. Ouyang A, Locke GR. Overview of neurogastroenterology, gastrointestinal motility, and functional GI disorders: classification, prevalence, and epidemiology. *Gastroenterol Clin N Am.* 2007;36:485–498.

18. Parkman HP. Digestive diseases training in gastrointestinal motility. *Dig Dis.* 2006;24:221–227.

19. Tack J. Gastric motor disorders. *Best Pract Res Clin Gastroenterol.* 2007;21(4):633–644.

20. Bouras EP, Scolapio JS. Gastric motility disorders management that optimizes nutritional status. *J Clin Gastroenterol.* 2004;38:549–557.

21. Rao SS, Hatfield R, Soffer E, et al. Manometric tests of anorectal function in healthy adults. *Am J Gastroenterol.* 1999;94:773–783.

22. Rao SS. Constipation: evaluation and treatment of colonic and anorectal motility disorders. *Gastroenterol Clin N Am.* 2007;36:687–711.

23. International Foundation for Functional Gastrointestinal Disorders (IFFGD). About GI motility. www.about gimotility.org. Accessed August 2, 2010.

24. Sabba M. Wireless capsule motility: comparison of the SmartPill GI monitoring system with scintigraphy for measuring whole gut transit. *Dig Dis Sci.* 2009;54(10):216.

25. Pearce CB, Duncan HD. Review: enteral feeding. Nasogastric, nasojejunal, percutaneous endoscopic gastrostomy, or jejunostomy: its indications and limitations. *Postgrad Med J.* 2002;78:198–204.

26. Gopalan S, Khanna S. Enteral nutrition delivery technique. *Curr Opin Clin Nutr Metab Care.* 2003;6(3):313–317.

27. Angus F, Burakoff R. The percutaneous endoscopic gastrostomy tube: medical and ethical issues in placement. *Am J Gastroenterol.* 2003;98(2):272–277.

28. Zopf Y, Rabe C, Bruckmoser T, Maiss J, Hahn EG, Schwab D. Percutaneous endoscopic jejunostomy and jejunal extension tube through percutaneous endoscopic gastrostomy: a retrospective analysis of success, complications and outcome. *Digestion.* 2009;79:92–97.

CHAPTER 3

Nutrition Assessment for Patients with Gastrointestinal Disorders

Mary E. Hise, PhD, RD, CNSC,
and Yolanda Cartwright, PhD, RD

Disorders of the gastrointestinal (GI) system can have an adverse impact on nutritional status by impairing ingestion, digestion, and absorption of food and nutrients, as well as by increasing nutritional losses and nutrient requirements (1). Nutritional status has a profound influence on morbidity and mortality from illness in hospitalized patients (2,3). In the clinical setting, nutrition assessment is a comprehensive evaluation of the nutritional status of an individual patient. As the first step of the Nutrition Care Process, nutrition assessment is defined as "a systematic method for obtaining, verifying, and interpreting data needed to identify nutrition-related problems, their causes, and significance" (4). Nutrition assessment involves an initial evaluation of the patient but is an ongoing process that guides the development of an individualized nutrition care plan to help maintain or improve the assessed status. The types of data collected during the assessment vary on a case-by-case basis, but are organized into five general categories (see Box 3.1) (4). No single method is ideal for nutrition assessment; use of a combination of methods is needed to effectively characterize nutritional status. All nutrition assessment methods provide indirect estimates of the process measured. Thus, the data obtained are usually compared to reference data to determine indicators of nutritional status.

Food/Nutrition-Related History

The food/nutrition-related history can include data related to dietary intake as well as diet-related information such as knowledge and beliefs about food and nutrition, medication and supplement use, and

---

BOX 3.1 Components of a Nutrition Assessment

Food/Nutrition-Related History
- Food and nutrient intake
- Medication and herbal supplement intake
- Knowledge/beliefs/attitudes
- Food availability
- Physical activity
- Nutrition quality of life

Biochemical Data, Medical Tests, and Procedures
- Laboratory data (eg, electrolytes, glucose, renal, liver, gastrointestinal profiles)
- Tests (eg, gastric emptying time, resting metabolic rate)

Anthropometric Measurements
- Height
- Weight
- Body mass index (BMI)
- Weight history
- Weight change

Nutrition-Focused Physical Findings
- Physical appearance
- Muscle and fat wasting
- Swallow function
- Appetite
- Affect

Client History
- Personal history (eg, age, gender, race, language, education)
- Medical/health/family history
- Treatments and complementary/alternative medicine use
- Social history (eg, socioeconomic status, housing situation)

Source: Data are from reference 4.

physical activity. Evaluation of usual dietary intake (ie, diet history) is an important part of the nutrition assessment. Commonly used methods for assessing dietary history include the following:

- Diet history
- 24-hour recall
- Food record/diary
- Food frequency questionnaire

Each method has advantages and disadvantages. In addition, the accuracy of these methods for predicting actual dietary intake is a matter of debate (5–7). Diet recall methods, such as the diet history and 24-hour recall, are commonly used in the clinical setting. The diet history is used to assess usual dietary intake over an extended period of time, such as the past month or the past year. The 24-hour recall method is used to estimate usual intake based on reported dietary intake in the past 24 hours. Multiple 24-hour recalls are sometimes used because one day of intake is not typically representative of usual intake (8). With food records, the types and amounts of food and beverages consumed for a predefined period of time, usually 1 to 7 days, are recorded and usual intake is estimated based on this information. Unlike the diet history and 24-hour recall methods, food records do not rely on memory. The food frequency questionnaire is a checklist with which respondents indicate how many times a day, week, or year they consume certain foods (depending on the dietary component of interest). Responses from the questionnaire are used to estimate dietary intake of the specific dietary parameter(s). The food frequency questionnaire is often used in the research setting. All of these data-gathering methods can provide valuable information regarding a patient's dietary intake, information that can then be compared to the patient's nutritional requirements to estimate adequacy of the diet.

Biochemical Data, Medical Tests, and Procedures

Biochemical tests using blood and urine provide quantitative data about nutritional status. They can supply useful information about recent nutrient intakes and nutrient deficiencies. However, because results of biochemical tests can be influenced by nonnutritional factors, such as medications, fluid status, and other metabolic processes (eg, stress), these findings should be evaluated in conjunction with other nutrition assessment methods. Biochemical assessment can include the following tests (4):

- Protein profile (ie, albumin, prealbumin, transferrin, C-reactive protein)
- Vitamin and mineral profiles
- Acid-base balance
- Electrolyte and renal profile
- Essential fatty acid profile
- Nutritional anemia profile (eg, hemoglobin, hematocrit, vitamin B-12, and folate)
- Lipid profile
- Gastrointestinal profile

Malabsorptive disorders are common with GI diseases. Malabsorption can involve defective digestion and absorption of carbohydrate, protein, fat, vitamins, and minerals, either in combination or independently. Biochemical tests and other procedures used in the diagnosis of malabsorptive disorders in patients with GI diseases are described in Chapter 5. Patients with malabsorptive disorders are at increased risk for vitamin and trace element deficiencies and, therefore, often require supplementation with a multivitamin, dependent on the location of the disorder (eg, vitamin B-12 supplementation is usually required for patients with disorders that affect the terminal ileum). See Table 3.1 for laboratory tests used for assessment of vitamin and trace element status (9–11).

TABLE 3.1 Assessment of Vitamin and Trace Element Status

Nutrient	Laboratory Assay	Normal Values[a]	Signs of Deficiency	Toxicity Symptoms
Water-Soluble Vitamins				
Thiamin	Whole blood	>1.7 mcg/dL	Beriberi, mental confusion, Wernicke's encephalopathy, congestive heart failure	(Rare) Irritability, headache, insomnia
Niacin	Urinary niacin metabolites	>1.6 mg per g of creatinine	Headaches, diarrhea, dermatitis, Pellagra, memory loss	Flushing, rash, irritation, vasodilation
Riboflavin	Urinary riboflavin	>80 mcg per g of creatinine	Mucositis, dermatitis, photophobia, cheilosis, normocytic anemia	Unknown
Folate	Serum folate	>6.0 ng/mL	Macrocytic anemia, diarrhea, lethargy	Unknown
Pyridoxine (B-6)	Plasma B-6 or urinary excretion of B-6 metabolite	>50 ng/mL or >3 mcmol/dL	Dermatitis, neuritis, microcytic anemia	Unknown
Pantothenic acid	Urinary pantothenic acid	>1 mg/dL	Fatigue, malaise, headache, insomnia	Diarrhea
Ascorbic acid	Plasma ascorbic acid	>0.3 mg/dL	Hemorrhaging skin, nose, GI tract, weakness, bleeding gums, impaired wound healing	Osmotic diarrhea, oxalate kidney stones, interferes with anticoagulation therapy
Cyanocobalamin (B-12)	Serum B-12[b]	>150 pg/mL	Megaloblastic anemia, neuropathy, stomatitis, glossitis, pernicious anemia	Unknown
Biotin	Serum biotin	0.5–2.7 ng/mL	Dermatitis, lethargy, anorexia, alopecia, paresthesias, conjunctivitis	Unknown
Choline	Plasma choline	>10 mcmol/L	Fatty liver, liver damage, elevated aminotransferase	Fishy body odor, sweating, salivation, hypotension
Fat-Soluble Vitamins				
A	Serum retinol	>30 mcg/dL	Night blindness, dermatitis, xerophthalmia, keratomalacia	Acute: nausea, vomiting, headache, dizziness, chronic peeling skin, gingivitis, alopecia
D	Serum 25-hydroxy vitamin D	78–100 nmol/L	Osteomalacia, rickets, muscle weakness	Excess bone and soft tissue calcification, kidney stones, and hypercalcemia

Continues

TABLE 3.1   Assessment of Vitamin and Trace Element Status *(Continued)*

Nutrient	Laboratory Assay	Normal Values[a]	Signs of Deficiency	Toxicity Symptoms
Fat-Soluble Vitamins *(continued)*				
E	Plasma alpha-tocopherol	>0.1–1.6 mcmol/L (5 mcg/mL)	Increased platelet aggregation hemolytic anemia, neuronal axonopathy, and myopathy	Impaired neutrophil function, thrombocytopenia
K	Serum phylloquinone	0.13–1.19 ng/mL	Bleeding, purpura, and bruising	Bruising, bleeding, jaundice
Trace Elements				
Zinc	Serum value[c]	50–150 mcg/dL	Dermatitis, hypogeusia, diarrhea, apathy, depression, impaired wound healing	Nausea, vomiting, headache
Selenium	Serum value	0.01–0.34 mcg/dL	Muscle weakness and pain, cardiomyopathy	Hair loss, dermatitis, brittle nails, tooth decay, fatigue
Manganese	Serum value	2–3 mcg/dL	Nausea, vomiting, dermatitis, changes in hair color, hypocholesterolemia	Extrapyramidal symptoms, encephalitis-like symptoms, hyperirritability
Chromium	Serum value	0.05–5 mcg/L	Glucose intolerance, peripheral neuropathy, increased serum cholesterol, hyperlipidemia, insulin resistance	Unknown
Copper	Serum value	70–150 mcg/dL	Neutropenia, microcytic anemia, osteoporosis, decreased hair and skin pigmentation, dermatitis	(Uncommon) Nausea, vomiting, epigastric pain, diarrhea
Molybdenum	Neutron	0.58–0.8 mcg/L	Tachycardia, tachypnea, altered mental status, vision changes, headache, nausea, vomiting	Increased copper excretion
Iodine[d]	Urine	<5 mcg/L	Hyperplasia of thyroid, goiter, reduced metabolic rate, hypercholesterolemia	Rhinorrhea, headache, parotitis, acne

[a]Reference ranges for adult patients.

[b]Metabolites that result from vitamin B-12 deficiency (ie, methylmalonic acid [MMA] and homocysteine) may be sensitive indicators of B-12 deficiency. Normal serum MMA levels are 0.08 to 0.56 mcmol/L, and normal homocysteine levels are 5 to 15 mcmol/L.

[c]During systematic inflammatory response syndrome (SIRS), serum zinc will decrease to about half normal and remain depressed until SIRS resolves.

[d]Serum thyroid-stimulating hormone (TSH) and free thyroxine (T4) can be used as initial screening. These surrogate markers for iodine deficiency can be used initially in place of a 24-hour urine iodine study.

Source: Data are from references 9, 10, and 11.

Anthropometric Measurements

Anthropometry includes measurements of body size, weight, and proportions. Anthropometric measurements used for nutrition assessment can include the following parameters (4):

- Height/length
- Weight
- Frame size
- Weight change
- Body mass index (BMI)
- Growth pattern indexes/percentile ranks
- Body compartment estimates (eg, fat mass, fat-free mass)

Anthropometric measures can be used, in conjunction with other assessment methods, as indicators of overall nutritional status. However, these measures are not useful for identifying specific nutrient deficiencies. Anthropometric assessments are particularly important in patients with GI disorders because wasting syndrome is a common adverse effect of the disease process (1).

Body Weight

Body weight provides a gross evaluation of overall fat and muscle stores. Ideal body weight (IBW) is often calculated using the Hamwi method (12):

- Males: 106 pounds for the first 5 feet, 6 pounds for each inch taller than 5 feet
- Females: 100 pounds for the first 5 feet, 5 pounds for each inch taller than 5 feet

Usual body weight (UBW) may be a more applicable parameter to use when evaluating patients with GI dysfunction. Although subject to patient memory, UBW provides a useful tool for assessing changes in weight status over time. IBW and UBW may be used to evaluate the degree of over- or undernutrition. Recent unintentional weight loss is a strong indicator of declining nutritional status (13). Weight loss of more than 10% of usual body weight within a 6-month period is considered clinically significant (14). Weight gain could indicate repletion of lean and fat tissue, overnutrition, or presence of edema. Percentages of IBW, UBW, and recent weight can all be used to evaluate weight status (15).

PERCENTAGE OF IDEAL BODY WEIGHT

To calculate a patient's percentage of IBW, divide current weight by IBW and multiply the result by 100. The results are interpreted as follows (15):

- Mild malnutrition: 80%–90% IBW
- Moderate malnutrition: 70%–80% IBW
- Severe malnutrition: <69% IBW

PERCENTAGE OF USUAL BODY WEIGHT

To calculate a patient's percentage of UBW, divide the current weight by UBW and multiply the result by 100. The results are interpreted as follows (15):

- Malnutrition: 85%–95% UBW
- Moderate malnutrition: 75%–84% UBW
- Severe malnutrition: <75% UBW

PERCENTAGE OF RECENT WEIGHT

To calculate a patient's percentage of recent weight, use the following formula:

$$\% \text{ Recent Weight} = [(\text{UBW} - \text{Current Weight})/\text{UBW}] \times 100$$

The results are interpreted as follows (15):

- *Significant weight loss* is defined as 1%–2% in 1 week; 5% in 1 month; 7.5% in 3 months; or 10% in 6 months.
- *Severe weight loss* is defined as weight loss that exceeds the preceding amounts.

Body Mass Index

BMI is commonly used to classify weight status and assess healthy weight, malnutrition, and obesity. It is calculated using relative weight for height, as shown in the following equations, and is significantly correlated with total body fat content (16).

$$\text{BMI} = \text{Weight (kg)}/\text{Height (m}^2)$$

$$\text{BMI} = [\text{Weight (lb)}/\text{Height (in)}^2] \times 703$$

Guidelines for interpretation of BMI in adults are presented in Table 3.2 (16). For children and adolescents ages 19 years and younger, assessment of BMI is age- and gender-specific. Refer to appropriate reference tables available from the Centers for Disease Control and Prevention (www.cdc.gov/growthcharts).

Body Composition

Historically, body composition (ie, fat and fat-free mass) has been estimated using skinfold measurements such as mid-arm circumference (MAC), mid-arm muscle circumference (MAMC), and skinfold thickness. Although not frequently used in the clinical setting, skinfold measurements (serial measures) can be used to evaluate changes in lean and fat mass over time in individual patients.

TABLE 3.2 Interpretation of Body Mass Index (BMI) in Adults

BMI	Classification
18.5–24.9	Normal weight
25.0–29.9	Overweight
30.0–34.9	Obesity grade I
35.0–39.9	Obesity grade II
≥40	Obesity grade III
17.0–18.4	Protein-energy malnutrition grade I
16.0–16.9	Protein-energy malnutrition grade II

Source: Data are from reference 16.

Waist Circumference

Waist circumference is an assessment of abdominal fat. Waist circumference is measured (in inches or centimeters) by placing a standard measuring tape around the bare abdomen just above the hip bone. Independent of BMI, a high waist circumference is a risk factor for several diseases, including diabetes, hyperlipidemia, hypertension, and cardiovascular disease (17). A waist circumference of more than 40 inches (102 cm) in men and more than 35 inches (88 cm) in women is associated with increased disease risk (17).

Nutrition-Focused Physical Findings

Nutrition-focused physical findings are described as "nutrition-related physical characteristics associated with pathophysiological states derived from a nutrition-focused physical examination, interview, or the medical record" (4). These findings are examined to assess overall physical appearance, muscle and subcutaneous fat wasting, swallow function, appetite, and affect. Both subjective and objective physical findings are assessed during the nutrition-focused physical examination, which includes evaluations of the following factors/systems (4):

- Overall appearance
- Body language
- Cardiovascular-pulmonary system (eg, edema, shortness of breath)
- Extremities, muscles, and bones
- Gastrointestinal system (mouth to rectum)
- Head and eyes
- Nerves and cognition
- Skin
- Vital signs (eg, blood pressure, heart rate, temperature)

A nutrition-focused physical examination may be useful in detecting nutrient deficiencies in patients with GI disorders. See Table 3.3 (next page) for clinical findings from the physical examination associated with nutrient deficiencies.

Client History

The client history includes information related to personal, medical, family, and social history with the potential to impact nutritional status. Box 3.2 (page 29) outlines the data to be included in the client history (4).

Assessment of Energy Requirements

Critically Ill Patients

Indirect calorimetry is used to calculate energy expenditure by measurement of respiration gas exchange (oxygen consumption and carbon dioxide production) and is considered the gold standard for assessing energy requirements, particularly in critically ill patients. Because indirect calorimetry is expensive and requires technical expertise, its use in the clinical setting is limited. Chapter 4 discusses the predictive equations recommended for use in the assessment of energy needs for critically ill patients.

TABLE 3.3   Clinical Findings from Physical Examination Associated with Nutrient Deficiencies

Clinical Findings	Possible Deficiency
Hair	
Alopecia	Protein
Dry, dull, lackluster, brittle, sparse	Protein, iron, zinc, essential fatty acids
Dyspigmentation	Biotin, protein
Flag sign (alternating bands of light and dark hair)	Protein
Skin and nails	
Xerosis	Vitamin A, essential fatty acids
Follicular hyperkeratosis	Vitamin A, essential fatty acids
Perifollicular petechiae	Vitamin C, vitamin K
Dermatitis	Essential fatty acids, niacin, zinc, riboflavin
Palor	Iron, folate, vitamin B-12
Nasolabial seborrhea	Niacin, riboflavin, vitamin B-6
Koilonychia	Iron
Eyes	
Xerophthalmia	Vitamin A
Bitot's spots	Vitamin A
Night blindness	Vitamin A
Angular palpebritis	Riboflavin
Mouth	
Cheilosis	Vitamin B-6, riboflavin, niacin
Angular stomatitis	Riboflavin, vitamin B-6, iron
Bleeding/spongy gums	Vitamin C
Magenta tongue	Riboflavin
Atrophic papillae	Iron, niacin, folate, vitamin B-12
Glossitis	Niacin, folate, iron, vitamin B-6, vitamin B-12
Dysgeusia	Zinc
Cardiovascular	
Irregular/abnormal rhythm/rate	Related to potassium excess or deficiency, calcium or phosphorus deficiency, or magnesium deficiency or excess
Musculoskeletal system	
Muscle wasting	Protein-energy malnutrition
Bow-legs	Vitamin D, calcium
Beading of ribs	Vitamin D, protein-energy malnutrition
Neurologic	
Mental confusion	Thiamin, vitamin B-12, vitamin B-6
Dementia	Niacin, vitamin B-12

BOX 3.2   Data to Include in a Client History

Personal History	**Medical History**	**Family/Social History**
• Age/gender/race	• Cardiovascular	• Socioeconomic status
• Language	• Endocrine/metabolism	• Living/housing situation
• Literacy factors	• Excretory	• Domestic issues
• Education	• Gastrointestinal	• Social and medical
• Role in family	• Gynecological	support
• Tobacco use	• Hematology/oncology	• Geographic location
• Physical disability	• Immune	of home
	• Musculoskeletal	• Occupation
	• Neurological	• Religion
	• Psychological	• History of recent crisis
	• Medical/surgical treat-	• Daily stress level
	ment or complementary	
	medicine	

Source: Data are from reference 4.

Non–Critically Ill Patients

In non–critically ill patients, basal energy expenditure (BEE) can be estimated using predictive equations, as an alternative to indirect calorimetry. The Harris-Benedict equation (18) is one of the oldest and most widely used predictive equations used to calculate BEE:

$$\text{Men: BEE} = 66 + (13.7 \times W) + (5 \times H) - (6.8 \times A)$$

$$\text{Women: BEE} = 655 + (9.6 \times W) + (1.7 \times H) - (4.7 \times A)$$

Where: W = body weight (kg), H = height (cm), and A = age (years).

In addition, estimated energy needs may be based upon resting metabolic rate (RMR) as calculated by the Mifflin-St. Jeor equation (19):

$$\text{Men: RMR} = (9.99 \times W) + (6.25 \times H) - (4.92 \times A) + 5$$

$$\text{Women: RMR} = (9.99 \times W) + (6.25 \times H) - (4.92 \times A) - 161$$

Where: W = body weight (kg), H = height (cm), and A = age (years).

This equation seems to be the most accurate for estimation of energy needs among obese and non-obese individuals who are not critically ill (20).

Assessment of Protein Requirements

Protein Requirements

In healthy individuals, the Recommended Dietary Allowance (RDA) for protein for men and women is 0.8 g/kg/d (21). Estimated protein requirements may be based on specific disease states and/or metabolic stress states, and may increase to levels of up to 2.0 g/kg/d, depending on level of hypermetabolism, stress, and exogenous losses (22). The body of a 70-kg man includes approximately 11 kg of protein, with about 43% of it in the form of skeletal muscle (23).

The rate of endogenous protein breakdown (catabolism) decreases during energy deprivation. An unstressed individual loses approximately 12 to 18 g protein per day after about 10 days of starvation, which equates to approximately 2 oz of muscle tissue (2 to 3 g of nitrogen). During metabolic stress, protein breakdown increases exponentially, to approximately 30 to 60 g/d postsurgery, 60 to 90 g/d with infection, 100 to 130 g/d with severe sepsis, and >175 g/d with burns or head injuries (24). In chronic illness, skeletal muscle becomes the largest single contributor to protein loss (25).

Nitrogen Balance

Nitrogen balance studies are sometimes used to evaluate the adequacy of protein intake. Nitrogen balance studies indicate the relationship between intake of protein and removal of nitrogen from the renal system. Positive nitrogen balance cannot confirm anabolism because it lacks the specificity of stable isotopic amino acid studies (26,27). The conversion factor commonly used for dietary protein is 6.25 g of nitrogen per g of protein. Accurate 24-hour urine collection is difficult to obtain, and significant error may consequently be introduced into nitrogen balance calculations.

$$\text{Nitrogen Balance} = \text{Nitrogen Intake} - \text{Nitrogen Losses}$$

$$\text{Nitrogen Intake} = \text{Protein Intake (g)}/6.25$$

$$\text{Nitrogen Losses} = \text{Urinary Urea Nitrogen (UUN [g])}$$
$$+ \text{Non-Urea Urinary Nitrogen Losses (1–2 g)} + \text{Fecal Nitrogen Losses (1–2 g)}$$

$$\text{Nitrogen Balance} = \frac{\text{(Protein Intake)}}{6.25} - \text{(UUN)} + 2\text{–}4 \text{ g}$$

Hepatic Transport Proteins

Historically, hepatic transport proteins have been used as markers of malnutrition. Low levels of these acute-phase proteins are correlated with morbidity and mortality (28). These proteins are useful prognostic indicators of severity of illness, but they should not be used routinely as the primary diagnostic marker of malnutrition. Synthesis of acute-phase proteins (eg, albumin, transferrin, prealbumin, and retinol-binding protein) decreases precipitously during inflammatory conditions. Positive acute-phase proteins (C-reactive protein) increase in concentration during acute and chronic inflammatory states. Elevation of C-reactive protein may be used to confirm inflammatory status (29,30).

Nutrition Assessment Tools

Numerous tools are available for general assessment of nutritional status. In the clinical setting, two of the most commonly used and validated assessment tools include the Subjective Global Assessment (SGA) and the Mini-Nutritional Assessment Short Form (MNA-SF).

The SGA (Figure 3.1) is a nutrition assessment tool used to measure nutritional status based on weight, dietary intake, GI symptoms, functional capacity, and physical examination findings (14). Nutritional status is categorized as well-nourished, moderate malnutrition, or severe malnutrition. The SGA was originally developed for patients with GI disease (14). It has since been validated and used clinically

A. History
   1. Weight change
      Overall loss in past 6 mos: amount = ___kg; % loss = ___
      Change in past 2 wks: ___increase, ___no change, ___decrease

   2. Dietary intake change (relative to normal)
      ___ No change
      ___ Change ___duration = # ___wks
      Type: ___suboptimal solid diet ___full liquid diet ___hypocaloric liquids ___starvation

   3. Gastrointestinal symptoms (that persisted for > 2 wks)
      ___ none ___ nausea ___ vomiting ___ diarrhea ___ anorexia

   4. Functional capacity
      __ No dysfunction (eg, full capacity)
      __ Dysfunction ___duration = #___wks
      Type: __ working suboptimally
             __ ambulatory
             __ bedridden

   5. Disease and its relation to nutritional requirements
      Primary diagnosis (specify) _____
      Metabolic demand (stress): ___no stress ___low stress ___moderate stress ___high stress

B. Physical (for each trait specify 0 = normal, 1+ = mild, 2+ = moderate, 3+ = severe)
   #_____loss of subcutaneous fat (triceps, chest)
   #_____muscle wasting (quadriceps, deltoids)
   #_____ankle edema
   #_____sacral edema
   #_____ascites

C. SGA Rating
   ___ A = Well-nourished
   ___ B = Moderately malnourished (or suspected of being malnourished)
   ___ C = Severely malnourished

FIGURE 3.1   Components of the Subjective Global Assessment (SGA). The appropriate category is selected with a checkmark, or a numerical value is entered where indicated by "#". Source: Reprinted with permission from reference 14: Detsky AJ, McLaughlin JR, Baker JP, et al. What is subjective global assessment of nutritional status? *JPEN J Parenter Enteral Nutr.* 1987;11:8–14.

Mini Nutritional Assessment
MNA®

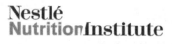

Last name:			First name:		
Sex:	Age:	Weight, kg:	Height, cm:	Date:	

Complete the screen by filling in the boxes with the appropriate numbers. Total the numbers for the final screening score.

Screening

A Has food intake declined over the past 3 months due to loss of appetite, digestive problems, chewing or swallowing difficulties?

0 = severe decrease in food intake
1 = moderate decrease in food intake
2 = no decrease in food intake   ☐

B Weight loss during the last 3 months

0 = weight loss greater than 3 kg (6.6 lbs)
1 = does not know
2 = weight loss between 1 and 3 kg (2.2 and 6.6 lbs)
3 = no weight loss   ☐

C Mobility

0 = bed or chair bound
1 = able to get out of bed / chair but does not go out
2 = goes out   ☐

D Has suffered psychological stress or acute disease in the past 3 months?

0 = yes   2 = no   ☐

E Neuropsychological problems

0 = severe dementia or depression
1 = mild dementia
2 = no psychological problems   ☐

F1 Body Mass Index (BMI) (weight in kg) / (height in m^2)

0 = BMI less than 19
1 = BMI 19 to less than 21
2 = BMI 21 to less than 23
3 = BMI 23 or greater   ☐

IF BMI IS NOT AVAILABLE, REPLACE QUESTION F1 WITH QUESTION F2.
DO NOT ANSWER QUESTION F2 IF QUESTION F1 IS ALREADY COMPLETED.

F2 Calf circumference (CC) in cm

0 = CC less than 31
3 = CC 31 or greater   ☐

Screening score (max. 14 points)

12 - 14 points: Normal nutritional status
8 - 11 points: At risk of malnutrition
0 - 7 points: Malnourished   ☐☐

References

1. Vellas B, Villars H, Abellan G, *et al.* Overview of the MNA® - Its History and Challenges. *J Nutr Health Aging.* 2006;**10**:456-465.
2. Rubenstein LZ, Harker JO, Salva A, Guigoz Y, Vellas B. Screening for Undernutrition in Geriatric Practice: Developing the Short-Form Mini Nutritional Assessment (MNA-SF). *J. Geront.* 2001; **56A**: M366-377
3. Guigoz Y. The Mini-Nutritional Assessment (MNA®) Review of the Literature - What does it tell us? *J Nutr Health Aging.* 2006; **10**:466-487.
4. Kaiser MJ, Bauer JM, Ramsch C, et al. Validation of the Mini Nutritional Assessment Short-Form (MNA®-SF): A practical tool for identification of nutritional status. *J Nutr Health Aging.* 2009; **13**:782-788.
® Société des Produits Nestlé, S.A., Vevey, Switzerland, Trademark Owners © Nestlé, 1994, Revision 2009. N67200 12/99 10M
For more information: www.mna-elderly.com

FIGURE 3.2   Mini-Nutritional Assessment Short Form (MNA-SF®). Source: Reprinted with permission from ®Société des Produits Nestlé S.A., Vevey, Switzerland, Trademark Owners. Copyright © Nestlé, 1994, Revision 2009. N67200 12/99 10M.

for many patient populations and is widely accepted as a practical and reliable tool for nutrition assessment (31).

The MNA-SF (Figure 3.2) is a six-question nutritional risk screening tool for older adults (32–35). A revision of the previously published, longer MNA tool, MNA-SF has been found to be valid and easy to use in studies of elderly patients in nursing homes and hospitals (32,35). The MNA-SF uses anthropometric measurements, general status, diet information, and subjective assessment (32). A score of fewer than 8 points (out of a maximum of 14) is regarded as an indication of malnutrition; 8 to 11 points indicate a risk for malnutrition; and more than 11 points indicate normal nutritional status (33,34).

Documenting Malnutrition

Malnutrition is a diagnosis known to be associated with poor outcomes in hospitalized and nonhospitalized individuals. A joint task force of the Academy of Nutrition and Dietetics and the American Society for Parenteral and Enteral Nutrition has recommended a standardized set of diagnostic characteristics to identify and document adult malnutrition (see Table 3.4 on pages 34–35) (36).

Conclusion

The GI tract is essential for the absorption and digestion of foods, and disorders of the GI system can have a significant impact on dietary intake and nutritional status. Nutrition assessment plays a vital role in identifying nutrition-related problems in patients with GI disorders and in developing appropriate nutrition interventions. A complete nutrition assessment includes evaluating dietary data, biochemical tests and procedures, anthropometric measures, nutrition-focused physical findings, and the personal/medical/social history with an ultimate goal of improving clinical outcomes in patients with GI disorders.

TABLE 3.4　Clinical Characteristics That Support a Diagnosis of Malnutrition[a]

Clinical Characteristic	Malnutrition in the Context of Acute Illness or Injury — Nonsevere (Moderate) Malnutrition	Malnutrition in the Context of Acute Illness or Injury — Severe Malnutrition	Malnutrition in the Context of Chronic Illness — Nonsevere (Moderate) Malnutrition	Malnutrition in the Context of Chronic Illness — Severe Malnutrition	Malnutrition in the Context of Social or Environmental Circumstances — Nonsevere (Moderate) Malnutrition	Malnutrition in the Context of Social or Environmental Circumstances — Severe Malnutrition
(1) Energy intake Malnutrition is the result of inadequate food and nutrient intake or assimilation; thus, recent intake compared to estimated requirements is a primary criterion defining malnutrition. The clinician may obtain or review the food and nutrition history, estimate optimum energy needs, compare them with estimates of energy consumed and report inadequate intake as a percentage of estimated energy requirements over time.	<75% of estimated energy requirement for > 7 days	≤50% of estimated energy requirement for ≥5 days	<75% of estimated energy requirement for ≥1 month	<75% of estimated energy requirement for ≥1 month	<75% of estimated energy requirement for ≥3 months	≤50% of estimated energy requirement for ≥1 month
(2) Interpretation of weight loss The clinician may evaluate weight in light of other clinical findings, including the presence of under- or over-hydration. The clinician may assess weight change over time reported as a percentage of weight lost from baseline.	*%* / *Time*: 1–2 / 1 wk 5 / 1 mo 7.5 / 3 mo	*%* / *Time*: >2 / 1 wk >5 / 1 mo >7.5 / 3 mo	*%* / *Time*: 5 / 1 mo 7.5 / 3 mo 10 / 6 mo 20 / 1 y	*%* / *Time*: >5 / 1 mo >7.5 / 3 mo >10 / 6 mo >20 / 1 y	*%* / *Time*: 5 / 1 mo 7.5 / 3 mo 10 / 6 mo 20 / 1 y	*%* / *Time*: >5 / 1 mo >7.5 / 3 mo >10 / 6 mo >20 / 1 y
(3) Body fat Loss of subcutaneous fat (eg, orbital, triceps, fat overlying the ribs).	Mild	Moderate	Mild	Severe	Mild	Severe

Physical findings: Malnutrition typically results in changes to the physical exam. The clinician may perform a physical exam and document any one of the physical exam findings below as an indicator of malnutrition.

Characteristic						
(4) Muscle mass Muscle loss (eg, wasting of the temples [temporalis muscle]; clavicles [pectoralis and deltoids]; shoulders [deltoids]; interosseous muscles; scapula [latissimus dorsi, trapezious, deltoids]; thigh [quadriceps] and calf [gastrocnemius]).	Mild	Moderate	Severe	Mild	Severe	
(5) Fluid accumulation The clinician may evaluate generalized or localized fluid accumulation evident on exam (extremities; vulvar/scrotal edema or ascites). Weight loss is often masked by generalized fluid retention (edema) and weight gain may be observed.	Mild	Moderate to severe	Severe	Mild	Severe	
(6) Reduced grip strength Consult normative standards supplied by the manufacturer of the measurement device.	N/A[b]	Measurably reduced	Measurably reduced	N/A[b]	Measurably Reduced	N/A[b]

[a]A minimum of two of the six characteristics above is recommended for diagnosis of either severe or nonsevere malnutrition. Height and weight should be measured rather than estimated to determine body mass index. Usual weight should be obtained to determine the percentage and to interpret the significance of weight loss. Basic indicators of nutritional status such as body weight, weight change, and appetite may substantively improve with refeeding in the absence of inflammation. Refeeding and/or nutrition support may stabilize but not significantly improve nutrition parameters in the presence of inflammation. The National Center for Health Statistics defines "chronic" as a disease/condition lasting 3 months or longer. Serum proteins such as albumin and prealbumin are not included as defining characteristics of malnutrition because recent evidence analysis shows that serum levels of these proteins do not change in response to changes in nutrient intake.

[b]N/A=not applicable.

Source: Adapted from reference 36: White VW, Guenter P, Jensen G, et al. Consensus statement of the Academy of Nutrition and Dietetics/American Society for Parenteral and Enteral Nutrition: characteristics recommended for the identification and documentation of adult malnutrition (undernutrition). *J Acad Nutr Diet.* 2012;112(5):730–738. Used with permission from Academy of Nutrition and Dietetics and Elsevier.

References

1. Fisher RL. Wasting in chronic gastrointestinal diseases. *J Nutr.* 1999;129(suppl):252S–255S.
2. Correia MI, Waitzberg DL. The impact of malnutrition on morbidity, mortality, length of hospital stay and costs evaluated through a multivariate model analysis. *Clin Nutr.* 2003;22:235–239.
3. Goiburu ME, Goiburu MM, Bianco H, et al. The impact of malnutrition on morbidity, mortality and length of hospital stay in trauma patients. *Nutr Hosp.* 2006;21:604–610.
4. *International Dietetics and Nutrition Terminology (IDNT) Reference Manual.* 4th ed. Chicago IL: Academy of Nutrition and Dietetics; 2013.
5. Schaefer EJ, Augustin JL, Schaefer MM, et al. Lack of efficacy of a food frequency questionnaire in assessing dietary macronutrient intakes in subjects consuming diets of known composition. *Am J Clin Nutr.* 2000;71:746–751.
6. Willett WC, ed. *Nutritional Epidemiology.* 2nd ed. New York, NY: Oxford University Press; 1998.
7. Buzzard IM, Faucett CL, Jeffery RW, et al. Monitoring dietary change in a low-fat diet intervention study: advantages of using 24-hour dietary recalls vs food records. *J Am Diet Assoc.* 1996;96:574–579.
8. Buzzard M. 24-hour recall and food record methods. In: Willett WC, ed. *Nutritional Epidemiology.* 2nd ed. New York, NY: Oxford University Press; 1998.
9. Strausburg KT. Nutrition/metabolic assessment. In: Teasley-Strausburg K, ed. *Nutrition Support Handbook.* Cincinnati, OH: Harvey Whitney; 1992.
10. Clark FS. Vitamin and trace elements. In: Gottschlich MM, ed. *The A.S.P.E.N. Nutrition Support Core Curriculum: A Case-Based Approach—The Adult Patient.* Silver Spring, MD: American Society for Parenteral and Enteral Nutrition; 2007.
11. Pesce-Hammond K, Wessel J. Nutrition assessment and decision making. In: Merrit R, ed. *The A.S.P.E.N. Nutrition Support Practice Manual.* Silver Spring, MD: American Society for Parenteral and Enteral Nutrition; 2005.
12. Hamwi G. Changing dietary concepts. In: Danowski TS, ed. *Diabetes Mellitus: Diagnosis and Treatment.* New York, NY: American Diabetes Association; 1964.
13. Kyle UG, Genton L, Pichard C. Hospital length of stay and nutritional status. *Curr Opin Clin Nutr Metab Care.* 2005;8:397–402.
14. Detsky AS, McLaughlin JR, Baker JP, et al. What is subjective global assessment of nutritional status? *JPEN J Parenter Enteral Nutr.* 1987;11:8–14.
15. Blackburn, GL, Bisttian, BR, Maini, BS, et al. Nutritional and metabolic assessment of the hospitalized patient. *JPEN J Parenter Enteral Nutr.* 1977;1:11–22.
16. *Clinical Guidelines on the Identification, Evaluation, and Treatment of Overweight and Obesity in Adults. The Evidence Report.* Washington, DC: National Heart, Lung and Blood Institute; 1998.
17. Chan JM, Rimm EB, Colditz GA, Stampfer MJ, Willett WC. Obesity, fat distribution, and weight gain as risk factors for clinical diabetes in men. *Diabetes Care.* 1994;17:961–969.
18. Harris JA, Benedict FG. *Biometric Studies of Basal Metabolism in Man.* Washington, DC: Carnegie Institution of Washington; 1919.
19. Mifflin MD, St Jeor ST, Hill LA, Scott BJ, Daugherty SA, Koh YO. A new predictive equation for resting energy expenditure in healthy individuals. *Am J Clin Nutr.* 1990;51(2):241–247.
20. Frankenfield DC, Roth-Yousey L, Compher C. Comparison of predictive equations for resting metabolic rate in healthy nonobese and obese individuals, a systematic review. *J Am Diet Assoc.* 2005;105:775–789.
21. Institute of Medicine. *Dietary Reference Intakes for Energy, Carbohydrate, Fiber, Fat, Fatty Acids, Cholesterol, Protein, and Amino Acids.* Washington, DC: National Academies Press; 2005:589.
22. A.S.P.E.N Board of Directors and Clinical Guidelines Task Force. Guidelines for the Use of Parenteral and Enteral Nutrition in Adult and Pediatric Patients. *JPEN J Parenter Enteral Nutr.* 2002;26(1 Suppl):1SA–138SA.
23. Lentner C. *Geigy Scientific Tables: Units of Measurement, Body Fluids, Composition of the Body, Nutrition.* Vol 1. 8th ed. West Caldwell, NJ: Ciba-Geigy Corporation; 1981.

24. Heimburger DC. Malnutrition and nutrition assessment. In: Fauci AS, Kasper DL, Longo DL, Braunwald E, Hauser SL, Jameson JL, eds. *Harrison's Principles of Internal Medicine*. 17th ed. New York, NY: McGraw-Hill; 2008:451.

25. Hansen RD, Raja C, Allen BJ. Total body protein in chronic diseases and in aging. *Ann N Y Acad Sci*. 2000;904:345–352.

26. Meesters RJ, Wolfe RR, Deutz NE. Application of liquid chromatography-tandem mass spectrometry (LC-MS/MS) for the analysis of stable isotope enrichments of phenylalanine and tyrosine. *J Chromatogr B Analyt Technol Biomed Life Sci*. 2009; 877(1–2):43–49. Epub 2008 Nov 14.

27. Tuvdendorj D, Chinkes DL, Zhang XJ, Ferrando AA, Elijah IE, Mlcak RP, Finnerty CC, Wolfe RR, Herndon DN. Adult patients are more catabolic than children during acute phase after burn injury: a retrospective analysis on muscle protein kinetics. *Intensive Care Med*. 2011;37(8):1317–1322. Epub 2011 Jun 7.

28. Fuhrman MP, Charney P, Mueller CM. Hepatic proteins and nutrition assessment. *J Am Diet Assoc*. 2004;104:1258–1264.

29. Kurtz EG, Ridker PM, Rose LM, Cook NR, Everett BM, Buring JE, Rexrode KM. Oral postmenopausal hormone therapy, C-reactive protein, and cardiovascular outcomes. *Menopause*. 2011;18(1):23–29.

30. Empana JP, Jouven X, Canouï-Poitrine F, et al. C-reactive protein, interleukin 6, fibrinogen and risk of sudden death in European middle-aged men: the PRIME study. *Arterioscler Thromb Vasc Biol*. 2010;30(10):2047–2052.]

31. Baker JP, Detsky AS, Wesson DE, et al. Nutritional assessment: a comparison of clinical judgment and objective measures. *N Engl J Med*. 1988;306:969–973.

32. Guigoz Y, Vellas B, Garry P. Assessing the nutritional status of the elderly: the Mini-Nutritional Assessment as part of the geriatric evaluation. *Nutr Rev*. 1996;54(Suppl 2):S59–S65.

33. Rubenstein LZ, Harker JO, Salva A, Guigoz Y, Vellas B. Screening for undernutrition in geriatric practice: developing the short-form mini-nutritional assessment (MNA-SF). *J Gerontol A Biol Sci Med Sci*. 2001;56:M366–M372.

34. Charlton KE, Kolbe-Alexander TL, Nel JH. Development of a novel nutrition screening tool for use in elderly South Africans. *Public Health Nutr*. 2005;8:468–479.

35. Kaiser MJ, Bauer JM, Ramsch C, et al. Validation of the Mini Nutritional Assessment Short-Form (MNA®-SF): a practical tool for identification of nutritional status. *J Nutr Health Aging*. 2009;13(9):782–788.

36. White VW, Guenter P, Jensen G, et al. Consensus statement of the Academy of Nutrition and Dietetics/American Society for Parenteral and Enteral Nutrition: characteristics recommended for the identification and documentation of adult malnutrition (undernutrition). *J Acad Nutr Diet*. 2012;112(5):730–738.

CHAPTER 4

Nutrition Assessment and Nutrient Requirements in Critical Care

Jennifer C. Lefton, MS, RD, CNSC, FAND,

Annette M. Carpenter, RD, CNSC,

and Jennifer R. Carter, RD, CNSC

This chapter focuses on nutrition assessment of critically ill patients and their nutrient requirements. Critical illness results in significant metabolic alterations (see Box 4.1) that ultimately result in net protein losses. Protein becomes a preferred energy source, and the losses cannot be corrected with nutrition support alone (1). One of the main goals of nutrition support is to minimize the amount of protein lost. Additional goals of nutrition support therapy are to maintain immune function, avoid metabolic complications, and attenuate the metabolic response to stress (2). See Chapter 3 for more general information about nutrition assessment, and refer to Chapters 19, 20, 21, and 22 for additional information on the use of enteral and parenteral nutrition.

Nutrition Assessment

Evaluating the nutritional status of critically ill patients is difficult because many of the usual assessment tools used are inaccurate or not validated in the critically ill. Nutrition assessment in the critical care setting should include evaluation of the patient's weight history and diet history prior to the critical illness as well as consideration of nutrition-related factors specific to the patient's particular disease or condition. The following sections touch briefly on issues specific to the assessment of critically ill patients. Refer to Chapter 3 for more information on the components of a nutrition assessment.

Nutrition-Related History

If available, diet history and intake prior to critical illness should be included in the assessment. Additionally, food allergies and intolerances should be documented.

BOX 4.1   Metabolic Changes During Critical Illness

Shock/resuscitation phase
- Low cardiac output
- Hypotension
- Poor tissue perfusion
- Reduced oxygen consumption

Acute catabolic phase
- Glycogenolysis
- Gluconeogenesis
- Proteolysis
- Increased oxygen consumption
- Increased CO_2 production
- Hypermetabolism
- Hyperglycemia
- Overall catabolism

Anabolic phase
- Energy expenditure returns to normal
- Normoglycemia
- Anabolism

Anthropometrics

Use caution when considering current body weight as an indicator of nutritional status. Weight measurements are often an inaccurate indicator of nutritional status because of fluid imbalances. It may also be difficult to obtain weight history data from critically ill patients, and family members often do not have the needed information.

Biochemical Data

Electrolytes and glucose tolerance should be evaluated in critically ill patients. Albumin and prealbumin are not reliable indicators of nutritional status in the critically ill. Albumin and prealbumin are negative acute-phase reactants, and serum levels will be low regardless of the patient's nutritional status and the nutrition support provided (2,3).

Diagnostic Tests

Relevant data from diagnostic tests may include results from indirect calorimetry, X-rays (to confirm proper placement of feeding tubes), or findings from other GI-related tests (eg, small bowel follow-through).

Findings from a Nutrition-Focused Physical Exam

Key findings from a physical exam may include evaluation of access sites for delivery of nutrition, fluid status and fluid intake and output, the presence or absence of wounds, vital signs, and results of an abdominal exam (4).

Energy Requirements

Determining the exact energy needs of the critically ill patient continues to be a challenge for clinicians. Underfeeding calories may result in impaired immune response and poor wound healing (5). Overfeeding calories may result in the following complications (6–10):

- Hyperglycemia
- Hyperinsulinemia

- Hypokalemia
- Hypophosphatemia
- CO_2 retention
- Pulmonary compromise
- Difficulty weaning off ventilator
- Hepatic steatosis
- Azotemia

Use of Indirect Calorimetry

Indirect calorimetry is the most accurate method to determine energy expenditure. However, many hospitals are unable to conduct the studies.

Use of Predictive Equations

Many clinicians rely on predictive equations to estimate energy needs. However, equations used in non–critically ill patients may not be appropriate for use when individuals are critically ill.

ESTIMATING ENERGY REQUIREMENTS FOR NONOBESE PATIENTS
According to the 2012 Academy of Nutrition and Dietetics Critical Illness Evidence-Based Nutrition Practice Guideline (4), the Penn State University (PSU) 2003b equation has the highest prediction accuracy and should be used in nonobese, critically ill, mechanically ventilated adults. See Box 4.2 for this equation (11).

ESTIMATING ENERGY REQUIREMENTS FOR OBESE PATIENTS
According to the 2012 Academy of Nutrition and Dietetics Critical Illness Evidence-Based Nutrition Practice Guideline (4), the PSU 2003b equation has the highest prediction accuracy in critically ill, mechanically ventilated adults with obesity who are younger than 60 years. However, for obese patients 60 years or older, the PSU 2010 equation has the highest prediction accuracy (4). See Box 4.2 for the PSU 2003b equation (11) and Box 4.3 for the PSU 2010 equation (12).

The Society of Critical Care Medicine (SCCM) and American Society for Parenteral and Enteral Nutrition (A.S.P.E.N.) suggest use of hypocaloric nutrition regimens (60%–70% of actual energy needs) for obese patients (body mass index [BMI] >30). As an alternative, they suggest estimating the needs of critically ill obese patients as follows (2):

- 11–14 kcal per kilogram of actual body weight *or*
- 22–25 kcal per kilogram of ideal body weight

Nutrient Requirements

Protein

Underfeeding protein results in greater protein losses and can slow wound healing. Protein needs for the nonobese critically ill patient range between 1.2 and 2 g protein per kilogram actual body weight (3). Some patients with large wounds (eg, burn patients) may require more than 2 g protein per kilogram.

BOX 4.2   Penn State 2003b Equation for Resting Metabolic Rate (RMR)

$$RMR = Mifflin\ (0.96) + V_E\ (31) + T_{max}\ (167) - 6,212$$

Where: RMR = energy expenditure; Mifflin = Mifflin-St Jeor RMR equation (see Chapter 3); V_E = minute ventilation (L/min); T_{max} = maximum temperature over previous 24 hours (degrees Celsius)

Source: Data are from reference 11.

BOX 4.3   Penn State University 2010 Equation for Resting Metabolic Rate (RMR)

$$RMR = Mifflin\ (0.71) + V_E\ (64) + T_{max}\ (85) - 3,085$$

Where: RMR = energy expenditure; Mifflin = Mifflin-St Jeor RMR equation (see Chapter 3); V_E = minute ventilation (L/min); T_{max} = maximum temperature over previous 24 hours (degrees Celsius).

Source: Data are from reference 12.

For obese patients (BMI 30–40), starting with at least 2 g protein per kilogram ideal body weight is recommended (3). For morbidly obese patients (BMI >40), starting with at least 2.5 g protein per kilogram ideal body weight is recommended (2).

Older adults may not tolerate as much protein. Azotemia due to high protein nutrition support regimens is more common in older adults. An increasing blood urea nitrogen (BUN) with a normal creatinine may be a sign that the patient is not tolerating the amount of protein given (13).

Carbohydrate

Insufficient carbohydrate intake can exacerbate protein catabolism. Excessive carbohydrate administration can result in hyperglycemia and higher insulin needs. Hyperglycemia can also cause a shift of potassium and phosphorus intracellularly, resulting in low serum levels (7). Higher amounts of carbohydrate intake have also been reported to cause CO_2 retention and respiratory distress (7–10).

The optimal amount of carbohydrate to provide is one that spares protein and minimizes hyperglycemia. For patients receiving parenteral nutrition, providing less than 4–5 mg/kg/min of carbohydrate is recommended (7). Patients with hyperglycemia or those who are malnourished should be started initially with less carbohydrate until tolerance to the nutrition regimen is established. Tolerance may be defined as near normal glucose levels and electrolyte levels (potassium, magnesium, and phosphorus) within normal ranges.

Fat

Inadequate intake of fat can contribute to negative energy balance and essential fatty acid deficiency. Typical recommendations suggest that between 20% and 35% of total energy should come from a fat source.

Provision of fat helps meet energy needs without having to provide excess carbohydrate. This is particularly of interest in parenteral nutrition patients. Essential fatty acid deficiency can occur in patients receiving fat-free total parenteral nutrition for 3 weeks (14). Excessive fat intake can lead to hypertriglyceridemia (7). See Chapter 20 for additional information on parenteral nutrition.

Propofol is a common sedative used in critical care settings. It is delivered in a fat emulsion and provides 1.1 kcal/mL. Energy provided from this medication should be included in assessment of the patient's overall energy intake.

Micronutrients

For critically ill patients on PN, care must be taken to provide adequate amounts of electrolytes, vitamins, and trace elements to meet the patients' requirements. Additional information on this topic is found in Chapter 20.

BOX 4.4   Parameters for Assessing Nutrition Support in the Critically Ill

Delivery of energy
- Determine daily intake.
- Monitor initiation, time to reach goal, and average intake delivered.

Patient position
- Head of bed should be inclined >45° to reduce incidence of aspiration pneumonia and gastric reflux.

Gastric residual volume (GRV)
- Enteral nutrition should be held if GRV ≥500 mL. It also can be held with GRV <500 mL in the presence of other signs of intolerance.

Abdominal assessment
- Intolerance may be indicated by increased abdominal distension, formula reflux or increased residuals, nausea, vomiting, diarrhea, and pain.

Fluid status
- Monitor daily intake and output, signs of fluid overload, weight, and presence of edema.

Laboratory data
- Assess daily: sodium, chloride, BUN, creatinine, bicarbonate, potassium, magnesium, phosphorus, and glucose.
- Assess weekly: UUN for nitrogen balance, LFTs, and triglycerides.

Other data
- Rate of wound healing
- Ventilator-weaning
- Functional status
- Stamina in therapy

Abbreviations: BUN, blood urea nitrogen; UUN, urinary urea nitrogen; LFT, liver function test.
Source: Data are from reference 4.

Ongoing Assessment of Patients on Nutrition Support

Critically ill patients on nutrition support must be regularly re-evaluated to ensure that the delivery of nutrition is adequate, safe, and appropriate. There is no single measure of nutritional adequacy. Therefore, several parameters should be evaluated when assessing the patient's response to nutrition therapy. Additionally, trends in serial measurements instead of one single measurement may be more useful in assessing the patients' response. Box 4.4 shows parameters used to evaluate nutrition therapy provision, tolerance, and adequacy (4).

Conclusion

Nutrition assessment in the critical care setting is challenging and requires understanding of the unique nutritional needs of the critically ill patient. The patient's nutritional status must be continually assessed and monitored to ensure that appropriate nutrition interventions are used to minimize protein losses. Indirect calorimetry is the preferred method of determining energy requirements. When indirect calorimetry is not practical, it is important to select the appropriate predictive equation for the critically ill patient. If oral intake is not possible or cannot provide adequate nutrition, nutrition support (enteral or parenteral nutrition) is required. Under these circumstances, regular evaluation of the nutrient delivery, potential physical signs and symptoms of complications, laboratory data, and other nutrition-related information is required.

References

1. Streat SJ, Beddoe AH, Hill GL. Aggressive nutritional support does not prevent protein loss despite fat gain in septic intensive care patients. *J Trauma.* 1987;27:262–266.
2. McClave SA, Martindale RG, Vanek VW, et al. Guidelines for the provision and assessment of nutrition support therapy in the adult critically ill patient: Society of Critical Care Medicine (SCCM) and American Society for Parenteral and Enteral Nutrition (A.S.P.E.N.). *JPEN J Parenter Enteral Nutr.* 2009;33:277–316.
3. Gabay C, Kushner I. Acute-phase proteins and other systemic responses to inflammation. *N Engl J Med.* 1999;340:448–454.
4. Academy of Nutrition and Dietetics. Critical Illness 2012 Evidence-Based Nutrition Practice Guideline. www.andevidencelibrary.com. Accessed November 13, 2013.
5. Cresci G, Martindale R. Nutrition support in trauma. In: Gottsclich MM, ed. *The Science and Practice of Nutrition Support: A Case-Based Core Curriculum.* Dubuque, IA: Kendall/Hunt Publishing; 2000:445–460.
6. Rosmarin D, Wardlaw G, Mirtallo J. Hyperglycemia associated with high, continuous infusion rates of total parenteral nutrition. *Nutr Clin Pract.* 1996;11:151–156.
7. Klein CJ, Stanek G, Wiles C. Overfeeding macronutrients to critically ill adults: metabolic complications. *J Am Diet Assoc.* 1998;98:795–806.
8. Askanazi J, Elwyn D, Silverberg P, Rosenbaum S, Kinney J. Respiratory distress secondary to high carbohydrate load: a case report. *Surgery.* 1980;87:596–598.
9. Covelli H, Black J, Olsen M, Beekman J. Respiratory failure precipitated by high carbohydrate loads. *Ann Intern Med.* 1981;95:579–581.
10. Dark D, Pingleton S, Kerby G. Hypercapnia during weaning: a complication of nutrition support. *Chest.* 1985;88:141–143.
11. Frankenfield D, Smith S, Cooney RN. Validation of 2 approaches to predicting resting metabolic rate in critically ill patients. *JPEN J Parenter Enteral Nutr.* 2004;28(4):259–264.
12. Frankenfield D. Validation of an equation for resting metabolic rate in older obese critically ill patients. *JPEN J Parenter Enteral Nutr.* 2011;35(2):264–269.

13. Frankenfield D, Cooney R, Mith J, Rowe W. Age-related differences in the metabolic response to injury. *J Trauma*. 2000;48:49–57.
14. Richardson T, Sgoutas D. Essential fatty acid deficiency in four adult patients during total parenteral nutrition. *Am J Clin Nutr*. 1975;28:258–263.

PART II

Nutrition and Gastrointestinal Tract Disorders

CHAPTER 5

Small Intestine Malabsorptive Disorders

Carol Rees Parrish, MS, RD,

Nora Rahn Baumgart, MS, RD, CNSC,

and Barbara J. Goodin, MS, RD, CDE

The process of digestion and absorption is a complex cascade of events. As with most other physiologic processes, it is not appreciated until it goes awry. This chapter focuses on the small bowel (SB) and disturbances with absorptive capacity. Malabsorption associated with disease states that are considered diseases of the gastrointestinal (GI) tract, such as Crohn's disease and celiac disease, are covered in the chapters devoted to those conditions (see Chapter 7 for information on Crohn's disease and Chapter 10 for discussion of celiac disease). Malabsorption that is the result of surgery is covered in Chapter 14.

The surface area of the SB is profound—2 million cm^2 (roughly the size of a doubles tennis court). The SB is so efficient in its role that more than 90% of foodstuffs are absorbed in the first 5 feet of SB (1,2). Furthermore, approximately 9 liters of exogenous and endogenous fluid are presented to the SB daily, with more than 90% reabsorbed (3). Table 5.1 (page 48) includes information about GI water movement (4).

Malabsorption

Adequate digestion and absorption rely on the coordinated activity of a multitude of factors, which include the following (5–7):

- Lipid emulsification in stomach to droplets less than 0.5mm in diameter
- Mechanical mixing of foodstuffs within the lumen of the bowel
- Enzyme production, secretion, and activity
- Proper mucosal surface and function (hydrolysis and epithelial transport)
- Adequate blood supply
- Intestinal motility
- Normal microbial ecology

TABLE 5.1 The GI Balance Sheet in the Normal Gut (Gastrointestinal Water Movement)

Source	Water, mL
Additions	
Diet	2,000
Saliva	1,500
Stomach	2,500
Pancreas/bile	2,000
Intestine	1,000
Total	**9,000**
Subtractions	
Colointestinal	8,900
NET STOOL LOSS	**100 mL**

Source: Reprinted with permission from reference 4: Parrish CR. The clinician's guide to short bowel syndrome. *Practical Gastroenterology.* 2005;29(9):67–106.

Malabsorption occurs when there is a net loss of nutrients in the patient consuming an adequate nutrient intake. It can express itself as any of the following:

- Unintentional weight loss
- Diarrhea
- Steatorrhea
- Gas
- Abdominal distension
- Bloating
- Fatigue
- Anorexia
- Hyperphagia
- Dehydration
- Electrolyte disarray
- Metabolic acidosis from bicarbonate loss
- Signs and symptoms of specific nutrient deficiencies
- Essential fatty acid deficiency

A defect in any aspect of digestion (maldigestion) or absorption (malabsorption), or a combination of the two (malassimilation), can precipitate a malabsorption syndrome. The broader term *malabsorption* is typically divided into three main types: luminal, mucosal, and postabsorptive. However, a fourth type that is a function of anatomical changes can be added (7). Box 5.1 lists potential causes of malabsorption.

Malabsorption in the Luminal Phase

The luminal phase refers to the mixing, hydrolysis, and solubilization of fat, protein, and carbohydrates within the small bowel lumen by pancreatic enzymes and bile salts. Maldigestion results from incomplete

---

BOX 5.1   Potential Causes of Malabsorption

Luminal
- Pancreatic insufficiency:
  - Chronic pancreatic disease
  - Pancreatic cancer
  - Cystic fibrosis
- Bile salt deficiency:
  - Primary biliary cirrhosis
  - Primary sclerosing cholangitis
  - Cirrhosis
  - Cholestatic process
  - External biliary drain
  - Obstruction below the common bile duct requiring decompression from above
- Microbial:
  - Small bowel bacterial overgrowth
  - Giardia
  - Whipple's disease
- Gastric hypersecretion:
  - Zollinger-Ellison syndrome
  - Short gut

Mucosal
- Celiac disease
- Crohn's disease
- Amyloidosis
- Scleroderma
- Radiation enteritis

Postabsorptive
- Lymphatic obstruction
- Lymphangiectasia
- Neoplasm (including lymphoma)

Anatomical
- Partial or total gastrectomy
- Short bowel syndrome
- Fistula
- Roux-en-Y gastric bypass
- Whipple's procedure
- Esophagectomy with gastric pull-up

---

breakdown of nutrients into their absorbable substrates. The osmotic load resulting from the inability of the intestine to absorb these nutrients often causes diarrhea. Bile acids are responsible for emulsification of fat by decreasing the surface area available for lipolytic action in preparation for digestion and absorption. They also play a role in the activation of lipase. The entire bile salt pool recycles twice per meal and up to 6 to 8 times per day (3). When bile salts are excluded from the intestine, up to 50% of ingested fat appears in the stool. A loss of more than 100 cm of terminal ileum can be associated with a relative bile salt deficiency because liver synthesis cannot keep up.

Malabsorption in the Mucosal Phase

The mucosal phase relies on the integrity of the brush-border membrane of intestinal epithelial cells to transport digested products from the lumen into the cells.

Malabsorption in the Postabsorptive Phase

Reassembled lipids and other key nutrients are transported via the lymphatic and portal circulation from epithelial cells to the rest of the body. Obstruction of the lymphatic system, both congenital and acquired, impairs the absorption of chylomicrons and lipoproteins, thereby causing fat malabsorption or a protein-losing enteropathy.

Of note, although diarrhea often accompanies malabsorption, it is not a prerequisite. High doses of narcotics may mask diarrhea as long as the narcotics are in use. Impaired absorption of a single nutrient is also possible (eg, vitamin B-12, lactose, fructose, or iron), but when the underlying insult is diffuse, then all nutrients may be at risk.

Malabsorption Related to Anatomical Changes

The degree of malabsorption related to surgery is dependent on the site and extent of the surgery (see Chapter 14). Gastric bypass procedures that are done for weight loss purposefully create malabsorption (see Chapter 15). Short bowel syndrome is a condition of severe malabsorption that is usually the result of extensive resection of the small bowel; it is described in detail in Chapter 8.

Diagnosing Malabsorption

There is no one test for malabsorption. Seeking the underlying etiology of the symptoms is the basis for the workup. In addition, if specific nutrient deficiencies are suspected, then obtaining available laboratory data is appropriate. It is common for patients to report weight loss at the onset of diarrhea. One of the first steps should be assessment of food intake. Classic malabsorption is highly suspected in a patient who comes to clinic with a food diary supporting a calorie intake that exceeds a reasonable calorie level for that individual. It is not uncommon, however, for patients to think they are eating a lot (or at least their usual intake) when, in fact, a food diary provides evidence that the patient's energy intake is suboptimal for their condition. Ruling out weight loss due to dehydration and/or chronic hyperglycemia are additional first assessments to make.

Osmotic vs Secretory Diarrhea

Osmotic diarrhea occurs when too much water is drawn into the bowel; it will stop when the offending food, fluid, or medication is stopped. Examples of osmotic offenders include lactose, sorbitol, lactulose, and bile salt or pancreatic insufficiency. Secretory diarrhea, by contrast, means that there is an increase in the active secretion into the bowel, or an inhibition of reabsorption from the bowel, that continues even when the patient has stopped all oral/enteral ingestion. It is typically defined as an output of 500 to 800 mL in 24 hours. Examples of the causes of secretory diarrhea include infectious agents and inflammation. A 24-hour fast can be used to evaluate whether the patient has osmotic vs secretory diarrhea. See Box 5.2 for additional information on the composition of stool and definitions of diarrhea.

Clinicians use a variety of tests for a malabsorption workup (see Box 5.3) (7,9–15). Some are more common than others. For example, the Schilling test (for malabsorption of vitamin B-12) and d-xylose test are not commonly used. In the era of curbing health care costs, it is even more incumbent on the clinician to order only what is necessary to devise a treatment plan; if the test result will not change the course of treatment, then its value in the care of that individual patient should be reevaluated.

Vitamin B-12 Status

Protein-bound cobalamin is freed by pepsin and acid and initially combines with the saliva R-proteins for safe passage. In the alkaline environment of the duodenum, R-proteins are hydrolyzed by pancreatic enzymes. The cleaved B-12 then binds preferentially to intrinsic factor, and this complex travels to the ileum where it is absorbed. The same is not true for synthetic (commercial) B-12. It does not require intrinsic factor or the ileum to be absorbed (13). As noted previously, the Schilling test is rarely performed anymore—most clinicians evaluate vitamin B-12 status by either obtaining a measure of serum B-12

BOX 5.2   Composition of Stool

What Is Stool?
Stool is ¾ water and ¼ solid matter that consists of the following:
- 30% dead bacteria
- 10%–20% fat
- 10%–20% inorganic matter
- 2%–3% protein
- 30% undigested roughage and other (food, bile pigment, sloughed epithelial cells)
- Stool becomes stool when it reaches the colon; prior to that it is called *effluent*.

What Is Diarrhea?
Definitions of diarrhea are often subjective. Various definitions include the following:
- Stool frequency (3 or more/d)
- Stool consistency (liquid)
- Stool volume (250 mL/d)
- Stool weight (typically >250 g/d)
- Patients often perceive diarrhea as a decrease in consistency.

BOX 5.3   Tests Commonly Used for Malabsorption

Basic assessment (7)
- Complete blood count (CBC).
- Electrolytes (including magnesium, phosphorus, calcium).
- Glucose.
- Liver function tests (these are tests of liver inflammation).
- Lipid profile.

Diagnosing essential nutrient deficiencies
- Vitamin K—PT/INR (clotting time) Need to measure directly, using vitamin K levels or PIVKA II (protein induced by vitamin K absence or antagonist II) levels.
- Vitamin D (as 25-OH vitamin D): Dual energy X-ray absorptiometry (DXA, previously DEXA) is used to measure bone mineral density.
- Vitamin A (retinol): Note: it is a negative acute-phase reactant (ie, it is bound to retinol-binding protein) (9–11).
- Vitamin E.
- RBC folate: Useful in the patient with celiac disease because it is absorbed in the duodenum where celiac disease originates; in those with small bowel bacterial overgrowth, RBC folate may be elevated.
- Iron, as ferritin (an acute-phase reactant).
- Essential fatty acids as triene:tetrene ratio is used as a marker of EFA deficiency. The ratio of eicosatrienoic acid:arachidonic acid ($20:3n$-$9:20:4n$-6) in plasma is elevated (a plasma triene:tetraene ratio of >0.4 suggests EFA deficiency) (12).
- Vitamin B-12, methylmalonic acid (13–15).

Source: Data are from references 7 and 9–15.

alone or assessing the serum B-12 level in combination with methylmalonic acid because evaluation of serum B-12 alone can miss 10% to 50% of B-12 deficiencies (14).

Stool Fat

Steatorrhea is a hallmark finding in patients with malabsorption. Fat malabsorption is diagnosed by excessive fecal fat content. The quantitative 72-hour fecal fat collection is considered the criterion standard as many disease processes result in fat malabsorption. Although commonly used by gastroenterologists, there has been a documented knowledge deficit in the execution of this test, leading to false negatives (16,17). For a list of important considerations when ordering a 72-hour fecal fat collection, see Box 5.4 (4). Qualitative tests are random spot samples—unlike the 72-hour fecal fat test in which the patient *must* consume fat for 2 to 3 days prior to the sample to make it valid (patients must ingest fat to malabsorb it). These tests include the acid steatocrit test and Sudan III stain of stool, but these tests are less reliable. Box 5.5 lists the instructions for a quantitative 72-hour fecal fat collection used by the University of Virginia Health System (UVAHS) Digestive Health Center (4). Table 5.2 (page 54) lists the fat content of selected foods.

D-xylose Tests

D-xylose tests have been used in the past to indicate malabsorption from mucosal dysfunction, although the test is actually a measure of permeability of the proximal SB. Patients are given a 25-g oral dose of

---

BOX 5.4   Important Considerations When Ordering a 72-hour Quantitative Fecal Fat Collection

1. Order a 100-g fat, regular diet.
2. If patient is hospitalized, ensure that the nutrition services department has such a diet and that because grams of fat are specified, it is not interpreted as a "low-fat" diet.
3. Inform the patient what constitutes fat and encourage them to eat it.
4. Do not make the patient NPO at midnight for a test—clear their inpatient calendar for the test (or get the procedures done, then start).
5. Record *all* fat ingested during collection period—start a calorie count for "grams of fat eaten" (not calories) to run concurrent with the 72-hour fecal fat collection. Enlist a dietitian to oversee this.
6. Inform the nursing staff that the diet records are as important as the stool collection.
7. Have the patient or family keep the records if they are reliable.
8. Consider nocturnal enteral infusion of a high-fat formula if the collection is absolutely necessary to document need for potential home TPN [total parenteral nutrition].
9. The cost of a 72-hour fecal fat collection:
   • Cost of nursing time
   • Sent out in most hospitals—turnaround time ~ 7–10 business days; > if it is over a holiday
   • Unpleasantness factor for patient (↑↑)

Source: Reprinted with permission from reference 4: Parrish CR. The clinician's guide to short bowel syndrome. *Practical Gastroenterology*. 2005;29(9):67–106.

BOX 5.5 University of Virginia Health System Digestive Health Center 100-Gram Fat Diet and Instructions for 72-Hour Fecal Fat Collection

1. Equipment needed:
   - Stool "hat" or specimen pan
   - Storage container (can or jug will be provided)
   - If the amount of stool exceeds the container given, you may use any container (preferably plastic or metal) with a screw on lid for the rest of the collection.
   - Stool does not need to be kept in the refrigerator or on ice
2. After 3 days of stool is collected, take it to the UVAHS Digestive Health Clinic.
3. 100-gram fat diet instructions to patient:
   - Start diet and follow for 4 days.
   - On the second morning, start stool collection and collect *all* stool for 3 days.
   - It is important that you eat about 100 grams of fat each day.
   - Also eat normal portions of other foods you would normally eat.
   - Please write down everything you eat and drink for the day, starting from the time you wake up in the morning until the time you go to sleep on the record sheet provided.
   - Be sure to include any sauces, etc, mayonnaise, butter or margarine added to your foods.
   - Do your best to guess the amount you have eaten.

Source: Reprinted with permission from reference 4: Parrish CR. The clinician's guide to short bowel syndrome. *Practical Gastroenterology.* 2005;29(9):67–106.

---

d-xylose. Urine is collected for 5 hours and 1- and 3-hour serum samples are obtained. Absorption is demonstrated if >4 g of d-xylose appears in the urine and >20 mg/dL and >18.5 mg/dL in the serum at 1 and 3 hours, respectively. Due to the many factors that alter d-xylose results, use of this test has waned considerably in clinical practice.

Treatment of Malabsorption

When possible, it is important to treat the underlying process that results in malabsorption. Nutrition therapy is directed at correcting nutritional deficiencies, hydration status, increasing weight for patients who are underweight, and monitoring bone health. Pancreatic insufficiency will require the addition of pancreatic enzymes or a low-fat diet (see Chapter 12 for additional information on pancreatic insufficiency). If patient has bile salt deficiency, then a lower fat diet will be necessary because bile salt replacement is not available at this time.

Use of Enteral and Parenteral Nutrition for Malabsorption

Many patients with malabsorption can tolerate, digest, and absorb standard enteral feedings if they are delivered on a continuous basis, which presents fewer nutrients per centimeter of mucosa than if the feedings are bolused. In those patients at risk of refeeding syndrome, assuming they have not received intravenous or parenteral calories, initiation of enteral feeding with careful monitoring of serum glucose, magnesium, and potassium can be a gross indicator that at least some absorption is taking place. To exhibit

TABLE 5.2   Fat Content of Selected Foods

Food Item	Serving Size	Fat, g
Avocado	⅛	5
Margarine, butter, lard, oil	1 teaspoon	5
Diet margarine	1 Tablespoon	5
Mayonnaise	1 teaspoon	5
Light mayonnaise	1 Tablespoon	5
Almonds	6 whole	5
Cashews	4 whole	5
Pecans	3 whole	5
Peanuts	20	5
Walnuts	4 halves	5
Peanut butter or almond butter	2 Tablespoons	15
Vegetable/cooking oil (corn, soybean, sunflower, corn, olive, etc)	1 teaspoon	5
Olives	10 small	5
Salad dressing, mayonnaise type	2 teaspoons	5
Salad dressing, oil varieties	1 Tablespoon	5
Bacon	1 slice	5
Sausage	2 links or 1 oz	10
Sour cream	2 Tablespoons	5
Heavy whipping cream	1 Tablespoon	5
Cream cheese	1 Tablespoon	5
Coffee creamer, liquid	2 Tablespoons	5
Coffee creamer, dry	1 Tablespoon	5
Cream, half & half (12%)	3 Tablespoons	5
2% milk or whole milk, white or chocolate	8 oz or 1 cup	10
Ice cream	½ cup	10
Yogurt, plain or flavored (low-fat)	8 oz or 1 cup	5
Corn chips	15	10
Corn bread, 2" × 2" × 1"	1 square	5
Muffin, plain or cornmeal, 2" diameter	1	5
Potato chips	15	15
Cheese	1 oz	10
Egg, whole	1	5
Hog dog	1	10
Meat (beef, lamb, pork, poultry, veal)	1 oz cooked	5
M&Ms chocolate	1 small bag	10
Hershey's Kisses or Chocolate bar	9 candies/1 small bar	13

refeeding syndrome, one must absorb nutrients and stimulate insulin release. There is little evidence to support the use of elemental products (18); however, a trial of a semi-elemental formula followed by an elemental formula would be appropriate before deciding to initiate parenteral nutrition (PN). The amount of medium-chain triglycerides (MCT) should be monitored because more than 30 g of MCT, alone or as an ingredient in some enteral products, has been shown to cause GI distress in *healthy* individuals (19).

A trial of an enteral product should be given enough time to determine whether the product is being absorbed (a 48- to 72-hour fecal collection may need to be repeated to assess the efficacy of the product). If the patient fails to absorb nutrients from the enteral feeding, PN should be initiated. See Chapters 19 and 20 for additional information on enteral and parenteral nutrition.

Diseases Frequently Associated with Malabsorption Syndromes

Pancreatic Disease and Pancreatic Insufficiency

Acute and chronic pancreatic diseases often result in significant malabsorption. Pancreatic conditions are discussed in detail in Chapter 12.

Cystic Fibrosis

Cystic fibrosis (CF) is primarily a pulmonary disease, but it can have a malabsorption component. The malabsorption that is associated with CF is multifactorial. Pancreatic insufficiency (PI) is associated with the most severe mutation of the CF gene. Those who are homozygous for the ΔF508 mutation, the most common mutation in the northern Europe and North America population, are very likely to have PI. Pancreatic insufficiency affects 85% of CF patients, and all of these patients have malabsorption (20). Pancreatic destruction begins in utero with the secretion of acidic fluid into the lumen of the pancreatic duct, leading to a precipitation of secreted proteins. Intraluminal obstruction of the ducts then causes progressive damage and atrophy (20). This obstructive process is the basis of newborn screening for CF. The measurement of serum trypsinogen in cord blood identifies CF in infants before signs of failure to thrive are apparent. High serum trypsinogen in newborns is the result of the release of enzymes into the circulation, owing to ductal obstruction and acinar cell damage (20). Diagnosis is confirmed through sweat chloride testing.

Altered pulmonary function is another feature of CF. There is a strong association between nutritional status and lung function in CF patients (21,22). This association has made the registered dietitian (RD) specializing in CF a key provider in ongoing care. Nutritional status is assessed at each clinic visit, along with pulmonary function. The RD assesses nutritional status by determining weight-for-length for infants and toddlers younger than 2 years of age; the body mass index (BMI) percentile for children and adolescents ages 2 to 20 years; or the BMI for adults. See Table 5.3 for the definition of nutritional failure in patients with CF and those at risk (22).

Children and adults with CF need 30% to 100% more energy intake compared to healthy populations matched for age and sex (22). After assessment, the RD needs to be able to provide guidance as to how to achieve and maintain this level of intake. To achieve adequate caloric intake, the CF diet includes as much as 50% of calories from fat. The challenge becomes one of balancing a "healthy" diet with one that meets the energy needs of the patient. The Cystic Fibrosis Foundation has established a Nutrition Consensus Report developed by physicians and RDs experienced in working with this population (22). The

TABLE 5.3 Definition of Nutritional Failure in Patients with Cystic Fibrosis and Those at Risk

Nutritional Status	Length or Height	Percentage of IBW All Ages	Weight-for-Length Percentile 0 to 2 Years	BMI Percentile 2 to 20 Years	Action
Acceptable	Normal growth	≥90%	>25th	>25th	Continue to monitor with usual care.
At-risk	Not at genetic potential	≥90%, with weight loss or plateau	10 to 25th	10 to 25th	Nutritional and medical evaluation; some, but not all in this category are at risk for nutrition failure.
Nutritional failure	<5%ile	<90%	<10th	<10th	Treat nutritional failure.

Source: Reprinted with permission from reference 22: Borowitz D, Baker RD, Stallings V. Consensus report on nutrition for pediatric patients with cystic fibrosis. *J Pediatr Gastroenterol.* 2002;35:246–249.

guidelines set out in the report are reviewed frequently and adjusted based on "best practice outcomes" from data fed into the population database from each CF center. Basic research, ongoing clinical trials, and clinical practice are all enhanced by the information provided through that database. It is the data from this model of cooperation that keeps pushing the boundaries of CF care and continues to increase life expectancy in this population.

ASSESSING NUTRITIONAL STATUS

Percentage of ideal body weight (IBW), although effective in many populations, does not identify a child with CF who is just beginning to fall behind. BMI percentile has been shown to be more sensitive to changes in lung function and is therefore a more effective predictor in identifying the early signs of malnutrition in children with CF (23). In children and adolescents ages 2 to 20 years, BMI is plotted on a growth curve by age. The ideal weight for height (ie, goal weight) is that which puts the BMI at the 50th percentile. Nutritional status is assessed every 3 months, during clinic visits. Clinic visits should include discussion of the following:

- Compliance with pancreatic enzymes
- Compliance with vitamin supplements
- Presence of symptoms of malabsorption
- Appetite
- Eating behaviors
- Enzyme dose with meals and snacks
- How enzymes are stored
- Meal and snack timing

The preceding information along with assessment of pulmonary status can be used to reverse a downward trend. Making the most of pancreatic enzyme replacement therapy (PERT) is essential to maintaining good nutritional status. Factors that may affect the efficacy of PERT include the following:

- Dosing of enzymes (see recommendations in following paragraph)
- Timing of enzymes
- Acidic gastric environment
- Slow gastric emptying
- Exposure of enzymes to heat during storage

Enzyme dosing is done most frequently based on units of lipase per kg of weight per meal or per feed (21,22). The enzyme dose should be reviewed at each clinic visit and adjusted when symptoms of malabsorption are present. If the enzyme dose is at the highest recommended level, then timing of the dose as well as compliance should be explored. Enzymes should be taken with meals, and no more than 30 minutes prior to eating in order to have maximum effectiveness. Enzymes stored in an exceptionally hot environment may lose efficacy. The pH of the intestinal lumen may also decrease efficacy. Decreased bicarbonate secretion and increased gastric acidity of CF may reduce enzyme activity by delaying the release of enzymes in the proximal duodenum. The enteric coating that protects the digestive enzyme is not dissolved until pH approaches 6. If this does not occur early in the duodenum, it may be helpful to add adjunct therapies such as proton pump inhibitors, H_2 blockers, or bicarbonate tablets, all of which help to increase the pH of gastric secretions higher in the duodenum, increasing the efficacy of enzymes (24). The Cystic Fibrosis Foundation has published a free, downloadable handout for patients on the use of pancreatic enzymes, which was reviewed and approved by the Pediatric Nutrition Dietetic Practice Group of the Academy of Nutrition and Dietetics (25). Additional information on this topic is also available in the Academy's Pediatric Nutrition Care Manual, in the Cystic Fibrosis subsection of Pulmonary Diseases (26).

Signs of PI and malabsorption include:

- Abdominal pain, cramping, bloating, and flatus
- Loose and frequent stools
- Steatorrhea
- Fat-soluble vitamin deficiency
- Poor weight gain and/or growth
- Presence of meconium ileus in newborns

The following tests should be used to document PI in CF (22):

- 72-hour fecal fat balance study
- Elevated immunoreactive trypsinogen (IRT) after 8 years of age
- Fecal elastase-1

Note: Fecal elastase-1 can be used as a marker for PI using an enzyme-linked immunosorbent assay (ELISA). The assay from ScheBo Biotech (Geiseen, Germany) is recommended for use in CF patients as it does not react with porcine elastase used in PERT. While there is argument as to the exact cut-off level for determining PI, there is evidence to support a level less than 100 mcg per gram of stool is indicative of PI (27).

Growth and weight expectations are based on best outcome correlates from the CF registry data. The guidelines in Box 5.6 have been determined to be associated with the best outcomes (21).

BOX 5.6   Recommendations for Growth and Weight in Cystic Fibrosis Care

- **Children <2 years of age**: Achieve weight-for-length ≥50th percentile by 2 years of age
- **Children and adolescents, ages 2–20 years**: Maintain body mass index (BMI) ≥50th percentile for age.
- **Adults**: Women maintain BMI ≥22.

Because we are seeing stronger correlations between healthy weight gain, good lung function, and prolonged life expectancy, there is a tendency toward more aggressive nutrition therapy. Use of BMI percentile in children is now the recommended measure to determine whether a patient is maintaining adequate nutritional status. Nutritional failure is treated with more frequent clinic visits, intensive nutrition counseling to increase calories and address feeding behavior problems, and possible enteral support with g-tube placement for nocturnal feeds.

Source: Data are from reference 21.

DISTAL INTESTINAL OBSTRUCTION SYNDROME

Distal intestinal obstruction syndrome (DIOS) is a recurrent obstruction starting in the ileocecal region and extending into the colon. It results from abnormal intestinal mucous, dysmotility, thickened secretions, and other unknown factors (28). Patients with a history of gastric surgery and dysmotility are at higher risk of developing DIOS. Possible causes of DIOS include the following (28):

- Dehydration
- Diet changes
- Medications that cause constipation
- Immobilization
- Respiratory infection
- Bacterial overgrowth
- Inadequate enzyme replacement therapy

DIOS is associated with right lower quadrant pain, and does not necessarily cause constipation. Once called "meconium ileus equivalent," it is seen in older children and adults with CF. Management of DIOS includes the following:

- Hydration
- Medications:
  - Stool softeners, laxatives (eg, docusate, senna, lactulose)
  - Osmotic agents (polyethylene glycol [Miralax])
  - Mucomyst (acetylcysteine) cocktail—ie, Mucomyst 10% (30–60 mL) added to 30–60 mL soda, orange juice, or mineral oil—taken orally every 8 hours for 24 hours
- Diet modification:
  - Adequate fluid intake
  - Regular meals and snacks with enzymes
  - Avoidance of grazing or binging
  - Adding fiber-containing foods unless slow motility noted
- Optimization of enzyme therapy

Abdominal radiography is used to determine the extent of obstruction as well as efficacy of the treatment regimen. In severe cases, an invasive procedure may be required to dissolve or resect the obstruction.

BONE HEALTH

As the CF population is growing older (current life expectancy is 32 years), we are seeing more adults with CF who have experienced increased bone fractures due to poor bone mineralization. Factors that contribute to bone disease include the following (29):

- Poor vitamin D absorption
- Poor nutritional status
- Physical inactivity
- Glucocorticoid therapy
- Delayed pubertal maturation
- Early hypogonadism
- Poor compliance with vitamin D or multiple vitamin supplement
- Increased serum cytokines from frequent lung inflammation increasing bone resorption and decreasing bone formation

Vitamin D deficiency is common among the CF population. Twenty-five hydroxyvitamin D levels are monitored annually, and low or low-normal levels are found in this population, regardless of season or latitude (29).

US CF guidelines advise that bone mass density be evaluated in all adults with CF at age 18 years, and in children older than 8 years of age with the following risk factors (29):

- Weight <90% IBW
- Forced expiratory rate <50% predicted
- Glucocorticoids >5 mg/d for more than 90 days
- Delayed puberty
- History of fracture

There is controversy about how best to improve vitamin D status in CF. As a result of their research, Khazai et al (30) suggest that cholecalciferol (vitamin D_3) is a more effective supplement than ergocalciferol (vitamin D_2). In adults, they found that oral supplementation with vitamin D_3 at 50,000 IU once a week for 12 weeks was an effective way to replenish stores (30). Current recommendations do not seem to be effective in preventing vitamin D deficiency; unfortunately, the many causal factors make a consensus difficult to achieve.

ENTERAL SUPPORT

The increased energy needs of the CF patient often lead to the need for nocturnal feedings to meet energy requirements. Because enteral support is usually a long-term therapy, G-tube placement is recommended. Enteral products do not need to be elemental, and should be as calorie-dense as tolerated by the patient without gastric upset.

Enzyme dosing for enteral feeds is usually done by starting with the full meal-dose of enteric-coated enzymes taken by mouth as the feeding begins, and a snack or half dose at or near the end of the feed. It is also a common practice to use a non-enteric-coated enzyme, such as Viokase powder, or crushed tablets added directly to the enteral formula if oral enzymes do not prevent symptoms of malabsorption.

This method may cause gastric discomfort if the caloric density of the enteral formula is more than 1.5 kcal/mL (21).

The following is the process for enzyme dosing in nocturnal continuous feeds:

- Calculate 2,000 units lipase per gram of fat in formula.
- Administer the full dose of enzymes at the beginning of the feed. (Patients may need a snack or ½ dose of enzymes near the end of the feed. If symptoms of malabsorption persist, adding Viokase powder at 2,000 units lipase per gram of fat directly to the bag of formula may improve absorption.)
- Shake bag well to distribute.
- Shake bag periodically through the feeding cycle to prevent clogging of tube when using calorie-dense formulas

The following are guidelines for starting nocturnal enteral feeds:

- Aim to provide one-third of estimated calorie needs via the night feed.
- Choose a formula that provides 1.0, 1.5 or, 2.0 kcal/mL. Elemental formulas may be needed only when there is history of intestinal resection or if symptoms of malabsorption are not resolved with enzyme therapy.
- Begin with two-thirds of desired volume at full strength.
- Calculate the rate and timing of feeds to provide the desired volume of product that fits into the patient's schedule.
- Determine enzyme dose:
    ○ Begin with the meal dose of enteric-coated enzyme orally before feed starts.
    ○ Add a snack-dose of enteric-coated enzyme at or near the end of feed.
- Monitor symptoms of malabsorption and tolerance.
- Increase feed rate until desired volume is achieved.
- Monitor weight gain.
- Add non-enteric-coated enzyme directly to feeding formula if symptoms of malabsorption occur.
- Continue to monitor and adjust formula until desired weight is achieved.

IMPORTANCE OF COMPREHENSIVE CARE

The effective management of malabsorption related to CF requires a comprehensive team of health care providers. The RD is a key member of the team, which also includes the physician, nurse, social worker, and respiratory therapist. The combined efforts of each team member are needed to adequately support patients with this complex disease. Ongoing clinical trials are continually adding new therapies, and it is the responsibility of each team member to stay educated about advances.

Celiac Disease

Celiac disease is an autoimmune disorder (not an allergy) that is the confluence of three factors: genetic predisposition, environmental exposure (ingesting gluten), and immunologically based mucosal inflammation resulting in a loss of villi and a flattening of the mucosa. The incidence of celiac disease seems to be rising, but it is difficult to determine whether the increasing numbers are due to better diagnosis. Although physicians have become more aware of the frequency of celiac disease, it is estimated that only

10% to 15% of current cases have been diagnosed (31). One reason celiac disease is so elusive is the myriad of signs and symptoms it can display in individuals (32–34). See Chapter 10 for more information.

Conclusion

The digestion and absorption of nutrients is a complex process. Malabsorption can occur when disease or surgery interferes with any of the many parts of this process. Diagnosis is often difficult, and treatment may be based primarily on the alleviation of symptoms. Diet is a critical part of the therapy for malabsorption.

References

1. Hecketsweiler P, Vidon N, Emonts P, et al. Absorption of elemental and complex nutritional solutions during a continuous jejunal perfusion in man. *Digestion.* 1979;19:213–217.
2. Barrett KE, Boitano S, Barman SM, Brooks HL. Overview of gastrointestinal function and regulation and digestion and absorption. In*: Review of Medical Physiology.* 23rd ed. New York, NY: Lange Medical Books/ McGraw Hill; 2010:467–478.
3. Harig JM. Pathophysiology of small bowel diarrhea. In: *American Gastroenterological Association Postgraduate Course.* Boston, MA: American Gastroenterological Association; 1993:199–203.
4. Parrish CR. The clinician's guide to short bowel syndrome. *Pract Gastroenterol.* 2005;29(9):67–106.
5. Owens SR, Greenson JK. The pathology of malabsorption: current concepts. *Histopathology.* 2007;50:64–82.
6. Sun W, Lo CM, Tso P. Intestinal lipid absorption. In: Yamada T, ed. *Yamada`s Textbook of Gastroenterology.* 5th ed. New York, NY: Wiley-Blackwell; 2009:445–463.
7. Schulzke J, Tröger H, Amasheh M. Disorders of intestinal secretion and absorption. *Best Pract Res Clin Gastroenterol.* 2009;23:395–406.
8. Farrell JJ. Overview and diagnosis of malabsorption syndrome. *Semin Gastrointest Dis.* 2002;13:182–190.
9. Stephensen CB. Vitamin A, infection, and immune function. *Ann Rev Nutr.* 2001;21:167–192.
10. Stephensen CB. When does hyporetinolemia mean vitamin A deficiency? *Am J Clin Nutr.* 2000;72:1–2.
11. Curran FJ, Sattar N, Talwar D, et al. Relationship of carotenoid and vitamins A and E with the acute inflammatory response in acute pancreatitis. *Br J Surg.* 2000;87:301.
12. Jeppesen PB, Christensen MS, Hoy CE, et al. Essential fatty acid deficiency in patients with severe fat malabsorption. *Am J Clin Nutr.* 1997;65:837–843.
13. Dali-Youcef NAE. An update on cobalamin deficiency in adults. *QJM.* 2009;102:17–28.
14. da Silva L, McCray S. Vitamin B-12: no one should be without it. *Pract Gastroenterol.* 2009;33:34.
15. Oh RBD. Vitamin B12 deficiency. *Am Fam Physician.* 2003;67:979–986.
16. Lust M, Nandurkar S, Gibson PR. Measurement of faecal fat excretion: an evaluation of attitudes and practices of Australian gastroenterologists. *Intern Med J.* 2006;36:77–85.
17. Dinning JP, Bowers JM, Trujillo MA. A standardized diet for performing fecal fat excretion studies. *Arch Intern Med.* 1997;157:245–246.
18. Makola D, Krenitsky J, Parrish CR. Enteral feeding in acute and chronic pancreatitis. *Gastrointest Endosc Clin N Am.* 2007;17:747–764.
19. Jeukendrup AE, Saris WH, Schrauwen P, et al. Metabolic availability of medium-chain triglycerides coingested with carbohydrates during prolonged exercise. *J Appl Physiol.* 1995;79:756–762.
20. Williams SK, ed. Virginia Department of Health: Virginia Newborn Screening Services Healthcare Practitioner Manual. 2006. www.vahealth.org/VNSP/documents/docs2006/PDF/VDH%20VNSS%20HCP%20 Manual%20-%20FINAL.pdf. Accessed April 1, 2014.
21. Stallings VA, Stark LJ, Robinson KA, et al. Evidence-based practice recommendations for nutrition-related management of children and adults with cystic fibrosis and pancreatic insufficiency: results of a systematic review. *J Am Diet Assoc.* 2008;108:832–839.

22. Borowitz D, Baker RD, Stallings V. Consensus report on nutrition for pediatric patients with cystic fibrosis. *J Pediatr Gastroenterol.* 2002;35:246–249.

23. Zhang Z, Lai HJ. Comparison of the use of body mass index percentiles and percentage of ideal body weight to screen for malnutrition in children with cystic fibrosis. *Am J Clin Nutr.* 2004;80:982–991.

24. Borowitz D, Durie PR, Clarke LL, et al. Gastrointestinal outcomes and confounders in cystic fibrosis. *J Pediatr Gastroenterol Nutr.* 2005;41:273–285.

25. Maguiness K, Casey S, Fulton J, et al. Nutrition: Pancreatic Enzyme Replacement in People with Cystic Fibrosis. Cystic Fibrosis Foundation. 2006. www.cff.org/UploadedFiles/LivingWithCF/StayingHealthy/Diet /EnzymeReplacement/Nutrition-Pancreatic-Enzyme-Replacement.pdf. Accessed July 2, 2014.

26. Cystic Fibrosis. Academy of Nutrition and Dietetics. Pediatric Nutrition Care Manual. www.nutritioncare manual.org. Accessed July 2, 2014.

27. Kalnins D, Durie PR, Pencharz P. Nutritional management of cystic fibrosis patients. *Curr Opin Clin Nutr Metab Care.* 2007;10:348–354.

28. Mascarenhas M. Treatment of gastrointestinal problems in cystic fibrosis. *Curr Treat Options Gastroenterol.* 2003;6:427–441.

29. Aris RM, Merkel PA, Bachrach LK, et al. Consensus statement: guide to bone health and disease in cystic fibrosis. *J Clin Endocrinol Soc.* 2005;90:1888–1896.

30. Khazai NB, Judd SE, Jeng L, et al. Treatment and prevention of vitamin D insufficiency in cystic fibrosis patients: comparative efficacy of ergocalciferol, cholecalciferol and UV light. *J Clin Endocrinol Metab.* 2009;94:2037–2043.

31. Armstrong MJ, Robins GG, Howdle PD. Recent advances in coeliac disease. *Curr Opin Gastroenterol.* 2009;25:100–109.

32. Farrell RJ KC. Celiac sprue. *N Engl J Med.* 2002;346:180–188.

33. Di Sabatino A, Corazza GR. Coeliac disease. *Lancet.* 2009;373:1480–1493.

34. Barker JM. Celiac disease: pathophysiology, clinical manifestations, and associated autoimmune conditions. *Adv Pediatr.* 2008;55:349–365.

CHAPTER 6

Common Gastrointestinal Symptoms

Kathy T. Barco, RD, CNSC, Mary Jo Alberino, RD, CNSC,
Kristen M. Roberts, MS, RD, LD, Jodi Wolff, MS, RD, LD, CNSC,
and Neha R. Parekh, MS, RD, LD, CNSC

Patients with diseases of the gastrointestinal (GI) tract may experience a wide variety of GI symptoms that adversely affect their ability to tolerate an adequate oral diet. Common GI symptoms include gas, bloating, nausea, vomiting, diarrhea, and constipation. Consideration should be given to the pathophysiology of the symptoms, because it plays a role in determining the most appropriate mode of treatment. Once the reasoning behind the therapy is established, appropriate dietary, medical, and behavioral modifications can often be optimized to treat the underlying disorder and potentially relieve the patient's symptoms.

Gas, Bloating, and Distention

The terms abdominal *gas*, *bloating*, and *distention* are often used interchangeably by both patients and medical personnel to describe GI complaints. The pathophysiology of these symptom(s) is complex and often poorly understood (1); however, clinicians have improved the definitions, diagnosis, and treatment of gas, bloating, and distention (2). The term *belching* or *eructation* is associated with aerophagia, whereas *flatulence* (*flatus*) is often used to describe intestinal gas that is passed via the anus.

Sources of Gas

Intestinal gas may be produced by bacteria in the bowel or by ingesting air during swallowing. The production of gas in the lumen of the small bowel results from the malabsorption of nutrients, especially carbohydrate, which provides a substrate for bacterial fermentation. The process of bacterial fermentation can increase the osmotic load within the GI tract, hasten or delay GI motility, and alter the bacterial flora of the bowel (3,4).

Aerophagia

DIAGNOSTIC CRITERIA AND ETIOLOGY

The diagnostic criteria for aerophagia include "troublesome repetitive belching at least several times a week and air swallowing that is objectively observed or measured." These criteria must be fulfilled for 3 months with symptom onset at least 6 months before diagnosis (5).

Patients rapidly swallow air into the esophagus with immediate proximal expulsion known as "supragastric belching" as measured by impedance monitoring (5–7). The patient may belch up to 20 times per minute. The belching is not related to meals and has no associated taste or scent.

Aerophagia is considered a behavioral disorder often seen in patients with anxiety. An organic etiology is rarely found (7). Patients with aerophagia also commonly report symptoms of abdominal bloating (8).

TREATMENT AND MANAGEMENT

There is no current evidence-based therapy for this disorder. Behavioral therapy and/or speech therapy is suggested to encourage small swallows and to eat slowly. Patients are encouraged to avoid chewing gum, drinking carbonated beverages, and sucking on candy. Medications such as simethicone and dimethicone are not helpful because an abnormal amount of intestinal gas is not present (7).

Bloating

Bloating affects up to 96% of patients with a functional GI disorder and 30% of the general population (9,10). There is no single cause for bloating (11).

Bloating is considered a subjective sensation of excessive gas/flatulence, fullness, abdominal hardness or tightness, or abdominal inflation or swelling (2,10). Bloating is episodic, usually occurring after meals and at the end of the day (12), and subsides or disappears overnight (10). Bloating is associated with gas trapping, loose bowel movements, and visceral hypersensitivity (2).

Impaired visceral reflexes may result in abnormal propulsion of both gas and nongaseous intestinal contents (12). Bloating in patients with a functional disorder is associated with diaphragmatic descent, abdominal-phrenic dyssynergia, and incoordinated abdominal accommodation (12).

Distention

DEFINITION AND ETIOLOGY

Distention is considered an objective finding associated with an increase in abdominal girth (2,10,12). Bloating associated with distention is a result of increased gas content and intra-abdominal volume that allows displacement of the abdominal wall (12). Intestinal dysmotility can cause distention through delayed small bowel and colonic transit and visceral hyposensitivity (10). Distention is more common in patients with constipation than diarrhea (10).

TREATMENT AND MANAGEMENT

The goal of treatment is to minimize symptoms and modify the microbiota of the GI tract with diet or probiotics (2). Dietary therapy involves avoiding gas-producing and fermentable foods (2,13).

The probiotic *Bifidobacterium lactis* DN-173-010 has been shown to accelerate GI transit in patients with constipation-associated irritable bowel syndrome (IBS), and improves distention and symptoms of bloating (11). Nonabsorbable antibiotics (rifaximin) have been found to be safe and effective for the treatment of abdominal bloating and flatulence (2,14).

Medications that accelerate transit may be useful in the treatment of distention (10). Prokinetics may improve symptoms of bloating, but may not decrease intestinal gas content (15). Consider antidepressants to reduce hypersensitivity in patients with functional disorders (2).

Diseases and Conditions Associated with Gas, Bloating, and Distention

The following diseases and conditions may be associated with nutrient malabsorption, resulting in increased gas production, bloating, and distention. Diagnosis and treatment for these conditions is beyond the scope of this review, but further information may be found in other chapters:

- Irritable bowel syndrome (IBS) (see Chapter 9)
- Malabsorptive disorders (see Chapter 5)
- Celiac disease (see Chapter 10)
- Short bowel syndrome (see Chapter 8)
- Small intestinal bacterial overgrowth (see Chapter 8)
- Gastric outlet obstruction (see Chapter 14)

Managing Functional GI Symptoms with Diet Modification

Diet may be modified to avoid or limit the following:

- Lactose (in milk and milk products) (4,13).
- Fructose (eg, in high-fructose corn syrup) (4,13).
- Raffinose (in vegetables) (4,13).
- Sorbitol (a sugar alcohol used in artificial sweetener) (4,13).
- Fermentable oligo-, di-, and monosaccharides, and polyols (FODMAPs), ie, short-chain, poorly absorbed carbohydrates (see Chapter 9 for a list of fermentable sources of FODMAPs, characteristics, and food sources). Malabsorption results in symptoms of both osmotic and fermentative etiology (ie, gas production, bloating, pain, and dysmotility) (2–4). Limit FODMAPs for 6 to 8 weeks and assess efficacy (2).
- Fiber: Soluble fiber is fermented in the colon and may be more gas-producing than insoluble fiber. Fiber increases volume and frequency of stools, but it may worsen symptoms in patients with gas and bloating (3). Fiber intake and treatment of constipation is discussed in greater detail later in this chapter.
- Carbonated beverages (3): Carbonation is the process of dissolving carbon dioxide into a solution. Bubbles are released as pressure is lowered and may contribute to intestinal gas.

Nausea and Vomiting

Vomiting is a forceful expulsion of gastric contents. Nausea is a sensation that often precedes vomiting, although patients may experience nausea without vomiting. Although nausea is very subjective, patients may describe the sensation as having an "upset stomach" or feeling "queasy" (16). Nausea and vomiting are common symptoms that can be quite distressing to patients. It is important to first assess the etiology of the nausea and vomiting to direct the type of treatment. Acute nausea and vomiting often quickly resolve, whereas chronic nausea and vomiting (lasting more than 1 month) may represent a more complex challenge (17).

Etiology

Common etiologies of nausea and vomiting include exogenous toxins, GI diseases, diseases of the central nervous system, and endocrine and metabolic causes (18). Exogenous toxins and/or adverse reactions to medications are among the most common causes of nausea and vomiting. Some common medications in this category include narcotics for pain control, chemotherapy agents, antibiotics, analgesics, and radiation therapy. GI diseases that may cause nausea and vomiting include mechanical obstruction (eg, gastric outlet obstruction or small bowel obstruction due to abdominal adhesions and strictures); motility disorders (eg, gastroparesis and chronic intestinal pseudo-obstruction); organic GI disorders (eg, cancer, peptic ulcer disease, hepatitis, Crohn's disease, and mesenteric ischemia); inflammatory conditions (eg, pancreatitis, cholecystitis, and appendicitis); and viral or bacterial infection of the GI tract or nongastro-intestinal infections, such as otitis media.

Nausea and vomiting can also be an adverse effect after surgery (18). Postoperative nausea and vomiting may be increased by the use of general anesthesia, the duration of surgery, the use of opiate medications after surgery, and the use of certain inhalation agents (19). Patients who undergo abdominal operations that alter the size of the stomach or length of the remaining bowel are at a greater risk of experiencing ileus and postoperative nausea and vomiting. Ileus is a nonmechanical insult that alters the bowel motility and is considered a normal physiologic response to abdominal surgery.

Impairments of the central nervous system, such as intracranial pressure, labyrinthine disorders, psychiatric disease, and seizure disorders, can provoke nausea and vomiting. Endocrine and metabolic causes, such as diabetic ketoacidosis, Addison's disease, pregnancy, and hypo- or hyperthyroidism, may cause nausea and vomiting due to multiple factors, such as the disruption of GI motor activity and hormonal responses.

Cyclic vomiting syndrome is a rare condition largely reported in children who experience recurrent acute episodes of nausea and vomiting. A variety of other conditions, such as cardiac disease and starvation, can also lead to nausea and vomiting.

Diagnostic Tests

Diagnostic tests for nausea and vomiting include the following:

- Abdominal radiographs
- Esophagogastroduodenoscopy
- Barium contrast studies: small-bowel follow-through
- Radioisotopic tests
- Scintigraphy
- Electrogastrography
- Antroduodenal manometry
- MRI, if a central nervous system etiology is suspected
- Psychological evaluation if nausea and vomiting are otherwise unexplained

Nutrition Therapy

Side effects of nausea and vomiting include dehydration, electrolyte imbalances, and nutritional deficiencies. Goals of treatment are to decrease the frequency and severity of nausea and vomiting, and maintain nutritional and hydration status (20). Nutritional deficiencies may result from chronic nausea and vomiting associated with inadequate nutritional intake. A physical examination can help document weight loss and identify signs of nutrient deficiency.

When vomiting stops, the patient should start with ice chips or clear liquids before attempting intake of other beverages or food. Once they can tolerate liquids, patients should then be encouraged to follow a low-fat, low-fiber diet. Fatty foods and high-fiber foods delay gastric emptying, which may worsen nausea. Patients should also be instructed to start with very small portions of one solid food item at a time to improve their tolerance (20). See Table 6.1 for a list of foods patients may eat after experiencing nausea and vomiting (20).

Initiation of nutrition support should be determined by the underlying etiology of the nausea and vomiting, adequacy of current nutritional intake, and the patient's nutritional status prior to development of nausea and vomiting. Well-nourished patients experiencing acute onset of nausea and vomiting expected to resolve in less than 7 days can be maintained on intravenous (IV) fluids without adverse effect on their nutritional status (21). Patients with upper GI diseases may benefit from the initiation of distal small bowel enteral feeding that bypasses the diseased or obstructed segment of bowel. Those who are unable to consume or absorb adequate oral or enteral nutrition may require a decompressive nasogastric tube for management of symptoms and parenteral nutrition to meet nutritional requirements (22). Dehydration and electrolyte imbalances are often present in patients with severe or prolonged nausea and vomiting. A standard chemistry profile and complete blood count should be obtained to assess for dehydration and hypokalemic metabolic alkalosis (18). Table 6.2 outlines the electrolyte composition of GI fluids (23).

TABLE 6.1 Recommended Foods for Managing Nausea and Vomiting

Food Group	Examples
Grains	Dry toast, crackers, rice, pretzels
Vegetables	Potato
Fruit	Banana, applesauce, juice, frozen fruit, popsicles
Milk and dairy	Yogurt, sherbet
Meats and eggs	Broth, low-fat meats, eggs

Source: Data are from reference 20.

TABLE 6.2 Electrolyte Composition of Gastrointestinal Fluids

Source	Sodium, mEq/L	Potassium, mEq/L	Bicarbonate, mEq/L	Chlorine, mEq/L
Pancreas	140	5	115	75
Bile	145	5	35	100
Duodenum	140	5	—	80
Ileum	140	5	30	104
Colon	60	30	—	40

Source: Data are from reference 23.

Medications

Pharmacologic approaches are primarily guided by clinical experience because there is a lack of literature on the use of medications in the treatment of nausea and vomiting. Antiemetics and prokinetics are used to help decrease frequency and severity of nausea and vomiting (19,22). Antiemetics suppress nausea and vomiting through the central nervous system. Many other drugs have antiemetic effects, but their use as a treatment for nausea and vomiting is often limited because of other side effects. Prokinetics are primarily used for dysmotility syndromes and have reported central nervous system and cardiovascular side effects, which limit their usefulness. See Box 6.1 for an explanation of the uses of three prokinetics (21).

Diarrhea

Diarrhea is a condition that contributes to mortality worldwide and therefore needs serious consideration for evaluation and treatment (24). Treatment begins with understanding the etiology of the symptoms.

Classification

Diarrhea can be classified by volume/frequency/consistency, acute vs chronic, and osmotic vs secretory. Acute diarrhea tends to be related to infection whereas chronic diarrhea is most likely related to

---

BOX 6.1   Prokinetics Used to Decrease Frequency and Severity of Nausea and Vomiting

Metoclopramide
- Peripheral and central dopamine antagonist.
- Stimulates gastric and duodenal motility.
- Short-term benefit; effects of the drug diminish within a few days.
- Long-term use (>3 months) and high doses of this drug are not permitted due to high incidence of adverse effects (hyperprolactinemia, central nervous system effects, and extrapyramidal effects).
- Dose: 5–30 mg 4 times per day; can be administered intraveneously or subcutaneously.

Erythromycin
- Antibiotic.
- Most potent agent that stimulates gastric emptying.
- Side effects are common.
- Prolonged use (>3–4 days) is associated with decreased efficacy, down-regulation of motilin receptors, tachyphylaxis, and possibility of antibiotic resistance.
- Dose:
  - Oral: 125–250 mg 4 times per day.
  - Intravenous: 0.75–3 mg/kg 3 times per day.

Domperidone
- Dose: 10–20 mg 4 times per day.
- Available from special compounding pharmacies in the United States; also available abroad and widely available in Canada.

Source: Data are from reference 21.

inflammatory bowel diseases, malabsorption syndromes, and chronic infections (25,26). Secretory diarrhea is related to increased secretions from the GI tract, and osmotic diarrhea refers to an increase in the osmotic pressure of the contents within the GI tract (27). See Chapter 5 for more information on the distinction between osmotic and secretory diarrhea.

Etiology

The pathophysiology of diarrhea is usually multifactorial. Thus, there are several differential diagnoses to consider when determining the etiology of diarrhea (see Box 6.2) (25–27). A complete medical and nutrition history is imperative to identify potential contributing factors leading to the onset of diarrhea (see Box 6.3).

Treatment

The management of diarrhea is complex and requires both medical and nutritional modifications in the plan of care (26). Dietary modifications should minimize the patient's symptoms and improve hydration (see Box 6.4 on page 70) (28–30). Table 6.3 (page 71) provides recommendations for meal planning (28). For further discussion of the management of malabsorption in the patient with short bowel syndrome, refer to Chapters 5 and 8.

BOX 6.2   Common Differential Diagnoses for Diarrhea

- Viral infections
- Bacterial infections
- Irritable bowel syndrome
- Crohn's disease
- Ulcerative colitis
- Malabsorption syndromes, such as lactose intolerance, chronic pancreatitis, celiac disease, and bacterial overgrowth of the small intestine

Source: Data are from references 25, 26, and 27.

BOX 6.3   Patient History Topics to Help Identify Potential Etiologies of Diarrhea

- Past medical history of diarrheal episodes and/or conditions of malabsorption
- Past surgical history affecting the gastrointestinal tract
- Recent travel history
- Any history of recent weight loss related to the onset of the diarrhea
- The presence of diarrhea and abdominal cramping while eating
- A review of the patient's current medications and any changes in medications and/or doses
- An evaluation of dietary intake
- An evaluation of sorbitol and xylitol content in the diet and/or in medications
- An assessment of the stool characteristics including the consistency, frequency, volume, color, smell, and presence of fat or grease
- Presence of excessive flatus

BOX 6.4   Management of Diarrhea Through Diet and Medications

- Dietary modifications aim to reduce foods that decrease gastrointestinal (GI) transit time and contribute to diarrhea, such as high-fat foods, sources of insoluble fiber, sugar alcohols, and caffeinated and/or high-sugar beverages:
  - High-fat foods and insoluble fiber stimulate the gastrocolic reflex, which decreases GI transit time.
  - Sugar alcohols are incompletely absorbed in the GI tract and have a laxative effect when taken in excess.
  - Caffeinated beverages can increase peristalsis, causing a food bolus to move through the GI tract faster and leading to diarrhea.
  - High-sugar beverages, such as regular soda and fruit juices, can contribute to an osmotic diarrhea.
- Fluid recommendations aim to prevent dehydration and may include the use of an oral rehydration solution (ORS)[a] to maximize the absorption of fluids in the GI tract. Refer to Chapter 8 for additional information on ORS.
- Medication recommendations aim to prolong transit through the GI tract and promote the absorption of nutrients into the intestinal lumen.
  - Antidiarrheals (ie, loperamide, diphenoxylate/atropine, codeine, paregoric, opium tincture, etc) decrease the motility of the GI tract.
  - Antisecretories (ie, famotidine, omeprazole, octreotide, etc) inhibit and/or diminish the production of gastric and intestinal secretions.
  - Soluble fiber supplements can absorb water in the GI tract, forming a gel-like consistency, which produces a thicker stool.
  - Pancreatic enzymes assist in the hydrolysis of fat, protein, and carbohydrates to improve digestion and absorption of these nutrients.

---

[a]ORS is an iso-osmolar mixture of water, salt, and sugar in a standard ratio used to prevent or treat dehydration.
Source: Data are from references 28, 29, and 30.

Constipation

Constipation is a common GI motility disorder defined as unsatisfactory defecation, characterized by infrequent stools, difficult stool passage, or both (31). It is generally defined as three or fewer spontaneous bowel movements per week.

Etiology

The etiology of constipation can be classified into two broad categories (32,33): (a) primary, idiopathic, or functional constipation, and (b) secondary constipation.

PRIMARY, IDIOPATHIC, OR FUNCTIONAL CONSTIPATION
Primary constipation is caused by physical or functional problems when no underlying disorder has been identified. Normal-transit constipation is the most common subtype of primary constipation. Patients perceive difficulty in evacuating their bowels despite stool passing through the colon at a normal rate.

TABLE 6.3 Food Choices for Managing Diarrhea

Food Group	Recommended Foods	Foods Not Recommended
Milk and Milk Products	Buttermilk Evaporated, fat-free, and low-fat milk Soy milk Yogurt with live active cultures Powdered milk Cheese Low-fat ice cream Sherbet	Whole milk Half-and-half Cream Sour cream Regular (whole milk) ice cream Yogurt with berries, dried fruit, or nuts
Meat and Other Protein Foods	Tender, well-cooked meat, poultry, fish, eggs, or soy foods made without added fat Smooth nut butters	Fried meat, poultry, or fish Luncheon meats, such as bologna or salami Sausage and bacon Hot dogs Fatty meats Nuts Chunky nut butters
Grains	White flour Bread, bagels, rolls, crackers, and pasta made from white or refined flour Cold or hot cereals made from white or refined flour	Whole wheat or whole grain breads, rolls, crackers, or pasta Brown or wild rice Barley, oats, and other whole grains Cereals made from whole grain or bran Breads or cereals made with seeds or nuts Popcorn
Vegetables	Most well-cooked vegetables without seeds or skins Potatoes without skin Lettuce Strained vegetable juice	Raw vegetables (except for lettuce) Fried vegetables Beets Broccoli Brussels sprouts Cabbage Cauliflower Collard, mustard, and turnip greens Corn Potato skins
Fruits	Fruit juice without pulp, except prune juice Ripe bananas Melons Canned soft fruits	All raw fruits except banana and melons Dried fruits, including prunes and raisins Fruit juice with pulp Canned fruit in heavy syrup Any fruits sweetened with sorbitol Prune juice
Fats	Fats include oil, butter, cream, cream cheese, margarine, and mayonnaise	Limit fats to less than 8 teaspoons per day
Beverages	Decaffeinated coffee Caffeine-free teas Soft drinks without caffeine Rehydration beverages	Beverages containing caffeine, including regular coffee, regular tea, colas, and energy drinks Limit beverages containing high-fructose corn syrup to 360 mL per day Avoid beverages sweetened with sorbitol Alcoholic beverages
Other		Sugar alcohols such as xylitol and sorbitol Honey

Source: Reprinted with permission from Academy of Nutrition and Dietetics. Diarrhea. In: Nutrition Care Manual. http://nutritioncaremanual.org.

Constipation is considered chronic if symptoms occur for 3 months. An international working committee developed the following standardized definition of functional constipation, known as the Rome III diagnostic criteria (32):

1. Constipation must include *2 or more* of the following, with the criteria fulfilled for the last 3 months with symptom onset at least 6 months prior to diagnosis:
   a. Straining during at least 25% of defecations
   b. Lumpy or hard stools in at least 25% of defecations
   c. Sensation of incomplete evacuation for at least 25% of defecations
   d. Sensation of ano-rectal obstruction/blockage for at least 25% of defecations
   e. Manual maneuvers to facilitate at least 25% of defecations
   f. Fewer than 3 defecations per week
2. Loose stools are rarely present without the use of laxatives.
3. There are insufficient criteria for IBS.

Slow-transit constipation occurs most commonly in women and is characterized by prolonged delay in passage of stool through the colon. Patients complain of infrequent bowel movements, limited urgency, or straining to defecate.

Ano-rectal dysfunction is characterized by inefficient coordination of the pelvic musculature in the evacuation mechanism. Patients with pelvic floor dysfunction frequently report straining of stools and feelings of incomplete evacuation.

SECONDARY CONSTIPATION

Secondary constipation may result from a variety of factors (see Box 6.5) (33,34). Lifestyle factors such as inactivity and inadequate dietary fiber or fluid intake are the most common causes. Diseases associated with constipation may include neurologic or metabolic disorders, mechanical obstructions, or endocrine disorders. Certain medications may also cause or contribute to constipation.

BOX 6.5   Secondary Causes of Constipation

- **Metabolic:** Hypercalcemia, hypokalemia, hypothyroidism, diabetes mellitus, scleroderma, amyloidosis
- **Neurologic:** Autonomic neuropathy, multiple sclerosis, Parkinson's disease, spinal cord injury, Hirschprung's disease
- **Psychogenic:** Anxiety, depression, eating disorders, dementia
- **Mechanical:** Colorectal cancer, adhesions, strictures, anal stenosis, anal fissures, rectocele, ascites
- **Medications:** Anticholinergics, antidepressants, antihistamines, anticonvulsants, anti-Parkinson's drugs, aluminum- or calcium-containing antacids, calcium channel blockers, calcium supplements, diuretics, iron, narcotics, nonsteroidal anti-inflammatory drugs, opioids, psychotropics
- **Lifestyle:** Inadequate fiber or fluid intake, inactivity, ignoring defecation urges, laxative abuse
- **Other:** Obesity, pregnancy, irritable bowel syndrome, celiac disease

---

Source: Data are from references 33 and 34.

Complications

In most cases, constipation is not serious. However, if chronic constipation is left untreated, it may lead to complications (35), such as the following:

- Hemorrhoids from straining or pushing
- Fecal impaction or obstruction
- Volvulus (twisting or looping of the bowel)
- Ulcers caused by hardened stool in the colon or rectum
- Rectal prolapse
- Anal fissures
- Fecal incontinence caused by pelvic floor dysfunction or inability to control rectal muscles
- Diarrhea (may occur when watery fecal matter moves around the blockage)

Constipation may be a sign of a more serious problem. Refer the patient to a physician for further evaluation if you note any of the following signs and symptoms (31):

- Age older than 50 years with recent onset of symptoms
- Weight loss of 10 pounds or more
- Hematochezia
- Positive fecal blood tests
- Abnormal blood tests (anemia)
- Strong family history of bowel cancer or inflammatory bowel disease

Treatment of Constipation

Identifying the etiology of each patient's constipation is essential for determining treatment and management plans. Patients should attempt dietary and lifestyle modifications prior to trying over-the-counter and prescription medications.

DIETARY MODIFICATIONS

Increasing dietary fiber is an important dietary modification for the treatment of constipation. Dietary fiber is the nondigestible portion of plants and is often categorized as soluble or insoluble.

- Soluble fiber attracts water and turns to gel, which acts to slow digestion. Sources of soluble fiber include oats, oat bran, barley, dried beans, legumes, flax seed, psyllium, and fruits such as oranges and apples. Most soluble fibers, with the exception of psyllium, do not have a laxative effect.
- Insoluble fiber absorbs water and adds bulk to stool, which accelerates fecal transit. Food sources include skins from fruits and vegetables, wheat bran, whole grains, and seeds. Insoluble fiber seems to be more effective than soluble fiber in treating constipation. However, due to the cholesterol-lowing benefits of soluble fiber, it is best to encourage a mixed-fiber diet as total daily fiber intake is increased.

The Adequate Intake (AI) for fiber is 25 g/d for women and 38 g/d for men (36). The AI is based on the level to protect against coronary heart disease and is not based on GI health. However, the Dietary

Reference Intake (DRI) development panel suggested that consuming the AI for fiber should prevent constipation when the individual is well hydrated (36). To avoid abdominal pain and discomfort that accompanies a sudden increase in fiber intake, fiber should be increased gradually, as tolerated, by 5 g per week up to 25 to 38 g/d. Refer to Table 6.4 for food recommendations to increase dietary fiber (37).

Prunes contain the sugar alcohol sorbitol, which has a laxative effect. Therefore, consumption of prunes may help to normalize bowel function (38).

To ensure adequate fluid intake, increase fluid intake to 6 to 8 cups per day. Additional fluid may be required as fiber intake is increased. Increasing fiber without increasing fluid can worsen constipation and may cause fecal obstruction. Research has not shown a clear benefit of increased fluid intake alone for the treatment of constipation unless there is evidence of dehydration (39).

LIFESTYLE MODIFICATIONS

One lifestyle modification is to increase or maintain regular exercise to keep the bowel active and improve blood supply. Thirty minutes of moderate-intensity aerobic activity 5 days per week is recommended to promote and maintain health (40).

Bowel training is also recommended for patients with constipation (41). Encourage patients to do the following:

- Allow adequate time sitting on the toilet for bowel movements.
- Have a bowel movement soon after waking in the morning or 30 minutes after a meal to take advantage of the body's natural gastrocolic reflex.
- Do not resist the urge to defecate because this can worsen constipation if done often.
- Monitor bowel habits with a daily journal to track frequency, stool characteristics, and abdominal symptoms.

PHARMACOLOGIC MODIFICATIONS

Patients should consult with their physician to discuss pharmacologic therapies if constipation persists despite dietary and lifestyle modifications. Research regarding effective medications in the treatment of constipation is limited. The American College of Gastroenterology Chronic Constipation Task Force has graded the medications according to the strength of the existing research, with Grade A medications having the strongest evidence to support their use in treating constipation (31).

- Osmotic laxatives such as polyethylene glycol and lactulose have been given a Grade A recommendation for improving stool frequency and consistency in patients with chronic constipation. (Grade A = Supported by two or more randomized controlled trials [RCT] with $P <.05$ without conflicting evidence from other RCTs, adequate sample sizes, and appropriate methodology.)
- The bulking agent psyllium increases stool frequency and has been given a Grade B recommendation. (Grade B = Based on evidence from one RCT or evidence from two or more RCTs with conflicting evidence; or supported by evidence from two or more RCTs with $P >.05$ or inadequate sample size and/or inappropriate methodology.)
- There are limited data regarding the use of stool softeners in the treatment of constipation, resulting in a Grade C recommendation (ie, recommendation is based on case series or nonrandomized trials with contemporaneous or historical controls). Stool softeners may be useful for patients with hemorrhoids or anal fissures who experience painful defecation.

See Table 6.5 (page 76) for a review of medications commonly used to treat constipation (33,41,42).

TABLE 6.4 Recommended Foods to Increase Dietary Fiber Intake

Food Group	Choose
Foods with at least 4 g Fiber per Serving	
Grains	⅓ to ½ cup high-fiber cereals: check Nutrition Facts labels and choose products with 4 or more grams (g) dietary fiber per serving
Dried beans	½ cup cooked red beans, kidney beans, large lima beans, navy beans, pinto beans, white beans, lentils, or black-eyed peas
Vegetables	1 artichoke (cooked)
Fruits	½ cup blackberries or raspberries 4 prunes (dried)
Foods with at least 1 to 3 g Fiber per Serving	
Grains	1 whole wheat bagel (3½-inch diameter) 1 slice whole wheat, cracked wheat, pumpernickel, or rye bread 2-inch square cornbread 4 whole wheat crackers 1 bran, blueberry, cornmeal, or English muffin ½ cup cereal with 1 g to 3 g fiber per serving (check Dietary Fiber on the product's Nutrition Facts label) 2 tablespoons wheat germ or whole wheat flour
Fruits	1 apple (3-inch diameter) ½ cup applesauce ½ cup apricots (canned) 1 banana ½ cup cranberries (fresh) 3 dates (whole) 2 medium figs (fresh) ½ cup fruit cocktail (canned) ½ grapefruit 1 kiwi fruit 1 orange (2½-inch diameter) 1 peach (fresh) or ½ cup peaches (canned) 1 pear (fresh) or ½ cup pears (canned) 1 plum (2-inch diameter) ¼ cup raisins ½ cup strawberries (fresh) 1 tangerine
Vegetables	½ cup bean sprouts (raw) ½ cup beets (diced, canned) ½ cup broccoli, brussels sprouts, or cabbage (cooked) ½ cup carrots ½ cup cauliflower ½ cup corn ½ cup eggplant ½ cup okra (boiled) ½ cup potatoes (baked or mashed) ½ cup spinach, kale, or turnip greens (cooked) ½ cup squash—winter, summer, or zucchini (cooked) ½ cup sweet potatoes or yams ½ cup tomatoes (canned)
Other	2 tablespoons almonds or peanuts 1 cup popcorn (popped)

Source: Reprinted with permission from Academy of Nutrition and Dietetics. High-Fiber Nutrition Therapy. In: Nutrition Care Manual. http://nutritioncaremanual.org.

TABLE 6.5 Medications Commonly Used to Treat Constipation

Type	Mechanism	Adverse Effects/Precautions
Bulking laxatives: methylcellulose (Citrucel)[a], polycarbophil (Fibercon)[b], psyllium (Metamucil)[c]	Soluble or insoluble fiber absorbs water from intestine, adds bulk, and softens stool	• May cause bloating, flatus • Take with adequate water to avoid intestinal obstruction
Stool softeners: docusate sodium (Colace)[d]	Allow water to enter bowel and moisten stool	• Use with caution in patients on low-salt diets
Osmotic laxatives: magnesium hydroxide (Milk of Magnesia)[e], magnesium citrate or sulfate, sodium phosphate (Phospho-Soda)[f], lactulose, sorbitol, polyethylene glycol (Miralax)[g]	Draw water into colon by creating an osmotic effect	• Flatulence, bloating, and abdominal cramping • Excessive absorption of magnesium, phosphate or sodium may result in electrolyte abnormalities in patients with cardiac or renal dysfunction • Acute phosphate nephropathy (Phospho-Soda)
Stimulant laxatives: bisacodyl (Dulcolax)[h], senna (Senokot)[i]	Cause rhythmic contraction of intestinal muscle, increasing motility	• Diarrhea • Cramping/abdominal pain • Fecal incontinence • Hypokalemia
Emollients: mineral oil	Soften and coat stool	• Long-term use may decrease absorption of fat-soluble vitamins • Anal seepage • Lipoid pneumonia in those at risk for aspiration
Chloride channel activator: lubiprostone (Amitiza)[j]	Activate type-2 chloride channels to enhance intestinal fluid secretion	• Nausea (common) • Diarrhea • Headache

Manufacturers: [a]GlaxoSmith Kline; [b]Wyeth; [c]Proctor & Gamble; [d]Purdue Products LP; [e]Bayer Consumer Products; [f]C.B. Fleet Company; [g]Shering-Plough; [h]Boehringer Ingelheim; [i]Purdue Products LP; [j]Sucampo Pharmaceuticals.
Source: Data are from references 33, 41, and 42.

Conclusion

Diet modification should be the first line of therapy for patients experiencing GI symptoms such as gas and bloating, nausea and vomiting, diarrhea, or constipation in a mild to moderate form. The management of patients with severe GI symptoms should begin with the correction of dehydration and electrolyte imbalances. A nutrition assessment and workup of the etiology will guide the timing and optimal route of nutrition intervention.

References

1. Quigley EM. Germs, gas, and the gut; the evolving role of the enteric flora in IBS. *Am J Gastroenterol.* 2006;101:334–335.
2. Whorwell PJ. Unraveling functional abdominal bloating and distension: the role of thoraco-abdominal accommodation and a physical sign to aid its detection. *Neurogastroenterol Motil.* 2012;24:301–304.
3. Sanjeevi A, Kirby DF. The role of food and dietary intervention in the irritable bowel syndrome. *Pract Gastroenterol.* 2008;64:33–42.

4. Barrett JS, Gibson PR. Clinical ramifications of malabsorption of fructose and other short-chain carbohydrates. *Pract Gastroenterol.* 2007;53:51–65.

5. Tack J, Talley NJ, Camilleri M, Holtmann G, Hu P, Malagelada J, Stanghellini V. Functional gastroduodenal disorders. *Gastroenterology.* 2006;130:1466–1479.

6. Bredenoord AJ, Weusten BL, Sifrim D, et al. Aerophagia, gastric, and supragastric belching: a study using intraluminal electrical impedance monitoring. *Gut.* 2004;53:1561–1565.

7. Bredenoord AJ, Smout AJ. Physiologic and pathologic belching. *Clin Gastroenterol Hepatol.* 2007;5:772–775.

8. Chitkara DK, Bredenoord AJ, Rucker MJ, Talley NJ. Aerophagia in adults: a comparison with functional dyspepsia. *Aliment Pharmacol Ther.* 2005;22:855–858.

9. Houghton LA, Whorwell PJ. Towards a better understanding of abdominal bloating and distension in functional gastrointestinal disorders. *Neurogastroenterol Motil.* 2005;17(4):500–511.

10. Houghton LA. Bloating in constipation: relevance of intraluminal gas handling. *Best Pract Res Clin Gastroenterol.* 2011;25:141–150.

11. Agrawal A, Whorwell PJ. Review article: abdominal bloating and distension in functional gastrointestinal disorders. Epidemiology and exploration of possible mechanisms. *Aliment Pharmacol Ther.* 2008;27(1):2–10.

12. Accarino A, Perez F, Azpiroz F, Quiroga S, Malagelada J. Abdominal distention results from caudo-ventral redistribution of contents. *Gastroenterology,* 2009;136:1544–1551.

13. Gibson PR, Shepherd SJ. Food choice as a key management strategy for functional gastrointestinal symptoms. *Am J Gastroenterol.* 2012;107:657–666.

14. Sharara AI, Aoun E, Abdul-Baki H, Mounzer R, Sidani S, ElHajj I. A randomized double-blind placebo-controlled trial of rifaximin in patients with abdominal bloating and flatulence. *Am J Gastroenterol.* 2006;101:326–333.

15. Accarino A, Perez F, Azpiroz F, Quiroga S, Malagelada JR. Intestinal gas and bloating: effect of prokinetic stimulation. *Am J Gastroenterol.* 2008;103(8):2036–2042.

16. Bender CM, McDaniel RW, Murphy-Ende K, Pickett M, Rittenberg CN, Rogers MP, Schneider SM, Schwartz RN. Chemotherapy-induced nausea and vomiting. *Clin J Oncol Nurs.* 2002;6(2):94–102.

17. Metz A, Hebbard G. Nausea and vomiting in adults—a diagnostic approach. *Aust Fam Physician.* 2007;36:688.

18. American Gastroenterological Association technical review on nausea and vomiting. *Gastroenterology.* 2001;120(1):263–286.

19. Apfel C, Korttila K, Abdalla M, et al. Preventing postoperative nausea and vomiting: a comprehensive comparison of treatments. *N Engl J Med.* 2004;350(2):3441–3451.

20. Academy of Nutrition and Dietetics. Nausea and vomiting. In: Nutrition Care Manual. http://nutritioncaremanual.org.

21. Debaise J."Motility Assessment and Management" Presented at Clinical Nutrition Week, Feb. 10, 2010, Las Vegas, NV.

22. Fraser RJ, Bryant L. Current and future prokinetic therapy to improve enteral feed intolerance in the ICU patient. *Nutr Clin Pract.* 2010;25(1):26–31.

23. Whitmire SJ. Fluids and electrolytes. In: Matarese LE, Gottschlich MM, eds. *Contemporary Nutrition Support Practice: A Clinical Guide.* Philadelphia, PA: Elsevier; 1998:130.

24. Bern C, Martines J, de Zoysa I, Glass R. The magnitude of the global problem of diarrheal disease: a ten-year update. *Bull World Health Organ.* 1992;70(6):705–714.

25. Musher D, Musher B. Contagious acute gastrointestinal infections. *N Engl J Med.* 2004;351:2417.

26. Fine K, Schiller L. AGA Technical review on the evaluation and management of chronic diarrhea. *Gastroenterology.* 1999;116(6):1464–1486.

27. Camilleri M. Chronic diarrhea: a review on pathophysiology and management for the clinical gastroenterologist. *Clin Gastroenterol Hepatol.* 2004;2:198–206.

28. Academy of Nutrition and Dietetics. Diarrhea. In: Nutrition Care Manual. http://nutritioncaremanual.org.

29. Hassoun H, Moore F. Electrolyte disorders. In: Cameron JL, ed. *Current Surgical Therapy.* 7th ed. Philadelphia, PA: Mosby; 2001:1315–1326.

30. Parekh N, Steiger E. Short bowel syndrome. *Curr Treat Opt Gastroenterol.* 2007;10:10–23.

31. American College of Gastroenterology Chronic Constipation Task Force. An evidence-based approach to the management of chronic constipation in North America. *Am J Gastroenterol.* 2005;100(suppl 1):S1–S4.

32. Longstreth GF, Thompson WG, Chey WD, Houghton LA, Mearin F, Spiller RC. Functional bowel disorders. *Gastroenterology.* 2006;130:1480–1491.

33. Eoff J, Lembo A. Optimal treatment of chronic constipation in managed care: review and roundtable discussion. *J Manag Care Pharm.* 2008;14(9 Suppl A):S4–S15.

34. Tariq SH. Constipation in long term care. *J Am Med Dir Assoc.* 2007;8(4):209–218.

35. Singh G, Kahler, et al. Constipation in adults: complications and comorbidities. *Gastroenterology.* 2005;128(suppl 2):A-154.

36. Institute of Medicine Food and Nutrition Board. *Dietary Reference Intakes: The Essential Guide to Nutrient Requirements.* Washington, DC: National Academies Press; 2006.

37. Academy of Nutrition and Dietetics. High-Fiber Nutrition Therapy. In: Nutrition Care Manual. http://nutritioncaremanual.org.

38. Grabitske HA, Slavin JL. Low-digestible carbohydrates in practice. *J Am Diet Assoc.* 2008;108:1677–1681.

39. Müller-Lissner SA, Kamm MA, Scarpignato C, Wald A. Myths and misconceptions about chronic constipation. *Am J Gastroenterol.* 2005;100:232.

40. Haskell W, Lee I-Min, Russell P, Powell K, et al. Physical activity and public health: updated recommendation for adults from the American College of Sports Medicine and the American Heart Association. *Circulation.* 2007;116:1081–1093.

41. Cash B, Chang L, Sabesin S, Vitat P. Update on the management of adults with chronic idiopathic constipation. *J Fam Pract.* 2007;56(6 Suppl Update):S14–S20.

42. Hsieh C. Treatment of constipation in older adults. *Am Fam Physician.* 2005;72:2277–2284.

CHAPTER 7

Inflammatory Bowel Disease

S. Devi Rampertab, MD, FACG, AGAF, and Amy C. Brown, PhD, RD

Inflammatory bowel disease (IBD) is a debilitating condition characterized by chronic intestinal inflammation. The two most common subtypes of IBD are Crohn's disease (CD) and ulcerative colitis (UC). As a result of the ongoing intestinal injury and loss of absorptive surface area, a number of micronutrient deficiencies and protein-energy malnutrition can occur. This chapter reviews the data that support identification of the specific dietary components that represent potential risk factors in the development of IBD and provides an overview of enteral and parenteral nutrition efficacy in the delivery of care for patients with IBD.

Clinical Presentation of IBD

UC and CD can occur at any age, but the onset is most often between the ages of 15 and 30 years.

In UC, the inflammation affects only the mucosal lining of the colon and rectum. It usually extends proximally from the rectum in a symmetrical, uninterrupted pattern to involve part or all of the large intestine. Diarrhea, abdominal pain, and hematochezia represent typical symptoms of UC.

In contrast, CD follows a patchy distribution with transmural inflammation that may involve any part of the gastrointestinal (GI) tract from mouth to anus. The most commonly affected areas are the small intestine and the colon; the rectum is usually spared. Patients with CD can experience significant weight loss and generalized malnutrition due to the loss of absorptive lining from the ongoing intestinal inflammation and injury. Another factor that differentiates CD from UC is that CD may also be complicated by fistula formation. The fistula output is high in protein and electrolytes, placing patients at risk for protein-energy malnutrition.

Diet in the Pathogenesis of IBD

It has been hypothesized that luminal antigens in the diet are an important factor in the immunopathogenesis of IBD. A possible relationship between presentation of hypersensitivity to cow's milk early in life and subsequent development of UC was postulated in a 1990 retrospective study (1). Since then, investigators have found that lactose sensitivity occurs in a much higher proportion of adult patients with IBD (approximately 70%) than was previously thought (2). Other studies have established a potential link between not breastfeeding and increased risk of CD (3,4) or UC (5).

As reported in several studies, an intake that is higher in refined sugar intake and high in overall carbohydrate precedes IBD development, although this outcome is more often associated with CD than UC (6–10). High levels of fat intake have been associated with an increased risk of IBD, and high fast-food consumption has been shown to predate both UC and CD (11). Studies dating back to the 1970s have reported an inverse relationship in that increased dietary intake of vegetables, fruits, fish, fiber, and omega-3 fatty acids contributes to lower risk of developing IBD (6,10,12,13).

The past 3 decades have seen a sharp increase in the number of patients in Japan with IBD. This substantial increase may be due to the Westernization of the Japanese diet, to a higher intake of total fat and animal fat with a raised ratio of omega-6 to omega-3 fatty acids. High intake of animal protein (excluding fish protein) is the strongest independent factor associated with the development of IBD (14).

The clinical usefulness of omega-3 fatty acids for patients with IBD involves regulating transcription factors, including peroxisome proliferator-activated receptors; inhibiting NF-κB; suppressing signaling of T-cells; reducing recruitment of inflammatory cells; and decreasing the release of pro-inflammatory cytokines IL-1β and TNF-α (15–17). Tissue cultures derived from biopsy specimens of patients with Crohn's colitis suggest that butyrate and other short-chain fatty acids decrease TNF-α and NF-κB production as well as cytokine messenger RNA expression, and may have an anti-inflammatory effect (18,19).

Despite the findings of the aforementioned studies, there is no consensus as to what role dietary patterns play and what sort of risk factors they represent in the development of IBD (20). Other risk factors for CD are listed in Box 7.1 (21–32).

Prevalence of Malnutrition and Nutrient Deficiencies Associated with IBD

Malnutrition is commonly associated with UC and CD. In a 2003 study, among 502 hospital medical admissions, patients with IBD had the highest prevalence (40%) of malnutrition in benign diseases (33). The rate of undernutrition in CD patients is reported to be 65% to 75% (34). In patients with active IBD, the reported prevalence rates of undernutrition and severe undernutrition are 25% to 70% and 1% to 32%, respectively (35).

Micronutrient deficiencies are relatively common in individuals with IBD, particularly in CD patients with active small bowel disease and/or multiple resections (36). Associated complications in these CD patients included anemia (iron, folate, and vitamin B-12 deficiencies), bone disease (calcium, vitamin D, and possibly vitamin K deficiencies), hypercoagulability (folate, vitamin B-6, and vitamin B-12 deficiencies), poor wound healing (zinc, vitamin A, and vitamin C deficiencies), and colorectal cancer risk (folate and possibly vitamin D and calcium deficiencies). Patients with IBD—particularly those with CD—are significantly affected by micronutrient deficiencies even when the disease is quiescent (37).

Among outpatients with IBD, weight loss is more common in the CD population than in the UC population. As many as 20% of CD patients in clinical remission have significantly reduced lean body mass and weigh 10% below ideal body weight (38). When the appropriate nutrition care is not provided to patients with long-standing CD, loss of visceral protein mass and impaired cellular immunity, which increase risk of infection and poor wound healing, are possible consequences (39).

Mechanisms of Malnutrition in IBD

There are multifactorial mechanisms for malnutrition in the patient population with IBD, including poor dietary intake, increased nutrient requirements, increased nutrient losses, nutrient malabsorption,

---

BOX 7.1   Risk Factors for Crohn's Disease

Risk factors
- Family history of the disease (22)
- Age of 15–35 or 55–65 years (23)
- Female sex (24)
- Urban dwellers (23)
- Smokers (25)
- Stress (26)
- Jewish heritage (27)
- Appendicitis[a] (28)
- High social, economic, educational, and/or occupational status (23)

Factors that may increase risk
- Use of nonsteroidal anti-inflammatory drugs (29), oral contraceptives (30), or antibiotics (31)
- Infectious bacterial and/or yeast agents (32):
  - *Listeria monocytogenes*
  - *Campylobacter*[b]
  - *Chlamydia trachomatis*
  - Clostridium[b]
  - *Cytomegalovirus*[b]
  - *Escherichia coli*
  - *Klebsiella pneumoniae*
  - *Mycobacterium paratuberculosis*
  - *Saccharomyces cerevisiae yersinia*[b]

---

[a]Significantly higher Crohn's disease risk during the first year following an appendectomy, but reached baseline levels within 5 years.
[b]Species not provided with genus.
Source: Adapted with permission from reference 21: Brown AC, Roy M. Does evidence exist to include dietary therapy in the treatment of Crohn's disease? *Expert Rev Gastroenterol Hepatol*. 2010;4(2):191–215. Data are from references 22–32.

medications, and surgery. Poor dietary intake, often directly caused by anorexia, is a common problem in IBD. Increases in both nutrient needs and losses in the affected mucosa are primary contributors to malnutrition in the IBD patient population. Because the IBD process is catabolic, causing rapid weight loss as well as fat and skeletal muscle mass loss from vomiting, diarrhea, intestinal protein loss, fistulae, and blood loss (which ultimately results in iron loss), nutrient requirements are higher in IBD patients. Increasing nutrients is particularly crucial when symptoms are exacerbated (40).

Poor nutrition, anorexia caused by several factors including cytokine release, and ongoing inflammation lead to growth impairment in IBD. Growth impairment can also develop as a complication from corticosteroid or surgical therapy. Approximately 40% to 50% of children with CD experience reduced growth velocity, linear growth retardation, and delayed pubertal growth (41).

The loss of mucosal integrity, which can be worsened by the medications used, is another major contributor to the development of malnutrition in the IBD patient population. For example, absorption of folic acid is minimized and folate blocked from metabolization to its active form (tetrahydrofolate) when a person takes the anti-inflammatory medication sulfasalazine. Corticosteroids are potent anti-inflammatory agents that also inhibit calcium absorption and result in increased urinary excretion of calcium and magnesium. Corticosteroids also alter the protein metabolism that causes muscle wasting (42). Cholestyramine alleviates diarrhea by binding bile acids, but because these acids are also important for adequate digestion of fat and fat-soluble vitamins, deficiencies of these vitamins can occur (43).

Bone Health in IBD

Osteopenia and osteoporosis—with prevalence among the IBD population of 50% and 15%, respectively—are concerns in the management of patients with IBD (44–48). The risk of fractures among patients with IBD, compared with age- and sex-matched controls, is 40% higher (49).

Bone thinning associated with IBD is often attributed to corticosteroid use; however, in 2002, researchers demonstrated the presence of osteopenia in newly diagnosed IBD patients before any steroid therapy was initiated (50). Age, body mass index, serum magnesium, and history of bowel resections may be better predictors than corticosteroid use for low bone mineral density (51,52).

Bone health is best supported by calcium and vitamin D supplementation. These nutrients are highly recommended for use in preventing and treating decreased bone density in patients with IBD (53).

The pediatric population is particularly at risk of decreased bone density. Schmidt and associates reported that IBD in childhood was associated with low bone mineral density and reduced bone mass accrual relative to muscle mass (54). The results of their cross-sectional cohort study of 80 IBD patients (median age 14.9 years, range 5 to 20 years; median disease duration of 3.4 years; 51 with UC, 26 with CD, 3 with unspecified colitis) and 80 control subjects suggest that careful follow-up and active preventive measures for IBD patients are warranted.

Managing Nutritional Deficiencies in IBD

Patients with IBD are at risk for a variety of nutritional deficiencies (see Table 7.1) that could be corrected or prevented with nutritional supplements; these supplements may also induce an anti-inflammatory effect.

Anemia

Anemia is common in IBD (estimated prevalence between 6% and 74%) (55). The prevalence of iron deficiency among IBD patients is estimated to range from 36% to 90% (56). Iron-deficiency anemia in people with IBD has multifactorial causes, including the presence of both iron deficiency and chronic GI blood loss. Thus, the prevalence of iron-deficiency anemia is higher in UC patients than in CD patients. Anemia may also be induced by medications. This effect is associated with mesalazine, sulfasalazine, azathioprine, and mercaptopurine. Iron therapy was reported to normalize elevated platelet counts in patients with IBD–associated anemia (57).

Vitamin B-12 and folate deficiencies—often detected among the patient population with IBD—may also lead to anemia (56). Insufficient levels of folic acid are typically found in IBD patients, so that nutrient should be monitored at least annually for all IBD patients (58). Medications (eg, sulfasalazine) that interfere with transport of folic acid, thereby resulting in malabsorption, potentially contribute to low levels of folate in IBD patients. Loss of surface area related to the primary disease or surgery may also play a role (59). Bacterial overgrowth, a complication of IBD, can result in depletion of vitamin B-12 because bacteria preferentially utilize vitamin B-12. Distal ileal resection or active disease of the ileum can also result in vitamin B-12 deficiency because vitamin B-12 is absorbed in the last 60 cm of ileum. Because the terminal ileum lacks a functional absorptive area, vitamin B-12 usually must be delivered subcutaneously.

Deficiencies in Fat-Soluble Vitamins

Decreased bile acid absorption may occur when ileal disease is present. Solubilization to facilitate absorption of lipids and fat-soluble vitamins (A, D, E, and K) is normally aided by bile acids. Malabsorption of bile acids results in poor absorption of lipids and fat-soluble vitamins. Vitamin D represents the fat-soluble vitamin most commonly deficient among IBD patients. A combination of vitamin D deficiency and calcium malabsorption, particularly when taking corticosteroids, has the potential to significantly alter bone density (60).

TABLE 7.1 Nutrient Deficiencies in Inflammatory Bowel Disease

| Deficiency | Frequency of Deficiency | | Treatment |
	Crohn's Disease	Ulcerative Colitis	
Negative nitrogen balance	69%	Unknown	Adequate energy and protein
Vitamin B-12	48%	5%	1,000 mcg/d for 7 d then once a month
Folate	67%	30%–40%	1 mg/d
Vitamin A	11%	Unknown	5,000–25,000 IU/d
Vitamin D	75%	35%	5,000–25,000 IU/d
Calcium	13%	Unknown	1,000–1,200 mg/d
Potassium	5%–20%	Unknown	Variable
Iron	39%	81%	300 mg Fe gluconate 3 times per day
Zinc	50%	Unknown	220 mg zinc sulfate 1 or 2 times per day

Source: Courtesy of Gerard E. Mullin, MD.

Zinc Deficiency

Zinc is an important cofactor for antioxidant defenses. Patients experiencing severe diarrhea or those who have intestinal fistulas are especially at risk for zinc deficiency. However, zinc deficiency may occur in CD patients regardless of those factors; it has been reported in 40% of that patient population (61).

The Role of Enteral Nutrition in IBD Treatment

Both the European Society for Parenteral and Enteral Nutrition (ESPEN) and American Society for Enteral and Parenteral Nutrition (A.S.P.E.N.) have published guidelines on enteral nutrition (EN) for patients with IBD (62,63). To improve the nutritional intake of undernourished patients, normal food with enteral nutrition—in the form of oral nutritional supplements and/or tube feeding—is indicated. Whereas EN should not be the sole therapy in treating adult CD patients, pediatric patients with active CD should receive EN as first-line therapy. For steroid-dependent CD patients in remission, an oral nutritional supplement is recommended. However, when UC is active or in clinical remission, EN is *not* recommended (64).

Enteral nutrition has been evaluated as primary therapy for CD in head-to-head trials. A recent Cochrane meta-analysis (65) and three other meta-analyses (64,66,67) demonstrated the higher rates of efficacy of steroid administration compared with EN. One meta-analysis found that EN and corticosteroids were equally effective in inducing remission in pediatric CD cases (RR 0.95; 95% CI 0.67–1.34) (68).

In contrast to the treatment approach in the United States, the first-line medical treatment for adult patients with CD in Japan is EN therapy, which is covered by the Japanese national health insurance plan (69). In general, approximately 3 to 5 weeks of treatment induces remission in approximately 85% of patients with active CD, and EN is often used in research to achieve remission before a new treatment is tested (70,71). Once remission is reached, patients begin the "slide method" in which a low-fat diet slowly replaces an elemental diet, nasogastric tube feeding during the night at home, and a low-fat diet (20 to 30 g per day) during the day (72). Possible side effects of liquid elemental diets are osmolar diarrhea, abdominal distension, colic, cholelithiasis, and pneumonia (due to pulmonary aspiration) (73).

In studies that examined the clinical usefulness of EN in maintaining remission in CD patients—whether induced medically or surgically—significant improvement in the rate of clinical remission was found in patients who had been treated with an elemental diet compared with those prescribed a low-fat or unrestricted diet (73–76).

There are no compelling data to identify the precise role of EN in treating patients with CD, but it is potentially useful as an auxiliary treatment for inducing and maintaining remission. Before EN can be definitively identified as truly effective in this line of treatment for CD, large randomized controlled trials are necessary. In the patient population with active UC, EN has not been extensively evaluated (77,78).

The Role of Parenteral Nutrition in IBD Treatment

Since total parenteral nutrition (TPN)—sometimes called central parenteral nutrition (CPN)—was first used in the treatment of IBD, its role has evolved. In the early years, TPN was used as the primary treatment for IBD because dietary antigens may stimulate the mucosal immune system and hypothetically worsen the disease. In patients with active CD, bowel rest along with TPN is as effective as corticosteroids at inducing remission, although the benefits of TPN are short lived (79).

Total parenteral nutrition also carries many associated risks. For this reason, it is not used as primary therapy for IBD.

There are limited indications for TPN in patients with IBD. The most common use of TPN in IBD patients occurs with short bowel syndrome resulting from extensive intestinal resection (see Chapter 8) (80). Other indications include fistulous disease of the intestine or leaks resulting from surgical complications (81); malabsorption causing failure to thrive from extensive small intestinal CD; and severe CD in which standard drug therapy is not improving outcomes as anticipated or EN is not tolerated (82). When extensive stenosing CD is present, short-term use of TPN and bowel rest may be indicated to limit the extent of resection or to deliver nutrition support until the disease responds to drug therapy.

Use of parenteral nutrition as primary therapy in UC is not supported by data (83).

Conclusion

Researchers have been focusing increasingly on diet for its role in triggering IBD and how it may be used in combination with traditional medical therapy to minimize adverse effects. Because nutritional deficiencies are common in patients with IBD, these patients should receive follow-up care from a registered dietitian as well as their digestive care specialist.

Enteral nutrition is highly beneficial in children with IBD. In the United States, the role of EN in the treatment of adults with IBD is more limited, whereas EN is commonly used in IBD treatment in Japan.

Parenteral nutrition has been shown to sustain patients while the gut heals and becomes capable of absorbing nutrients, thus allowing for a transition to more aggressive therapy. In patients with extensive small bowel CD, parenteral nutrition may be life-sustaining.

For more on existing clinical guidelines, we refer you to our prior reviews on the subject (21,84).

References

1. Glassman MS, Newman LJ, Berezin S, et al. Cow's milk protein sensitivity during infancy in patients with inflammatory bowel disease. *Am J Gastroenterol.* 1990;85:838–840.
2. Eadala P, Matthews SB, Waud JP, Green JT, Campbell AK. Association of lactose sensitivity with inflammatory bowel disease—demonstrated by analysis of genetic polymorphism, breath gases and symptoms. *Aliment Pharmacol Ther.* 2011;34(7):735–746.

3. Koletzko S, Sherman P, Corey M, et al. Role of infant feeding practices in development of Crohn's disease in childhood. *BMJ.* 1989;298:1617–1618.

4. Corrao G, Tragnone A, Caprilli R, et al. Risk of inflammatory bowel disease attributable to smoking, oral contraception and breastfeeding in Italy: a nationwide case-control study. Cooperative Investigators of the Italian Group for the Study of the Colon and the Rectum (GISC). *Int J Epidemiol.* 1998;27:397–404.

5. Thompson NP, Montgomery SM, Wadsworth ME, et al. Early determinants of inflammatory bowel disease: use of two national longitudinal birth cohorts. *Eur J Gastroenterol Hepatol.* 2000;12:25–30.

6. Thornton JR, Emmett PM, Heaton KW. Diet and Crohn's disease: characteristics of the pre-illness diet. *Br Med J.* 1979;2:762–764.

7. Mayberry JF, Rhodes J, Newcombe RG. Increased sugar consumption in Crohn's disease. *Digestion.* 1980;20:323–326.

8. Mayberry JF, Rhodes J, Allan R, et al. Diet in Crohn's disease: two studies of current and previous habits in newly diagnosed patients. *Dig Dis Sci.* 1981;26: 444–448.

9. Tragnone A, Valpiani D, Miglio F, et al. Dietary habits as risk factors for inflammatory bowel disease. *Eur J Gastroenterol Hepatol.* 1995;7:47–51.

10. Reif S, Klein I, Lubin F, et al. Pre-illness dietary factors in inflammatory bowel disease. *Gut.* 1997;40:754–760.

11. Persson PG, Ahlbom A, Hellers G. Diet and inflammatory bowel disease: a case-control study. *Epidemiology.* 1992;3:47–52.

12. Martini GA, Stenner A, Brandes WJ. Diet and ulcerative colitis. *Br Med J.* 1980;280:1321.

13. Amre DK, D'Souza S, Morgan K, et al. Imbalances in dietary consumption of fatty acids, vegetables, and fruits are associated with risk for Crohn's disease in children. *Am J Gastroenterol.* 2007;102:2016–2025.

14. Andersen V, Olsen A, Carbonnel F, Tjønneland A, Vogel U. Diet and risk of inflammatory bowel disease. *Dig Liver Dis.* 2012;44(3):185–194.

15. Whiting CV, Bland PW, Tarlton JF. Dietary n-3 polyunsaturated fatty acids reduce disease and colonic pro-inflammatory cytokines in a mouse model of colitis. *Inflamm Bowel Dis.* 2005;11(4):340–349.

16. Zhang P, Kim W, Zhou L, et al. Dietary fish oil inhibits antigen-specific murine Th1 cell development by suppression of clonal expansion. *J Nutr.* 2006;136(9):2391–2398.

17. Caughey GE, Mantzioris E, Gibson RA, et al. The effect on human tumor necrosis factor alpha and interleukin 1 beta production of diets enriched in n-3 fatty acids from vegetable oil or fish oil. *Am J Clin Nutr.* 1996;63(1):116–122.

18. Segain JP, Raingeard de la Bletiere D, Bourrelle A, et al. Butyrate inhibits inflammatory responses through NFkappaB inhibition: Implications for Crohn's disease. *Gut.* 2000;47(3):397–403.

19. Huda-Faujan N, Abdulamir AS, Fatimah AB, et al. The impact of the level of the intestinal short chain fatty acids in inflammatory bowel disease patients versus healthy subjects. *Open Biochem J.* 2010;4:53–58.

20. Loftus EV. Clinical epidemiology of inflammatory bowel disease: Incidence, prevalence, and environmental influences. *Gastroenterology.* 2004;126:1504–1517.

21. Brown AC, Roy M. Does evidence exist to include dietary therapy in the treatment of Crohn's disease? *Expert Rev Gastroenterol Hepatol.* 2010;4(2):191–215.

22. Baumgart DC, Carding SR. Inflammatory bowel disease: cause and immunobiology. *Lancet.* 2007;369(9573):1627–1640.

23. Appleyard CB, Hernández G, Rios-Bedoya CF. Basic epidemiology of inflammatory bowel disease in Puerto Rico. *Inflamm Bowel Dis.* 2004;10(2):106–111.

24. Gupta N, Bostrom AG, Kirschner BS, et al. Gender differences in presentation and course of disease in pediatric patients with Crohn's disease. *Pediatrics.* 2007;120(6):e1418–e1425.

25. Seksik P, Nion-Larmurier I, Sokol H, Beaugerie L, Cosnes J. Effects of light smoking consumption on the clinical course of Crohn's disease. *Inflamm Bowel Dis.* 2009;15(5):734–741.

26. García-Vega E, Fernandez-Rodriguez C. A stress management programme for Crohn's disease. *Behav Res Ther.* 2004;42(4):367–383.

27. Ben-Horin S, Avidan B, Yanai H, et al. Familial clustering of Crohn's disease in Israel: prevalence and association with disease severity. *Inflamm Bowel Dis.* 2009;15(2):171–175.

28. Kaplan GG, Jackson T, Sands BE, et al. The risk of developing Crohn's disease after an appendectomy: a meta-analysis. *Am J Gastroenterol.* 2009;103(11):2925–2931.

29. Bjarnason I, Peters TJ. Intestinal permeability, non-steroidal anti-inflammatory drug enteropathy and inflammatory bowel disease: an overview. *Gut.* 1989;30:22–28.

30. Ekbom A, Montgomery SM. Environmental risk factors (excluding tobacco and microorganisms): critical analysis of old and new hypotheses. *Best Pract Res Clin Gastroenterol.* 2004;8(3):497–508.

31. Prantera C, Scribano ML. Antibiotics and probiotics in inflammatory bowel disease: why, when, and how. *Curr Opin Gastroenterol.* 2009;25(4):329–333.

32. Danese S, Fiocchi C. Etiopathogenesis of inflammatory bowel diseases. *World J Gastroenterol.* 2006;12(30):4807–4812.

33. Pirlich M, Schutz T, Kemps M, et al. Prevalence of malnutrition in hospitalized medical patients: impact of underlying disease. *Dig Dis.* 2003;21(3):245–251.

34. Vaisman N, Dotan I, Halack A, Niv E. Malabsorption is a major contributor to underweight in Crohn's disease patients in remission. *Nutrition.* 2006;22(9):855–859.

35. Mijač DD, Janković GL, Jorga J, Krstić MN. Nutritional status in patients with active inflammatory bowel disease: prevalence of malnutrition and methods for routine nutritional assessment. *Eur J Intern Med.* 2010;21(4):315–319.

36. Hwang C, Ross V, Mahadevan U. Micronutrient deficiencies in inflammatory bowel disease: from A to zinc. *Inflamm Bowel Dis.* 2012;18(10):1961–1981.

37. Filippi J, Al-Jaouni R, Wiroth JB, et al. Nutritional deficiencies in patients with Crohn's disease in remission. *Inflamm Bowel Dis.* 2006;12:185–191.

38. Jahnsen J, Falch JA, Mowinckel P, et al. Body composition in patients with inflammatory bowel disease: a population-based study. *Am J Gastroenterol.* 2003;98(7):1556–1562.

39. Seidman EG. Nutritional management of inflammatory bowel disease. *Gastroenterol Clin N Am.* 1989;18:129–155.

40. Razack R, Seidner DL. Nutrition in inflammatory bowel disease. *Curr Opin Gastroenterol.* 2007;23(4):400–405.

41. Heyman MB, Garnett EA, Wojcicki J, et al. Growth hormone treatment for growth failure in pediatric patients with Crohn's disease. *J Pediatr.* 2008;153(5):651–658.

42. Sapone N, Pellicano R, Simondi D, et al. A 2008 panorama on osteoporosis and inflammatory bowel disease. *Minerva Med.* 2008;99(1):65–71.

43. Jacobson TA, Armani A, McKenney JM, Guyton JR. Safety considerations with gastrointestinally active lipid-lowering drugs. *Am J Cardiol.* 2007;99(6A):47C–55C.

44. Silvennoinen JA, Karttunene TJ, Niemela SE, et al. A controlled study of bone mineral density in patients with inflammatory bowel disease. *Gut.* 1995;37:71–76.

45. Fries W, Dinca M, Luisetto G, et al. Calcaneal ultrasound bone densitometry in inflammatory bowel disease: a comparison with double energy x-ray absorptiometry. *Am J Gastroenterol.* 1998;93:2339–2344.

46. Bernstein CN. Calcium and bone issues in inflammatory bowel disease. *Gastroenterol Int.* 1997;10:71–77.

47. Compston JE. Review article: osteoporosis, corticosteroids and inflammatory bowel disease. *Aliment Pharmacol Ther.* 1995;9:237–250.

48. Robinson RJ, Iqbal SJ, Abrams K, et al. Increased bone resorption in patients with Crohn's disease. *Aliment Pharmacol Ther.* 1998;12:699–705.

49. Bernstein CN, Blanchard JF, Leslie W, et al. The incidence of fracture among patients with inflammatory bowel disease. *Ann Int Med.* 2000;133:795–799.

50. Lamb EJ, Wong T, Smith DJ, et al. Metabolic bone disease is present at diagnosis in patients with inflammatory bowel disease. *Aliment Pharmacol Ther.* 2002;16(11):1895–1902.

51. Habtezion A, Silverberg MS, Parkes R, et al. Risk factors for low bone density in Crohn's disease. *Inflamm Bowel Dis.* 2002;8(2):87–92.

52. Jong DJ, Corstens FHM, Mannaerts L, et al. Corticosteroid induced osteoporosis: does it occur in patients with Crohn's disease? *Am J Gastroenterol.* 2002;97(8):2011–2015.

53. Bernstein CN, Leslie WD, Leboff MS. American Gastroenterology Association medical position statement: guidelines on osteoporosis in gastrointestinal diseases. *Gastroenterology.* 2003;124(3):791–794.

54. Schmidt S, Mellström D, Norjavaara E, Sundh V, Saalman R. Longitudinal assessment of bone mineral density in children and adolescents with inflammatory bowel disease. *J Pediatr Gastroenterol Nutr.* 2012;55(5):511–618.

55. Kulnigg S, Gasche C. Systematic review: managing anaemia in Crohn's disease. *Aliment Pharmacol Ther.* 2006;24:1507–1523.

56. Bayraktar UD, Bayraktar S. Treatment of iron deficiency anemia associated with gastrointestinal tract diseases. *World J Gastroenterol.* 2010;16(22):2720–2725.

57. Kulnigg-Dabsch S, Evstatiev R, Dejaco C, Gasche C. Effect of iron therapy on platelet counts in patients with inflammatory bowel disease-associated anemia. *PLoS One.* 2012;7(4):e34520.

58. Goh J, O'Morain CA. Review article: nutrition and adult inflammatory bowel disease. *Aliment Pharmacol Ther.* 2003;17(3):307–320.

59. Mason JB. Folate, colitis, dysplasia, and cancer. *Nutr Rev.* 1989;47(10):314–317.

60. Lichtenstein GR. Management of bone loss in inflammatory bowel disease. *Semin Gastrointest Dis.* 2001;12(4):275–283.

61. Valberg LS, Flanagan PR, Kertesz A, et al. Zinc absorption in inflammatory bowel disease. *Dig Dis Sci.* 1986;31:724–731.

62. Lochs H, Dejong C, Hammarqvist F, et al. ESPEN guidelines on enteral nutrition: gastroenterology. *Clin Nutr.* 2006;25:260–274.

63. Druyan ME, Compher C, Boullata JI, et al. Clinical guidelines for the use of parenteral and enteral nutrition in adult and pediatric patients: applying the GRADE system to development of A.S.P.E.N. clinical guidelines. *JPEN J Parenter Enteral Nutr.* 2012;36(1):77–80.

64. Fernandez-Banares F, Cabre E, Esteve-Comas M, et al. How effective is enteral nutrition in inducing clinical remission in active Crohn's disease? A meta-analysis of the randomized clinical trials. *JPEN J Parenter Enteral Nutr.* 1995;19:356–364.

65. Zachos M, Tondeur M, Griffiths AM. Enteral nutritional therapy for induction of remission in Crohn's disease. *Cochrane Database Syst Rev.* 2007:CD000542.

66. Griffiths AM, Ohlsson A, Sherman PM, et al. Meta-analysis of enteral nutrition as a primary treatment of active Crohn's disease. *Gastroenterology.* 1995;10:1056–1067.

67. Messori A, Trallori G, D'Albasio G, et al. Defined-formula diets versus steroids in the treatment of active Crohn's disease: a meta-analysis. *Scand Gastroenterol.* 1996;31:267–272.

68. Heuschkel RB, Menache CC, Megerian JT, Baird AE. Enteral nutrition and corticosteroids in the treatment of acute Crohn's disease in children. *J Pediatr Gastroenterol Nutr.* 2000;31:8–15.

69. Matsui T, Sakurai T, Yao T. Nutritional therapy for Crohn's disease in Japan. *J Gastroenterol.* 2007;40(Suppl 16):S25–S31.

70. Axelsson C, Jarnum S. Assessment of the therapeutic value of an elemental diet in chronic inflammatory bowel disease. *Scand J Gastroenterol.* 1977;12(1):89–95.

71. Göschke H, Buess H, Gyr K, et al. [Elementary diet as an alternative to parenteral feeding in severe gastrointestinal diseases.] *Schweiz Med Wochenschr.* 1977;107(2):43–49.

72. Yamamoto T, Nakahigashi M, Saniabadi AR. Review article: diet and inflammatory bowel disease—epidemiology and treatment. *Aliment Pharmacol Ther.* 2009;30(2):99–112.

73. Yamamoto T, Nakahigashi M, Saniabadi AR, et al. Impacts of long-term enteral nutrition on clinical and endoscopic disease activities and mucosal cytokines during remission in patients with Crohn's disease: a prospective study. *Inflamm Bowel Dis.* 2007;13:1493–1501.

74. Yamamoto T, Nakahigashi M, Umegae S, et al. Impact of long-term enteral nutrition on clinical and endoscopic recurrence after resection for Crohn's disease: a prospective, non-randomized, parallel, controlled study. *Aliment Pharmacol Ther.* 2007;25:67–72.

75. Verma S, Kirkwood B, Brown S, et al. Oral nutritional supplementation is effective in the maintenance of remission in Crohn's disease. *Dig Liver Dis.* 2000;32:769–774.
76. Takagi S, Utsunomiya K, Kuriyama S, et al. Effectiveness of an "half elemental diet" as maintenance therapy for Crohn's disease: a randomized-controlled trial. *Aliment Pharmacol Ther.* 2006;24:1333–1340.
77. Klaassen J, Zapata R, Mella JG, et al. Enteral nutrition in severe ulcerative colitis. Digestive tolerance and nutritional efficiency [in Spanish with English abstract]. *Rev Med Chil.* 1998;126:899–904.
78. Gonzalez-Huix F, Fernandez-Banares F, Esteve-Comas M, et al. Enteral versus parenteral nutrition as adjunct therapy in acute ulcerative colitis. *Am J Gastroenterol.* 1993;88:227–232.
79. Graham TO, Kandil HM. Nutritional factors in inflammatory bowel disease. *Gastroenterol Clin North Am.* 2002;31(1):203–218.
80. Ekema G, Milianti S, Boroni G. Total parenteral nutrition in patients with short bowel syndrome. *Minerva Pediatr.* 2009;61(3):283–291.
81. Evans JP, Steinhart AH, Cohen Z, McLeod RS. Home total parenteral nutrition: an alternative to early surgery for complicated inflammatory bowel disease. *J Gastrointest Surg.* 2003;7(4):562–566.
82. Grivceva Stardelova K, Misevska P, Zdravkovska M, Trajkov D, Serafimoski V. Total parenteral nutrition in treatment of patients with inflammatory bowel disease. *Prilozi.* 2008;29(1):21–43.
83. Schulz RJ, Bischoff SC, Koletzko B. Working group for developing the guidelines for parenteral nutrition of the German Association for Nutritional Medicine. Gastroenterology Guidelines on Parenteral Nutrition, Chapter 15. *Ger Med Sci.* 2009;7:Doc13.
84. Brown AC, Rampertab SD, Mullin GE. Existing dietary guidelines for Crohn's disease and ulcerative colitis. *Expert Rev Gastroenterol Hepatol.* 2011;5(3):411–425.

CHAPTER 8

Short Bowel Syndrome

Laura E. Matarese, PhD, RDN, LDN, CNSC, FADA, FAND, FASPEN, and Hossam M. Kandil, MD, PhD

Intestinal failure (IF) is a condition resulting from obstruction, dysmotility, surgical resection, congenital defect, or disease-associated loss of absorption characterized by the inability to maintain protein-energy, fluid, electrolyte, or micronutrient balance (1). Short bowel syndrome (SBS), one of the most common forms of IF, results from surgical resection, congenital defect, or disease-associated loss of absorption. The etiology of the malabsorption that results from SBS is multifactorial and involves the following:

- Changes in motility
- Increased gastric secretions
- Osmotic stimulation from hypertonic fluids and fatty acids
- Deconjugated bile salts
- Bacterial overgrowth
- Lactose intolerance
- Fatty acid irritation of the colon

The causes of SBS vary for adults and children (see Box 8.1). Regardless of the cause, the physiologic consequences and treatment options remain the same.

The management of the patient with SBS is complex. Generally, after bowel resection, the patient is on short-term parenteral nutrition (PN). If possible, bowel rehabilitation and surgical reconstruction should be considered to avoid long-term PN. Some long-term PN patients may eventually become candidates for intestinal or multivisceral transplantation.

Factors Affecting Absorption in Short Bowel Syndrome

The severity of malabsorption in individuals with SBS is determined by the following:

- Amount of intestine resected
- Site of the resection
- Ability of the intestine to undergo adaptive hyperplasia

BOX 8.1   Causes of Short Bowel Syndrome in Children and Adults

Children
- Abdominal tumors
- Apple peel anomaly
- Crohn's disease
- Congenital SBS
- Gastroschisis
- Hirschsprung's disease
- Intestinal atresia
- Necrotizing enterocolitis
- Radiation enteritis
- Trauma

Adults
- Crohn's disease
- Chronic intestinal pseudo-obstruction
- Complications of bariatric surgery
- Extensive surgical resection
- Hypercoagulable states
- Malignancy
- Radiation enteritis
- Strangulated hernia
- Small bowel fistulas
- Surgical bypass
- Trauma
- Volvulus

Immediately after surgical resection, the bowel begins to adapt both structurally and functionally. This generally occurs over a 2- to 3-year period (2,3).The remnant bowel will compensate for a reduction in surface area by increasing the length and diameter of the remaining intestine, by villous hypertrophy, and by altering motility and hormonal response.

The length of the remaining bowel is one of the most important factors—the more bowel that remains, the greater the absorption. Small bowel resections decrease transit time through the intestine and reduce the normal rate of mixing of food with digestive enzymes and the contract time of nutrients with the mucosal surface. The normal length of the small bowel in the adult ranges from 365 to 600 cm, and the length of the large bowel is 50 cm. The minimum amount of intestine required to be autonomous from PN is estimated to be 60 to 90 cm of small bowel with a portion of the colon, or 150 cm of small bowel if the colon is absent. This illustrates the importance of the colon and its role as an absorptive organ.

The site of the resection will also impact absorption. Resection of the jejunum will have less of a detrimental effect on intestinal motility when compared to an equivalent length of ileal resection (3). The more distal portions of the intestine tend to increase the transit time of chyme through the previous segments of bowel. In the small bowel, this effect is most prominent for the ileum. Unless more than 75% has been resected, patients with an end-jejunostomy will have adequate absorption (3) because they have preserved absorption of vitamin B-12 and bile salts and good ileal adaptation. Overall transit time is normal, but gastric emptying of liquids is increased. Digestive secretions contribute to stoma losses. Sodium and water losses may be high. Dietary sodium and oral rehydration solutions (ORS) can help control stoma output. Fat absorption is constant. The consequences of an ileal resection are more severe (3). Patients who have undergone an ileal resection may have the following:

- Adequate calorie and fluid absorption but malabsorption of bile salt and vitamin B-12
- Poor jejunal adaptation and very rapid intestinal transit
- Increased fluid losses and shorter transit times if the patient has an ileal resection and loses the ileocecal valve
- Bile acid malabsorption resulting in bile salt pool depletion, which then leads to fat and fatty acid malabsorption
- Decreased calcium, zinc, and magnesium absorption

If the colon is in continuity, there is the potential for increased colonic oxalate absorption and increased secretion from malabsorbed bile salts and fatty acids. There is also an increased risk of small intestinal bacterial overgrowth (SIBO) if the ileocecal valve is no longer present.

When an intestinal resection results in an enterocolic anastomosis, sodium and water balance is often positive. Diarrhea may be due to unabsorbed fatty acids of bile salts if enterohepatic circulation is maintained. Carbohydrate malabsorption can cause an osmotic diarrhea and D-lactic acidosis. Colonic fermentation of unabsorbed carbohydrate can result in energy absorption along with a reduced stool pH.

The extent of resection determines the degree of clinical severity. The physiologic consequences of extensive small bowel resection can be quite severe (3,4). These patients often experience the following:

- Substantial fluid and electrolyte losses
- Nutrient malabsorption
- Gastric acid hypersecretion
- Vitamin B-12 and bile salt malabsorption
- Rapid gastric emptying and intestinal transit
- SIBO

The ileocecal valve and colon have an even greater tendency to increase (slow) intestinal transit time. The colon is important for the absorption of fluid, electrolytes, and nutrients such as short-chain fatty acids (SCFA) (5,6).

An intact stomach, pancreas, and liver are all important for digestion. Therefore, any previous surgeries or disease of these organs can impact absorption for the patient with SBS.

The health of the remaining intestinal mucosa will also affect absorption. Patients with active Crohn's disease, ulcerative colitis, or radiation enteritis in the remnant bowel may not absorb fluid, electrolytes, and other nutrients as well as those with healthy mucosa. See Chapter 7 for more information on Crohn's disease and ulcerative colitis.

Management of Short Bowel Syndrome

Dietary Modification

Dietary modification in the management of SBS aims to minimize GI symptoms, optimize absorption, and provide a stimulus to enhance intestinal adaptation and minimize parenteral nutrient requirements (7,8). The general tactics for dietary modification are as follows:

- Patients should consume small frequent meals, minimize concentrated sugars, and maximize complex carbohydrates.
- In some circumstances, it may help to limit fluid intake with solids and take sips of fluids between meals.
- Antidiarrheal medications are used to prolong intestinal transit.
- Commercial fiber supplementation is used as needed to slow intestinal transit, gelatinize ostomy effluent, and provide a substrate for the production of short chain fatty acids in the colon.
- Patients should take vitamin and mineral supplements.

The dietary modification plan is based on the presence or absence of the colon. Table 8.1 outlines the appropriate diet modification for SBS based on whether the colon is present or absent (9). Table 8.2 presents oral vitamin/mineral supplements recommendations for patients with SBS (7).

TABLE 8.1 Diet Modifications for Short Bowel Syndrome

	Colon Present	Colon Absent
Carbohydrate, % of kcal/d	50%–60%	40%–50%
Protein, % of kcal/d	20%	20%
Fat, % of kcal/d	20%–30%	30%–40%
Meals per day	5–6	4–6
Oxalates	Avoid	No restriction
Fluids	Isotonic/hypo-osmolar fluids	Isotonic, high-sodium fluids
Soluble fiber, g/d	5–10	5–10
Lactose	As tolerated	As tolerated

Source: Data are from reference 9.

TABLE 8.2 Oral Vitamin/Mineral Supplements for Patients with Short Bowel Syndrome

Nutrient	Strength	Dose
Vitamins A, D, and E	Vitamin A: 25,000 IU/tablet Vitamin D: 1,000 IU/tablet Vitamin E: 400 IU/tablet	1 tablet/d
Calcium	500–600 mg/tablet	1–2 tablets TID
Magnesium lactate	84 mg/tablet	1–2 tablets TID
Magnesium gluconate	1,000 mg/tablet (or liquid)	1–3 tablets TID
Potassium chloride	20 mg/tablet	1–2 tablets/d
Phosphorus (NeutraPhos)	250 mg/package	1 package TID
Sodium bicarbonate	650 mg/tablet	1 tablet TID
Chromium	100 mcg/tablet	1–2 tablets TID
Copper	3 mg/tablet	1–2 tablets/d
Selenium	200 mcg/tablet	1 tablet/d
Zinc sulfate	220 mg/tablet	1–3 tablets/d

Abbreviation: TID = 3 times per day.
Source: Data are from reference 7.

Management of Fluids

The typical volume of fluid entering the intestine is approximately 8.8 liters per day and is derived from oral intake and endogenous GI secretions (10). Most of the fluid that passes through the intestine is absorbed. Only about 150 to 200 mL passes in stool. The small intestine's maximum reabsorptive capacity is 12 liters and the colon's is 5 liters (11). When the maximum reabsorptive capacity of the colon is exceeded, as in the case of SBS (due to decreased intestinal fluid absorption, increased secretion, or both), diarrhea will result.

The factors determining capacity for intestinal fluid absorption include the following:

- Surface area (residual healthy tissue vs damaged tissue)
- Mucosal integrity

- Motility (contact time: faster motility = less contact time for absorption)
- Luminal osmolarity (unabsorbed solutes in lumen of the gut draw in water and electrolytes from the plasma)

Impairment of any one or all of these factors can result in diarrhea. Positive fluid balance is generally achieved when bowel length approaches 90 cm.

The discovery of the sodium-glucose cotransporter and clinical studies in patients with cholera led to the development of oral rehydration solutions (ORS) that are used to treat diarrhea in developing countries. Maximum absorption of sodium and water occurs from a solution containing between 90 and 120 mM of sodium per liter and 56 mM of glucose per liter (12). Several ORS are commercially available (see Table 8.3); their sodium and carbohydrate contents vary considerably. ORS can also be made with individual components or simple household ingredients (see Box 8.2 on page 94).

Most sport drinks are *not* appropriate for patients with SBS because of the high glucose content and low electrolyte content of these products. Other drinks that are low in sodium, such as water and fruit juices, will cause sodium to move from the blood into the lumen of the bowel. Hypertonic juices (which are rich in fructose) also draw water into the jejunum lumen, thereby increasing fluid loss. Because the bowel is shortened, sodium and water are lost in the ostomy effluent.

Medications

Adjunctive medical therapy is used to control symptoms and maximize absorption (13). For a list of medications used to treat SBS, see Table 8.4 (page 95).

ANTIDIARRHEAL MEDICATIONS

Antidiarrheal medications slow intestinal transit and are generally given 30 to 60 minutes prior to meals.

TABLE 8.3 Commercially Available Oral Rehydration Solutions (ORS)

	Carbohydrate, g/L	Sodium, mEq/L	Potassium, mEq/L	Bicarbonate, mEq/L	Osmolality, mOsm/L
World Health Organization ORS					
Standard formula	20	90	20	30	310
Reduced-osmolality formula	13.5	75	20	30	245
Rehydration solutions					
CeraLyte 70[a]	40	70	20	30	235
CeraLyte 90[a]	40	90	20	30	260
Equalyte[b]	30	78	22	30	305
Jianas Brothers ORS[c]	20	90	20	10	300
Liquilyte[d]	25	45	20	30	250
Pedialyte[b]	25	45	20	30	300
Rehydralyte[b]	25	75	20	30	300
Sport drink					
Gatorade[e]	60	20	3		340

Manufacturers: [a]Cera Products; [b]Ross; [c]Jianas Brothers; [d]Gerber; [e]PepsiCo.

BOX 8.2   Oral Rehydration Solution (ORS) Recipes

I. Basic ORS Recipe
1 liter (4½ cups) water
¾ teaspoon table salt
3 tablespoons sugar (sucrose)
1 teaspoon baking powder
   (or ½ teaspoon baking soda)
½ teaspoon 20% potassium chloride[a]
   or salt substitute[b]
Sugar-free artificial flavoring or sweetener

II. Grape or Cranberry Juice ORS
½ cup 100% grape or cranberry juice
3½ cups water
½ teaspoon table salt

III. Apple Juice ORS
1 cup apple juice
3 cups water
½ teaspoon table salt

IV. Orange Juice ORS
½ teaspoon table salt
½ teaspoon baking soda
8 teaspoons sugar
1 cup orange juice (unsweetened) without
   the pulp
1 liter (4½ cups) water

V. Gatorade-Based ORS
2 cups Gatorade (do not use reduced-calorie
   products)
2 cups water
½ teaspoon table salt

---

[a]By prescription
[b]Concentration: 7–14 mEq potassium per gram; 1 teaspoon weighs 5 g (⅙ oz) = 35–70 mEq potassium.

ACID BLOCKERS

Acid blockers, including H_2 antagonists and proton pump inhibitors, are used to reduce gastric hyperacidity that occurs within the first 6 months after a massive small bowel resection. They work by different mechanisms. H_2 antagonists inhibit histamine stimulation of the H_2 receptor in gastric parietal cells, which in turn reduces gastric acid secretion, gastric volume, and hydrogen concentrations. Proton pump inhibitors decrease gastric acid secretion by inhibiting parietal cell H+/K+-ATP pump.

OCTREOTIDE

Octreotide, a somatostatin analog, is an inhibitory hormone (somatostatin) produced by neuroendocrine cells throughout the GI tract and pancreas. It is effective in controlling hypersecretory states and severe diarrhea and slows jejunal transit. Significant side effects include increased risk for the following:

- Cholelithiasis
- Maldigestion
- Pseudo-obstruction
- Inhibition of intestinal adaptation (animal models)

CLONIDINE

Clonidine is an α2-adrenergic receptor antagonist that has been shown to reduce output fecal and stomal in patients with SBS (14,15).

TABLE 8.4 Medications for Short Bowel Syndrome

Medication	*Dose and Administration Notes*
Antidiarrheals	
Loperamide (Imodium) (OTC)	2–4 mg PO, 3–4 times per day, 1 hour before meals; minimal side effects
Diphenoxylate with atropine (Lomotil)	2.5–5 mg PO, 3–4 times per day, 1 hour before meals
Codeine phosphate	30–60 mg PO, 1 hour before meals
Opium tincture (1% morphine anhydrous)	10–20 drops PO, 1 hour before meals
H$_2$ blockers	
Famotidine (Pepcid)	40 mg PO or IV per day
Ranitidine (Zantac)	150–300 mg PO, twice a day; or 300 mg PO, once daily; or 50 mg IV, every 6–8 hours
Cimetidine (Tagamet)	400 mg PO or IV, 4 times per day
Proton pump inhibitors	
Omeprazole (Prilosec)	40 mg PO, twice per day
Lansoprazole (Prevacid)	30 mg IV, once per day, for up to 7 days
Esomeprazole (Nexium)	40 mg PO, twice per day
Pantoprazole (Protonix)	40 mg IV or PO, 1–2 times per day
Somatostatin analogue	
Octreotide	50–250 mcg, 3 times per day (subcutaneously)
LAR Depo-Octreotide	1 injection/mo
α2-adrenergic receptor antagonist	
Clonidine	0.1–0.3 mg PO, up to 3 times per day
Pancreatic enzymes	
Pancrelipase (Viokase)	1–8 tablets PO, with meals
Choleretic	
Ursodeoxycholic acid (Actigall)	300 mg PO, twice per day
Bile acid therapy	
Cholestyramine	2–4 g PO, up to 4 times per day
Colestipol	10–15 g PO, twice per day
Antimicrobials	
Augmentin	500 mg PO, twice per day
Levofloxacin (Levaquin)	500 mg/d PO
Metronidazole (Flagyl)	250 mg PO, 3 times per day
Ciproflaxin (Cipro)	500 mg PO, twice per day
Rifaximin (Xifaxan)	400 mg PO, 3 times per day

Source: Data are from reference 13.

PANCREATIC ENZYMES

Patients with SBS have rapid intestinal transit and, therefore, have reduced mixing of pancreatic enzymes with food. Theoretically, supplementing pancreatic enzymes may help with digestion. Use uncoated, rapid-release preparations, one to eight capsules with meals and snacks.

BILE ACID SEQUESTRATES

Bile acid sequestrates are used to increase fat absorption. They bind bile acids in the intestine, producing an insoluble complex, which is excreted in the stool. The use of bile acid sequestrates also results in partial removal of bile acids from the enterohepatic circulation, which prevents reabsorption. It is important to note that these medications also bind and impede the absorption of a variety of nutrients, including the fat-soluble vitamins. Bile acid supplements may worsen diarrhea in some patients.

ANTIBIOTICS AND PROBIOTICS

Patients with SBS often have SIBO due to impaired peristalsis. SIBO can be treated with antibiotics or probiotics to restore the natural flora. For short-term treatment of 1 to 2 weeks, antibiotics are more effective than probiotics. The use of antibiotics for treating SIBO has certain disadvantages, including the following:

- Recurrence of symptoms after treatment is discontinued
- The need for a prolonged or repeated course of treatment in some patients
- Long-term side effects of the antibiotics such as diarrhea, impaired immunity, changes in gut microflora, and the emergence of bacteria that are resistant to the antibiotics

Compared with antibiotics, there is less concern about the long-term side effects or the emergence of resistant bacteria with probiotics. These probiotics are unregulated and generally not covered by third-party payers. One option is to initially treat with a short course of antibiotics and then switch to long-term treatment with probiotics.

GROWTH FACTORS

Several growth factors have been evaluated for the treatment of SBS. Currently, recombinant human growth hormone (Zorbtive) and Teduglutide (Gattex), an analog of GLP-2, are FDA-approved for the treatment of SBS. Zorbtive is generally given over a 28-day course in combination with modified diet with or without oral glutamine. Gattex is a daily injection.

Surgical Reconstruction

Attempts at intestinal rehabilitation with diet and adjunctive medication will sometimes fail. For these patients, surgical options for preventing dehydration and malnutrition should be considered. Surgical intestinal rehabilitation or autologous gastrointestinal reconstruction is used to restore intestinal continuity by re-anastomosing isolated loops of bowel to provide more absorptive surface, lengthen, taper, or relieve obstructions. In some instances, it may be necessary to slow transit by utilizing a reversed segment. See Box 8.3 for an explanation of the surgical management of SBS.

Only a small number of patients will be candidates for these reconstructive procedures. However, for these patients, GI reconstruction may provide autonomy from PN.

BOX 8.3   Surgical Management of Short Bowel Syndrome

A. Surgical reconstruction
- Strictureplasty
- Salvage out-of-circuit bowel
- Colon preservation
- Repair fistulas instead of excision

B. Slow intestinal motility of dilated bowel
- Tapering enteroplasty
- Longitudinal intestinal lengthening and tailoring (Bianchi)
- Transverse intestinal lengthening (Kimura and Georgeson)
- Serial transverse enteroplasty procedure (STEP)

C. Slow intestinal transit—non-dilated bowel
- Valves
- Reverse segments
- Colon interposition

D. Replacement
- Small bowel/multivisceral transplantation

Long-Term Parenteral Nutrition

When rehabilitation efforts fail, patients can also be supported with long-term PN. Central parenteral nutrition (CPN) has been considered a standard life-saving therapy for more than 3 decades. Long-term CPN is costly and has appreciable risks, such as life-threatening bloodstream infections. See Chapter 22 for information on home parenteral nutrition.

Small Bowel Transplantation

Small bowel transplantation with or without other viscera should be considered in those who are candidates. Survival rates have been improving over the last decade.

Conclusion

The management of patients with SBS is complex and requires a comprehensive, multidisciplinary approach with meticulous attention to detail. Specific and meticulous nutrition intervention can facilitate weaning from PN. The use of certain nutrients or nonnutritive components of foods may also benefit some patients. When nutritional autonomy cannot be achieved through efforts in a rehabilitation program and home PN fails, small bowel transplantation should be considered. The ultimate goal is to improve the nutritional status of these patients through the safest, most efficacious method that will improve the quality of their lives.

References

1. O'Keefe SJ, Buchman AL, Fishbein TM, Jeejeebhoy KN, Jeppesen PB, Shaffer J. Short bowel syndrome and intestinal failure: consensus definitions and overview. *Clin Gastroenterol Hepatol.* 2006;4(1):6–10.

2. Jeppesen PB, Mortensen PB. Experimental approaches: dietary and hormone therapy. *Best Pract Res Clin Gastroenterol.* 2003;17(6):1041–1054.

3. Nightingale JM, Lennard-Jones JE. The short bowel syndrome: what's new and old? *Dig Dis.* 1993;11(1):12–31.

4. Nightingale JM, Kamm MA, van der Sijp JR, et al. Disturbed gastric emptying in the short bowel syndrome. Evidence for a "colonic brake." *Gut.* 1993;34(9):1171–1176.

5. Royall D, Wolever TM, Jeejeebhoy KN. Evidence for colonic conservation of malabsorbed carbohydrate in short bowel syndrome. *Am J Gastroenterol.* 1992;87(6):751–756.

6. Jeppesen PB, Mortensen PB. The influence of a preserved colon on the absorption of medium chain fat in patients with small bowel resection. *Gut.* 1998;43(4):478–483.

7. Matarese LE, Steiger E. Dietary and medical management of short bowel syndrome in adult patients. *J Clin Gastroenterol.* 2006;40(5 Suppl 2):S85–S93.

8. Matarese LE, O'Keefe SJ, Kandil HM, Bond G, Costa G, Abu-Elmagd K. Short bowel syndrome: clinical guidelines for nutrition management. *Nutr Clin Pract.* 2005;20(5):493–502.

9. Byrne TA, Veglia L, Camelio M, et al. Beyond the prescription: optimizing the diet of patients with short bowel syndrome. *Nutr Clin Pract.* 2000;15(6):306–311.

10. Fordtran JS, Locklear TW. Ionic constituents and osmolality of gastric and small-intestinal fluids after eating. *Am J Dig Dis.* 1966;11(7):503–521.

11. Levitan R, Fordtran JS, Burrows BA, Ingelfinger FJ. Water and salt absorption in the human colon. *J Clin Invest.* 1962;41:1754–1759.

12. Lennard-Jones JE. Oral rehydration solutions in short bowel syndrome. *Clin Ther.* 1990;12(Suppl A):129–137; discussion 138.

13. Steiger E. Guidelines for pharmacotherapy, nutritional management, and weaning parenteral nutrition in adult patients with short bowel syndrome: introduction. *J Clin Gastroenterol.* 2006;40(Suppl 2):S73–S74.

14. McDoniel K, Taylor B, Huey W, et al. Use of clonidine to decrease intestinal fluid losses in patients with high-output short-bowel syndrome. *JPEN J Parenter Enteral Nutr.* 2004;28(4):265–268.

15. Buchman AL, Fryer J, Wallin A, Ahn CW, Polensky S, Zaremba K. Clonidine reduces diarrhea and sodium loss in patients with proximal jejunostomy: a controlled study. *JPEN J Parenter Enteral Nutr.* 2006;30(6):487–491.

CHAPTER 9

Irritable Bowel Syndrome

Bani Chander Roland, MD,
and Gerard E. Mullin, MD, CNSP, FACN, AGAF

Irritable bowel syndrome (IBS) is a disorder characterized by altered bowel movements and abdominal pain that affects 10% to 15% of the US population (1). IBS is diagnosed in women more often than in men by a ratio of approximately 2 to 1. It results in a poor quality of life and has significant adverse economic impact, with associated absenteeism from work and health care costs measured in the billions of dollars annually (2).

The pathophysiology of IBS is complex and involves altered enteric neurotransmitters, imbalances in the gut microbiota, neuroendocrine disruption, visceral hypersensitivity, altered permeability, motility, chronic stress, and a maladaptive psychological component (3–7). The resulting chronic symptoms include constipation, diarrhea, abdominal pain and/or discomfort, distension, and flatulence. IBS can be diagnosed by the following Rome III criteria (8):

- Symptoms that have developed at least 6 months prior.
- Abdominal pain or discomfort that have been present for at least 3 days per month for 3 months, and that should be associated with two or more of the following:
  - Improvement with defecation
  - Onset associated with a change in stool frequency
  - Onset associated with a change in form (appearance) of stool

However, the diagnosis is often one of exclusion given that other conditions, such as Crohn's disease, celiac disease, and small intestinal bacterial overgrowth (SIBO), frequently involve overlapping symptoms. Dietary modifications are among the primary treatments to alleviate gastrointestinal (GI) symptoms and improve overall health in this challenging patient population (9).

Etiology

There are three main subtypes of IBS: constipation-predominant (IBS-C), diarrhea-predominant (IBS-D), and mixed (IBS-M). Known triggers for the flare-up of IBS symptoms include stress, infections, antibiotics, nonsteroidal anti-inflammatory medications, and surgery. However, symptoms are most commonly provoked by specific foods (4). As compared to the general population, individuals with IBS report more food sensitivities and intolerances. According to double-blind challenge methodologies, approximately two-thirds of patients with IBS have at least one food intolerance, and some have multiple intolerances (10). Foods rich in carbohydrate, fatty foods, caffeinated beverages, alcohol, and hot spices are most frequently reported to cause symptoms (11). The most common allergens are dairy products (40% to 44%) and grains (40% to 60%) (12). A number of elimination diet trials have shown benefit (13–20). Elimination of foods based upon IgG-antibody testing has proved to be beneficial in most patients and shown to improve both IBS global symptoms and quality of life in several studies (14,15,19,21). Most research on elimination of foods for the management of IBS has concentrated on fermentable carbohydrates, and we outline the evidence about elimination trials of fermentable carbohydrates in the following sections.

Lactose

Lactose is a disaccharide that is enzymatically digested to monosaccharides, glucose, and galactose by the intestinal brush border enzyme lactase. It is fermented by colonic bacteria to short-chain fatty acids, hydrogen, methane, carbon dioxide, and other gases. These gases have been postulated to precipitate symptoms in individuals with IBS.

Patients with IBS have also been shown to have a higher prevalence of SIBO than control subjects, and malabsorbed carbohydrates may be rapidly fermented into gases, causing symptoms of gas, distention, and bloating (22). Delivery of lactose to the intestinal lumen may additionally exert an osmotic effect and result in more luminal water, increasing the liquidity of intestinal contents and resulting in more rapid intestinal transit time. Typical GI symptoms that result from lactose malabsorption include abdominal cramping, bloating, flatulence, and diarrhea.

In a study of 60 participants with IBS and 60 controls, Yang et al found that the patients with IBS experienced GI symptoms following lactose ingestion more frequently than control subjects (23). In another case-control study with 82 IBS subjects and 102 healthy control subjects, Farup and colleagues determined that 38% of IBS patients had symptoms after the ingestion of lactose products, as compared with 20% of the healthy controls ($P = .01$) (24). In a 4-month-long, double-blind, crossover, therapeutic clinical trial involving 12 individuals with IBS, Lisker et al concluded that lactase supplementation does not improve symptoms in patients with IBS who ingest lactose products (25). Heizer and colleagues have suggested in a recent review of subjects with IBS that patients with IBS and known lactose intolerance show improvement with dietary restriction (26).

Fructose

Fructose is naturally found in honey, fruits, and table sugar, and it is present in many foods and beverages as high-fructose corn syrup. The human intestine does not have a specific enzyme for digestion or transport of fructose. Fructose relies on glucose transporters for absorption, which can easily be overwhelmed with a large fructose load (more than 25 g) and result in GI symptoms. The typical American consumes more than 50 g fructose daily (27).

In a case-control study of 25 women with IBS and 25 health control subjects, fructose intolerance was observed more frequently in subjects with IBS as compared with the control subjects (52% vs 16%; $P = .01$), and patients clearly benefitted from dietary restriction (28). Shepherd and associates conducted a double-blinded, randomized, quadruple-arm, placebo-controlled rechallenge trial and concluded that restriction of fructose and fructans was beneficial in resolving symptoms in IBS (11).

FODMAPs

Fermentable oligo-, di-, and monosaccharides and polyols (FODMAPs) represent a family of poorly absorbed, short-chain carbohydrates, which are highly fermentable in the presence of gut bacteria. Lactose (disaccharide), fructose (monosaccharide), fructans, and galactans are the major FODMAPs consumed in the standard American diet.

Fructans are long polymers of fructose with a glucose terminal end. Fructans with more than 10 molecules of fructose in a chain are known as *inulins*, and those with fewer than 10 fructose molecules in a chain are referred as *fructo-oligosaccharides* (FOS) or *oligofructose*. The latter are highly fermentable. Wheat-based products and onions account for most fructan intake in typical Western diets.

Galactans (eg, stacchyose and raffinose) are chains of fructose with one galactose molecule on the end. They act similarly to fructans. Foods rich in galactans include legumes (eg, soy and other beans, chickpeas, lentils), cabbage, and brussels sprouts.

Sugar alcohols, such as sorbitol, are polyols. They are digested and absorbed poorly in the upper GI tract and produce hyperosmolarity in the intestinal lumen and are subsequently fermented by the gut microbiota.

In a single-blind, crossover intervention trial involving 15 patients with IBS and 15 healthy control subjects, subjects ingesting a diet high in FODMAPs had higher levels of breath hydrogen and methane, reflecting bacterial fermentation (29). In 2012, Barrett and Gibson reviewed studies on FODMAP restriction in IBS and concluded that they have shown beneficial results (30). Foods higher and lower in FODMAPs are shown in Table 9.1.

Wheat

Ingestion of wheat can be problematic in patients with IBS for several reasons. Wheat is a FODMAP food because it is high in fructans. Wheat is also among the top eight food allergens in the Western diet. Many people are also sensitive to gluten, the protein in wheat. Interestingly, patients with IBS have a four-fold higher prevalence of celiac disease than individuals without IBS (31). (See Chapter 10 for more information on celiac disease.)

IBS-D patients with celiac disease–associated serum antibodies and HLA-DQ2 expression normalized their GI symptoms score when they followed a gluten-free diet (32). In a double-blind, placebo-controlled challenge, ingestion of wheat-filled capsules provoked IBS-like GI symptoms (33). Gluten-enriched bread

TABLE 9.1 FODMAP Content of Foods

FODMAP Content	*Fructose*	*Polyols*	*Lactose*	*Fructans*
Higher	Apples, pears, watermelon, honey, artichoke, high-fructose corn syrup	Sugar alcohols, avocado, mushrooms	Milk, yogurt, soft cheese	Wheat, rye, garlic, onions, asparagus, soy, legumes, cruciferous vegetables
Lower	Citrus fruits, berries, bananas, grapes, honeydew, cantaloupe, kiwi	Glucose, sucralose, aspartame, Stevia	Rice milk, almond milk, hard cheese	Rice, corn, potatoes, quinoa, squash, lettuce, cucumbers, string beans

provoked significantly more IBS-like GI symptoms in healthy individuals in a double-blind controlled trial (34). In a prospective study of 13 patients with IBS, 77% of the participants improved when they followed a very low–carbohydrate (20 g/d) diet (35).

Dietary Management and Supplement Use

A diet to manage IBS can eliminate potential triggers or involve use of foods or food-based supplements that provide a therapeutic benefit. The following dietary supplements may provide symptomatic improvement in patients with IBS.

Fiber Supplements

There are multiple systematic reviews and meta-analyses for the use of fiber in IBS (36–38). Overall, fiber seems to offer benefit specifically for patients who have IBS with constipation. Soluble fiber has been shown to have a tendency toward greater global symptom improvement as compared with insoluble fiber (38). Soluble fibers include psyllium or ispaghula, partially hydrolyzed guar gum, FOS, oligosaccharides, and calcium polycarbophil. Insoluble fibers common in the food supply are wheat bran, corn bran, and defatted ground flaxseed. Oat bran is a 50-50 mixture of soluble and insoluble fiber.

Nutraceutical Supplements

Most patients with IBS use at least one form of complementary and alternative medicine (CAM). Dietary supplements are the CAM modality most commonly used by IBS patients. Dietary supplements that have been studied for IBS management include Chinese herbs, Iberogast (a liquid extract of nine Western-based herbs that is formulated in Germany), artichoke extract, melatonin, and peppermint oil (39). For additional information on nutraceuticals, refer to Chapter 24.

PEPPERMINT OIL
Peppermint oil has a long tradition of use for IBS (40), and one large meta-analysis has demonstrated that it is beneficial for alleviating symptoms (41). This supplement has a number of effects on GI motility, immunity, and inflammation that may benefit patients with IBS, including its blockade of calcium channels, which are spasmolytic.

TRADITIONAL CHINESE MEDICINE
Most studies of the use of traditional Chinese medicine to treat IBS have been conducted in Asia. Of the 75 randomized trials identified in a literature search, only 5 trials of TCM therapies for IBS were considered to be high quality (42–46). Interestingly, of these high-quality trials, 4 of 5 (using different TCM therapies) showed benefit for IBS, as did a meta-analysis of 12 studies of Tong xie yao fang (TXYF), a type of TCM prepared from 4 herbs (47).

In one randomized double-blind placebo-controlled trial of 116 patients, both standard and individualized Chinese herbal medicine significantly improved bowel symptoms (42). The benefit of individualized herbal treatment was maintained at 14 weeks after completion of treatment.

Padma Lax, a complex Tibetan herbal formula, was evaluated for safety and effectiveness in treating IBS-C in a 3-month, double-blind randomized pilot study. Compared with participants who took a placebo, those in the Padma Lax group were improved in constipation, severity of abdominal pain, daily activities, incomplete evacuation, abdominal distension, and flatus/flatulence (43).

Leung et al reported the results of a clinical trial of 119 individuals with Rome II confirmed IBS-D who were randomly assigned to receive a standard concoction of TCM extracts that contained 11 herbs or a placebo with a similar appearance and taste for 8 weeks after a 2-week run-in period. There was no difference in symptom score and quality-of-life assessment between the two groups (44).

Wang and colleagues evaluated the effect of 24-g Shugan Jianpi granule (SJG) on the number of gut mucosal serotonin-positive cells (5-HT+C) in 24 patients with IBS and found that SJG decreased the number of 5-HT+C; additionally, this effect of SJG was enhanced with the concomitant use of the herb Smecta (15 g three times a day) (45).

The efficacy of TXNG in IBS-D patients was evaluated in a prospective, randomized, double-blind placebo-controlled trial. In the TXNG group, 82.7% of the participants reported decreased IBS-related pain, compared with 39.3% in the placebo group. Furthermore, the frequency and duration of abdominal pain were significantly reduced in the TXNG group compared with the placebo group. Improvement in IBS-related diarrhea was observed in 86.2% of participants in the TXNG group and 42.9% of subjects in the placebo group. Neither the effective time of IBS-related pain nor the effective time of IBS-related diarrhea was significantly different between the two groups. However, the participants in the TXNG group had notably shorter IBS-related pain alleviation and IBS-related diarrhea alleviation times (46).

Note: Some TCM products have been contaminated with heavy metals. Clinicians should warn patients to exercise caution when pursuing TCM therapies.

IBEROGAST

There is strong scientific support for the use of Iberogast for GI disorders (48). In a double-blind, randomized, placebo-controlled multi-center trial, Madisch et al (49) investigated the effects of Iberogast in 208 patients with IBS and found that Iberogast herbal preparations STW 5 (standard Iberogast) and STW 5-II (Iberogast minus four herbs) improved the symptoms of participants. Iberogast has been shown to influence immunity, inflammation, and motility modulation that may benefit individuals with IBS (50).

MELATONIN

Melatonin, a precursor to serotonin, is the principle neurotransmitter that modulates GI motility. Melatonin urinary metabolites have been shown to be deficient in patients with IBS (51,52). Sleep disorders, depression, anxiety, and dysregulation of the motility are commonly seen in patients with IBS (53). These disorders are known to be improved by melatonin, forming the rationale for investigation of its potential efficacy on IBS. Melatonin in IBS has shown efficacy at 3 mg/d, with improvements in IBS symptoms, pain, and visceral hypersensitivity (54–56).

ARTICHOKE LEAF EXTRACT

Treatment with artichoke leaf extract has been shown to decrease IBS symptoms in one large study of 208 adults. A significant shift ($P < .001$) in self-reported usual bowel pattern away from "alternating constipation/diarrhea" toward "normal" was observed. There was also a significant 20% improvement in the total quality-of-life score after treatment with artichoke leaf extract (57).

PREBIOTICS AND PROBIOTICS

Prebiotics are defined as nondigestible, fermentable food components that result in the selective stimulation of growth and/or activity of one or a limited number of microbial genera/species in the gut microbiota that confer health benefits to the host. The most commonly used prebiotics are inulin-type fructans (inulin, oligofructose, FOS) and galacto-oligosaccharides (GOS). The human GI tract does not produce enzymes capable of digesting these prebiotic compounds. Therefore, they reach the colon and are fermented by the microbiota. Four controlled trials of prebiotics for IBS have been conducted, with three of the trials showing benefit for low-doses (3 to 5 g/d), whereas high doses caused bloating, gas, and worsening of symptoms (58).

Probiotics are dietary supplements containing live microorganisms that, when ingested, exert a beneficial effect on the host. Among the most commonly used and studied species are *Lactobacillus, Bifidobacteria,* multistrain bacterial species, and *Saccharomyces boulardii* (59–61). Probiotics may improve IBS by regulating immunity, inflammation, motility, and permeability, and the gut microbiota (62). Meta-analyses support the use of probiotics in IBS. However, many questions remain about strain-specificity, dose, and duration of therapy (58,63,64). Concerns have been raised that the use of probiotics in the setting of SIBO may perpetuate microbial populating of the proximal gut (65). See Chapter 25 for additional information regarding probiotics.

Conclusion

Irritable bowel syndrome is an enigmatic disorder that involves a number of pathophysiological mechanisms that produce chronic GI symptoms. Given the relatively high known prevalence of celiac disease in IBS, every patient with IBS should be screened for celiac disease. SIBO is also common in patients with IBS, and referral for hydrogen and methane breath testing should be considered if a patient experiences gas, bloating, abdominal discomfort, or flatulence.

The registered dietitian should also be aware of the influence of diet and nutritional supplements on the course of illness. A careful dietary history to discern whether food intolerances are provoking symptoms should be performed on every IBS patient. Elimination of foods high in lactose, fructose, and wheat should be considered if they are suspected to be causing IBS symptoms. Soluble fiber may be useful as a prebiotic and may regulate IBS symptoms. Finally, nutraceutical supplements are commonly used by IBS patients, who may experience benefit from their use. Probiotics, low-dose prebiotics, peppermint oil, Iberogast, and melatonin may be useful adjuncts in selected patients. Large-scale studies on the influence of food and food-based supplements in IBS are warranted.

References

1. Choung RS, Locke GR. Epidemiology of IBS. *Gastroenterol Clin North Am.* 2011;40(1):1–10.
2. Maxion-Bergemann S, Thielecke F, Abel F, Bergemann R. Costs of irritable bowel syndrome in the UK and US. *Pharmacoeconomics.* 2006;24(1):21–37.
3. Feng B, La JH, Schwartz ES, Gebhart GF. Irritable bowel syndrome: methods, mechanisms, and pathophysiology. Neural and neuro-immune mechanisms of visceral hypersensitivity in irritable bowel syndrome. *Am J Physiol Gastrointest Liver Physiol.* 2012;302(10):G1085–G1098.
4. Camilleri M, Lasch K, Zhou W. Irritable bowel syndrome: methods, mechanisms, and pathophysiology. The confluence of increased permeability, inflammation, and pain in irritable bowel syndrome. *Am J Physiol Gastrointest Liver Physiol.* 2012;303(7):G775–G785.
5. Zhou Q, Verne GN. New insights into visceral hypersensitivity—clinical implications in IBS. *Nat Rev Gastroenterol Hepatol.* 2011;8(6):349–355.
6. O'Malley D, Quigley EM, Dinan TG, Cryan JF. Do interactions between stress and immune responses lead to symptom exacerbations in irritable bowel syndrome? *Brain Behav Immun.* 2011;25(7):1333–1341.
7. Hasler WL. Traditional thoughts on the pathophysiology of irritable bowel syndrome. *Gastroenterol Clin North Am.* 2011;40(1):21–43.
8. Drossman DA, Chang L, Bellamy N, et al. Severity in irritable bowel syndrome: a Rome Foundation Working Team report. *Am J Gastroenterol.* 2011;106(10):1749–1759; quiz 60.

9. Eswaran S, Tack J, Chey WD. Food: the forgotten factor in the irritable bowel syndrome. *Gastroenterol Clin North Am*. 2011;40(1):141–162.

10. Jones VA, McLaughlan P, Shorthouse M, Workman E, Hunter JO. Food intolerance: a major factor in the pathogenesis of irritable bowel syndrome. *Lancet*. 1982;2(8308):1115–1117.

11. Shepherd SJ, Parker FC, Muir JG, Gibson PR. Dietary triggers of abdominal symptoms in patients with irritable bowel syndrome: randomized placebo-controlled evidence. *Clin Gastroenterol Hepatol*. 2008;6(7):765–771.

12. Simonato B, De Lazzari F, Pasini G, Polato F, et al. IgE binding to soluble and insoluble wheat flour proteins in atopic and non-atopic patients suffering from gastrointestinal symptoms after wheat ingestion. *Clin Exp Allergy*. 2001;31(11):1771–1778.

13. Yang CM, Li YQ. [The therapeutic effects of eliminating allergic foods according to food-specific IgG antibodies in irritable bowel syndrome]. *Zhonghua Nei Ke Za Zhi*. 2007;46(8):641–643.

14. Drisko J, Bischoff B, Hall M, McCallum R. Treating irritable bowel syndrome with a food elimination diet followed by food challenge and probiotics. *J Am Coll Nutr*. 2006;25(6):514–522.

15. Zar S, Mincher L, Benson MJ, Kumar D. Food-specific IgG4 antibody-guided exclusion diet improves symptoms and rectal compliance in irritable bowel syndrome. *Scand J Gastroenterol*. 2005;40(7):800–807.

16. Hunter JO. Food elimination in IBS: the case for IgG testing remains doubtful. *Gut*. 2005;54(8):1203.

17. Zar S, Benson MJ, Kumar D. Food-specific serum IgG4 and IgE titers to common food antigens in irritable bowel syndrome. *Am J Gastroenterol*. 2005;100(7):1550–1557.

18. Floch MH. Use of diet and probiotic therapy in the irritable bowel syndrome: analysis of the literature. *J Clin Gastroenterol*. 2005;39(5 Suppl 3):S243–S246.

19. Atkinson W, Sheldon TA, Shaath N, Whorwell PJ. Food elimination based on IgG antibodies in irritable bowel syndrome: a randomised controlled trial. *Gut*. 2004;53(10):1459–1464.

20. Zar S, Kumar D, Kumar D. Role of food hypersensitivity in irritable bowel syndrome. *Minerva Med*. 2002;93(5):403–412.

21. Aydinlar EI, Dikmen PY, Tiftikci A, et al. IgG-based elimination diet in migraine plus irritable bowel syndrome. *Headache*. 2013;53(3):514–525.

22. Pyleris E, Giamarellos-Bourboulis EJ, Tzivras D, et al. The prevalence of overgrowth by aerobic bacteria in the small intestine by small bowel culture: relationship with irritable bowel syndrome. *Dig Dis Sci*. 2012;57(5):1321–1329.

23. Yang J, Deng Y, Chu H, et al. Prevalence and presentation of lactose intolerance and effects on dairy product intake in healthy subjects and patients with irritable bowel syndrome. *Clin Gastroenterol Hepatol*. 2013;11(3):262–268.

24. Farup PG, Monsbakken KW, Vandvik PO. Lactose malabsorption in a population with irritable bowel syndrome: prevalence and symptoms. A case-control study. *Scand J Gastroenterol*. 2004;39(7):645–649.

25. Lisker R, Solomons NW, Perez Briceno R, Ramirez Mata M. Lactase and placebo in the management of the irritable bowel syndrome: a double-blind, cross-over study. *Am J Gastroenterol*. 1989;84(7):756–762.

26. Heizer WD, Southern S, McGovern S. The role of diet in symptoms of irritable bowel syndrome in adults: a narrative review. *J Am Diet Assoc*. 2009;109(7):1204–1214.

27. Vos MB, Kimmons JE, Gillespie C, Welsh J, Blanck HM. Dietary fructose consumption among US children and adults: the Third National Health and Nutrition Examination Survey. *Medscape J Med*. 2008;10(7):160.

28. Reyes-Huerta JU, de la Cruz-Patino E, Ramirez-Gutierrez de Velasco A, Zamudio C, Remes-Troche JM. [Fructose intolerance in patients with irritable bowel syndrome: a case-control study]. *Rev Gastroenterol Mex*. 2010;75(4):405–411.

29. Ong DK, Mitchell SB, Barrett JS, et al. Manipulation of dietary short chain carbohydrates alters the pattern of gas production and genesis of symptoms in irritable bowel syndrome. *J Gastroenterol Hepatol*. 2010;25(8):1366–1373.

30. Barrett JS, Gibson PR. Fermentable oligosaccharides, disaccharides, monosaccharides and polyols (FODMAPs) and nonallergic food intolerance: FODMAPs or food chemicals? *Therap Adv Gastroenterol*. 2012;5(4):261–268.

31. Ford AC, Chey WD, Talley NJ, et al. Yield of diagnostic tests for celiac disease in individuals with symptoms suggestive of irritable bowel syndrome: systematic review and meta-analysis. *Arch Intern Med.* 2009;169(7):651–658.

32. Wahnschaffe U, Schulzke JD, Zeitz M, Ullrich R. Predictors of clinical response to gluten-free diet in patients diagnosed with diarrhea-predominant irritable bowel syndrome. *Clin Gastroenterol Hepatol.* 2007;5(7):844–850; quiz 769.

33. Carroccio A, Mansueto P, Iacono G, et al. Non-celiac wheat sensitivity diagnosed by double-blind placebo-controlled challenge: exploring a new clinical entity. *Am J Gastroenterol.* 2012;107(12):1898–1906.

34. Biesiekierski JR, Newnham ED, Irving PM, et al. Gluten causes gastrointestinal symptoms in subjects without celiac disease: a double-blind randomized placebo-controlled trial. *Am J Gastroenterol.* 2011;106(3):508–514; quiz 515.

35. Austin GL, Dalton CB, Hu Y, et al. A very low-carbohydrate diet improves symptoms and quality of life in diarrhea-predominant irritable bowel syndrome. *Clin Gastroenterol Hepatol.* 2009;7(6):706–708e1.

36. Ruepert L, Quartero AO, de Wit NJ, et al. Bulking agents, antispasmodics and antidepressants for the treatment of irritable bowel syndrome. *Cochrane Database Syst Rev.* 2011(8):CD003460.

37. Quartero AO, Meineche-Schmidt V, Muris J, Rubin G, de Wit N. Bulking agents, antispasmodic and antidepressant medication for the treatment of irritable bowel syndrome. *Cochrane Database Syst Rev.* 2005(2):CD003460.

38. Ford AC, Talley NJ, Spiegel BM, et al. Effect of fibre, antispasmodics, and peppermint oil in the treatment of irritable bowel syndrome: systematic review and meta-analysis. *BMJ.* 2008;337:a2313.

39. Pirotta M. Irritable bowel syndrome: the role of complementary medicines in treatment. *Aust Fam Physician.* 2009;38(12):966–968.

40. Grigoleit HG, Grigoleit P. Peppermint oil in irritable bowel syndrome. *Phytomedicine.* 2005;12(8):601–606.

41. Pittler MH, Ernst E. Peppermint oil for irritable bowel syndrome: a critical review and meta-analysis. *Am J Gastroenterol.* 1998;93(7):1131–1135.

42. Bensoussan A, Talley NJ, Hing M, et al. Treatment of irritable bowel syndrome with Chinese herbal medicine: a randomized controlled trial. *JAMA.* 1998;280(18):1585–1589.

43. Sallon S, Ben-Arye E, Davidson R, et al. A novel treatment for constipation-predominant irritable bowel syndrome using Padma Lax, a Tibetan herbal formula. *Digestion.* 2002;65(3):161–171.

44. Leung WK, Wu JC, Liang SM, et al. Treatment of diarrhea-predominant irritable bowel syndrome with traditional Chinese herbal medicine: a randomized placebo-controlled trial. *Am J Gastroenterol.* 2006;101(7):1574–1580.

45. Wang ZJ, Li HX, Wang JH, Zhang F. Effect of Shugan Jianpi granule on gut mucosal serotonin-positive cells in patients with irritable bowel syndrome of stagnated Gan-qi attacking Pi syndrome type. *Chin J Integr Med.* 2008;14(3):185–189.

46. Wang G, Li TQ, Wang L, et al. Tong-xie-ning, a Chinese herbal formula, in treatment of diarrhea-predominant irritable bowel syndrome: a prospective, randomized, double-blind, placebo-controlled trial. *Chin Med J (Engl).* 2006;119(24):2114–2119.

47. Bian Z, Wu T, Liu L, et al. Effectiveness of the Chinese herbal formula TongXieYaoFang for irritable bowel syndrome: a systematic review. *J Altern Complement Med.* 2006;12(4):401–407.

48. Ottillinger B, Storr M, Malfertheiner P, Allescher HD. STW 5 (Iberogast ®): a safe and effective standard in the treatment of functional gastrointestinal disorders. *Wien Med Wochenschr.* 2013;163(3–4):65–72.

49. Madisch A, Holtmann G, Plein K, Hotz J. Treatment of irritable bowel syndrome with herbal preparations: results of a double-blind, randomized, placebo-controlled, multi-centre trial. *Aliment Pharmacol Ther.* 2004;19(3):271–279.

50. Patrick L. Gastroesophageal reflux disease (GERD): a review of conventional and alternative treatments. *Altern Med Rev.* 2011;16(2):116–133.

51. Radwan P, Skrzydlo-Radomanska B, Radwan-Kwiatek K, Burak-Czapiuk B, Strzemecka J. Is melatonin involved in the irritable bowel syndrome? *J Physiol Pharmacol.* 2009;60(Suppl 3):67–70.

52. Wisniewska-Jarosinska M, Chojnacki J, Konturek S, et al. Evaluation of urinary 6-hydroxymelatonin sulphate excretion in women at different age with irritable bowel syndrome. *J Physiol Pharmacol.* 2010;61(3):295–300.

53. Thor PJ, Krolczyk G, Gil K, Zurowski D, Nowak L. Melatonin and serotonin effects on gastrointestinal motility. *J Physiol Pharmacol.* 2007;58(Suppl 6):97–103.

54. Lu WZ, Song GH, Gwee KA, Ho KY. The effects of melatonin on colonic transit time in normal controls and IBS patients. *Dig Dis Sci.* 2009;54(5):1087–1093.

55. Sanchez-Barcelo EJ, Mediavilla MD, Tan DX, Reiter RJ. Clinical uses of melatonin: evaluation of human trials. *Curr Med Chem.* 2010;17(19):2070–2095.

56. Lu WZ, Gwee KA, Moochhalla S, Ho KY. Melatonin improves bowel symptoms in female patients with irritable bowel syndrome: a double-blind placebo-controlled study. *Aliment Pharmacol Ther.* 2005;22(10):927–934.

57. Joy JF, Haber SL. Clinical uses of artichoke leaf extract. *Am J Health Syst Pharm.* 2007;64(18):1904, 1906–1909.

58. Whelan K. Probiotics and prebiotics in the management of irritable bowel syndrome: a review of recent clinical trials and systematic reviews. *Curr Opin Clin Nutr Metab Care.* 2011;14(6):581–587.

59. Quigley EM. Bacterial flora in irritable bowel syndrome: role in pathophysiology, implications for management. *J Dig Dis.* 2007;8(1):2–7.

60. Quigley EM, Bytzer P, Jones R, Mearin F. Irritable bowel syndrome: the burden and unmet needs in Europe. *Dig Liver Dis.* 2006;38(10):717–723.

61. Quigley EM, Flourie B. Probiotics and irritable bowel syndrome: a rationale for their use and an assessment of the evidence to date. *Neurogastroenterol Motil.* 2007;19(3):166–172.

62. Marteau P. Probiotics in functional intestinal disorders and IBS: proof of action and dissecting the multiple mechanisms. *Gut.* 2010;59(3):285–286.

63. McFarland LV, Dublin S. Meta-analysis of probiotics for the treatment of irritable bowel syndrome. *World J Gastroenterol.* 2008;14(17):2650–2661.

64. Moayyedi P, Ford AC, Talley NJ, et al. The efficacy of probiotics in the treatment of irritable bowel syndrome: a systematic review. *Gut.* 2010;59(3):325–332.

65. Mullin GE. Probiotics and digestive disease. *Nutr Clin Pract.* 2012;27(2):300–302.

CHAPTER 10

Celiac Disease

S. Devi Rampertab, MD, FACG, AGAF

Celiac disease—also known as *celiac sprue*, *non-tropical sprue*, or *gluten-sensitive enteropathy*—is an autoimmune disorder that results from close interaction of genetic, environmental, and immunologic components. In individuals who are genetically predisposed, the ingestion of certain sequences of amino acids found in wheat, rye, or barley (ie, "gluten") triggers an immune response that results in inflammation, villous atrophy, and crypt hyperplasia in the small intestine.

Although the classic gastrointestinal (GI) symptoms of celiac disease are abdominal pain, diarrhea, and weight loss, these are experienced by a minority of patients with celiac disease; many patients are completely asymptomatic. Some patients who are asymptomatic may be incidentally diagnosed with celiac disease.

Eliminating gluten from the diet is the mainstay of treatment for patients with celiac disease. In some cases, treatment may also involve elimination of related proteins, such as casein (a milk protein) and avenin (which is found in oats).

Epidemiology

Based on serologic screening tests, celiac disease in the United States and Europe affects approximately 1% of the population (1–5) and is predominantly diagnosed in females (2.9 to 1). In a study that examined characteristics of the disease, patients experienced symptoms for a mean of 11 years before receiving a celiac disease diagnosis because clinicians could not always identify celiac disease; this is particularly true when the patient experiences atypical manifestations (6). The "Celiac Iceberg" theory (see Figure 10.1) illustrates this concept by stating that for every case of celiac disease diagnosed on clinical suspicion (tip of the iceberg), many more remain undiagnosed (area submerged in water) (7).

Pathogenesis

Genetic Factors

Celiac disease is linked to specific HLA haplotypes; 95% of this patient population will be diagnosed as HLA-DQ2 positive, and most of the other 5% will be identified as HLA-DQ8 positive (8). Concordance

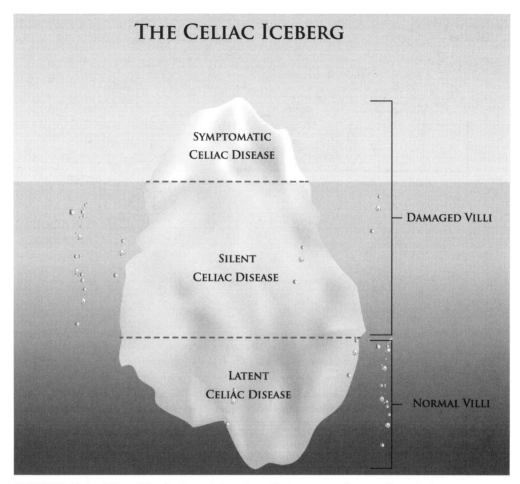

FIGURE 10.1   The celiac iceberg. Note that all the groups (latent, silent, and symptomatic) manifest the HLA DQ2/DQ8 subtype. See reference 7 for additional information about this theory. © Can Stock Photo Inc. www.canstockphoto.com.

rates are much higher in monozygotic twins (70%) when compared to HLA-matched siblings (30%) (9). Celiac disease diagnoses are found in approximately 10% of the first-degree relatives of an affected individual (6).

The Role of Gluten

Gluten—the inciting agent of celiac disease—is a protein that naturally occurs in wheat, barley, and rye. The alcohol-soluble fraction of gluten—gliadin—induces celiac symptoms. The gliadin molecules that have not been digested can enter the lamina propria and interact with antigen-presenting cells (APC).

Mucosal Immune Responses

Figure 10.2 (page 110) presents the immunological processes that cause celiac disease–associated mucosal damage. The tissue transglutaminase (TTG) enzyme is responsible for deamidation, which is the conversion of glutamine residues on the gliadin protein to glutamic acid, thereby facilitating binding of gliadin to the APC. Once gliadin binds to the APC, deamidated gliadin is presented by HLA-DQ2 and/or HLA-DQ8 molecules to CD4 T cells. This process yields cytokines, which induce production of

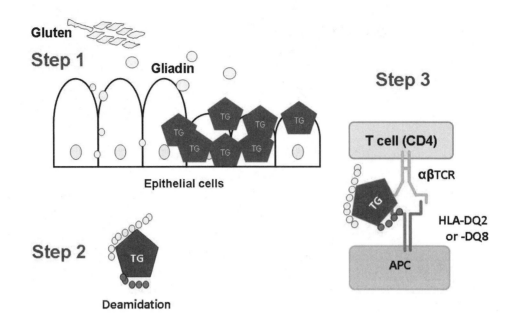

FIGURE 10.2   Pathophysiology of celiac disease. Gluten is broken down into gliadin. Gliadin moves from the lumen into the mucosa via leaky tight junctions between the epithelial cells. The enzyme tissue transglutaminase (TG) converts glutamine residues on the gliadin protein into glutamic acid (red circular molecules on cartoon), a critical process known as deamidation. This results in a negative charge, which favors binding and presentation by the HLA-DQ2 and DQ8 molecules on the antigen-presenting cell (APC) in the lamina propria. The APC then presents this deamidated gliadin to the T cells, triggering an inflammatory reaction that targets the mucosa of the small intestine.

antibodies to gliadin, TTG, and endomysium, and the eventual development of mucosal damage—villous atrophy, crypt hyperplasia—that defines patients with celiac disease (10,11).

Environmental Factors

Epidemiological studies suggest that breastfeeding may offer protective properties that prevent celiac disease development in infants (12). The timing of introducing gluten into an infant's diet also seems to play an important role. Data suggest that the most beneficial timing for introducing gluten into the diet to render protection from celiac disease development is between ages 4 and 6 months (13).

Clinical Manifestations

There is a wide range of intestinal tract symptoms and extra-intestinal manifestations along the expansive clinical spectrum of celiac disease. Mistaken diagnoses of irritable bowel syndrome (IBS) are common in celiac disease patients reporting vague GI symptoms; for that reason, ruling out celiac disease in patients who have been diagnosed with IBS is crucial (6). See Chapter 9 for more information on IBS.

Based on the presence or absence of symptoms, celiac disease can be classified into the following clinical subtypes:

- *Symptomatic/classic:* For patients with "symptomatic" or "classic" celiac disease, manifestations of the illness include chronic diarrhea, abdominal distension and pain, weakness, and occasional malabsorption marked by steatorrhea, weight loss, failure to thrive, bloating, flatulence, and a range of nutrient and mineral deficiency states.

- *Atypical:* "Atypical" celiac disease—which is being diagnosed more frequently—presents with extra-intestinal manifestations, including anemia, osteoporosis, short stature, infertility and neurological deficits (14). Box 10.1 lists some of the associated disorders of celiac disease.
- *Latent/silent:* None of the classic or atypical symptoms are experienced by patients diagnosed with "latent," or "silent," celiac disease. In these cases, the disease is inadvertently detected during endoscopy or serologic studies for unrelated health care purposes.

Hematologic Manifestations

Because involvement of the proximal duodenum (the primary site for dietary iron absorption) is nearly universal in persons with celiac disease, iron-deficiency anemia is common among this patient population. Occult bleeding may occur in 40% to 50% of celiac disease patients (15). Vitamin B-12 deficiency may also play a role when anemia develops in patients with celiac disease (16). Following a strict gluten-free diet typically addresses these nutrient deficiencies.

Dermatologic Manifestations

Patients with celiac disease are at increased risk for dermatitis herpetiformis, an extremely pruritic bullous skin lesion that is closely associated with celiac disease. The rash is usually present on the extensor surfaces of the major joints—including elbows and knees—as well as back and buttocks (17). Among the patients who develop dermatitis herpetiformis, 90% will not experience GI symptoms. Dapsone may help as therapy; however, the mainstay of treatment is strict avoidance of gluten.

BOX 10.1   Disorders Associated with Celiac Disease

Endocrine
- Type 1 diabetes mellitus
- Autoimmune thyroid disorders
- Addison's disease
- Reproductive disorders
- Alopecia aereata

Neurologic
- Cerebellar ataxia
- Neuropathy
- Epilepsy
- Migraine

Cardiac
- Idiopathic dilated cardiomyopathy
- Autoimmune myocarditis

Hepatic
- Primary biliary cirrhosis
- Autoimmune hepatitis
- Autoimmune cholangitis

Other
- Iron-deficiency anemia
- Osteoporosis
- IgA deficiency
- Intestinal lymphoma
- Autoimmune atrophic gastritis
- Sjögren's syndrome
- Turner syndrome
- Down syndrome
- Dental enamel defects
- Recurrent aphthous
- Psoriasis
- Stomatitis

Neurologic Manifestations

It is believed that 6% to 10% of celiac disease patients will develop neurologic complications, such as peripheral neuropathy and cerebellar ataxia (18). Although epilepsy, myelopathy, myopathy, dementia, and psychiatric illness have been reported in patients with celiac disease, incidence of these conditions is rare (19).

Hepatic Manifestations

Hepatic involvement—ranging from mild asymptomatic elevation in serum transaminases to severe liver failure—may occur in patients with celiac disease. Among those with diagnosed sprue, a rise in amino-transferases may be observed in approximately 15% to 55%; conversely, approximately 10% of patients with unexplained increases in transaminases have celiac disease (20). These elevations reverse on a strict gluten-free diet.

Bone Disease

Patients with celiac disease are predisposed to developing bone disease as evidenced by an increase in osteopenia/osteoporosis, bone deformities, bone pain, and fractures (21). The causes of bone disease are multifactorial and include calcium and vitamin D deficiency, due to diseased small intestinal mucosal lining, preventing adequate absorption; precipitation of ingested calcium with unabsorbed intraluminal fats that are excreted in the stool; and elevated bone turnover, in an effort to preserve a positive calcium balance.

Endocrine Disorders

Type 1 diabetes and autoimmune thyroid disease, which are observed in 5% to 10% of patients with celiac disease, represent the most common comorbid endocrine disorders in this patient population (22).

Infertility

Reduced fertility is common among both men and women with celiac disease. Women with celiac disease also have substantially higher rates of miscarriage, stillbirth, perinatal deaths, and intrauterine growth retardation (23–25). Risks for some of these events are lowered when patients follow a gluten-free diet (23).

Diagnosis

Celiac disease is often difficult to diagnose due to its wide range of clinical symptoms and presentations.

Serologic Testing

Serological studies (see Table 10.1) are the initial steps in evaluating patients with symptoms indicative of celiac disease (26); screen those whose laboratory tests reveal abnormalities that could be attributed to malabsorption (eg, folate or iron deficiency) and individuals at high risk (eg, first-degree relatives with celiac disease, type 1 diabetes, Down syndrome, Turner syndrome, and other associated conditions) who may or may not have celiac disease symptoms (27,28).

TABLE 10.1 Serum Tests for the Diagnosis of Celiac Disease

Test	Sensitivity (Range)	Specificity (Range)	Comments
IgA anti-TTG antibodies	>95.0% (73.9%–100%)	>95.0% (77.8%–100%)	Recommended as first-level screening test
IgG anti-TTG antibodies	Widely variable (12.6%–99.3%)	Widely variable (86.3%–100%)	Useful in patients with IgA deficiency
IgA aniendomysial antibodies	>90% (82.6%–100%)	98.2% (94.7%–100%)	Useful in patients with an uncertain diagnosis
IgG DGP	>90.0% (80.1%–98.6%)	>90.0% (86.0%–96.9%)	Useful in patients with IgA deficiency and in young children
HLA-DQ2 or HLA-DQ8	91.0% (82.6%–97.0%)	54.0% (12.0%–68.0%)	High negative predictive value

Abbreviations: DGP, deamidated gliadin peptides; HLA, human leukocyte antigen; IG, immunoglobulin; TTG, tissue transglutaminase.
Source: Reprinted from reference 26: Fasano A, Catassi C. Celiac disease. *N Engl J Med.* 2012;367(25):2419–2426. Copyright © 2012 Massachusetts Medical Society. Reprinted with permission from Massachusetts Medical Society.

The antigliadin antibodies (IgA and IgG) have sensitivity and specificity between 80% and 90%. Due to a positive predictive value of less than 30% in most populations, these antibodies are no longer recommended to diagnose celiac disease (28–30).

More recently, antibodies to deamidated gliadin peptide (DGP), the product of gliadin deamidation via intestinal transglutaminase, have been developed. The combined sensitivity and specificity for IgA and IgG anti-DGP are greater than 80% and greater than 95%, respectively (31). Although anti-DPG performs well, TTG antibody outperforms it and remains the preferred serological test for the diagnosis and/or exclusion of celiac disease.

Anti-endomysial IgA antibody (anti-EMA) is based on indirect immunofluorescence, requiring either monkey esophagus or human umbilical cord tissue as a substrate, and uses TTG as the target antigen. Although its sensitivity is greater than 90% and its specificity is 97% to 100%, anti-EMA is not considered the best test for diagnosing celiac disease because it is very costly, time-consuming, and operator-dependent with high interobserver and intersite variability (26,31,32).

Testing for IgA anti-TTG is currently the initial serological test of choice in patients suspected of having celiac disease because it is much cheaper, faster, and less-operator dependent as compared to anti-EMA testing. In addition, the high sensitivity and specificity of IgA anti-TTG compare well with that of anti-EMA (26,31).

IgG anti-TTG is also available. However, its diagnostic utility is limited by the wide variation in sensitivity and specificity, so it is reserved for use in patients with selective IgA deficiency (26).

Titers of endomysial and transglutaminase antibodies correlate with the degree of mucosal damage. Therefore, false-negative serologies could be seen in the presence of partial villous atrophy or in patients who have already started on a gluten-free diet.

Detection of selective IgA deficiency is 10 times more likely in the celiac disease patient population than in the normal population. Because IgA-derived antibodies would yield a false-negative result in this context, screening these individuals using IgG-based antibodies—such as IgG anti-gliadin or the preferred antibodies IgG anti-DGP and IgG anti-TTG—is necessary (27,31,33).

Upper Endoscopy and Histological Assessment

Serological testing has high sensitivity and specificity for the diagnosis of celiac disease, is readily available, and carries minimal risk, but upper endoscopy with biopsy of the small intestine remains the gold standard for the diagnosis of celiac disease (27,28,34). It is recommended that four to six biopsies of the proximal small bowel be taken because of the patchy nature of the disease (35,36). Duodenal bulb biopsies should be part of the specimen collection since a number of studies have shown that duodenal bulb biopsies can sometimes be the only evidence of villous atrophy (37,38).

Biopsy should always be performed in patients who test positive for a serological marker for celiac disease (34). However, a recent guideline put forth by the European Society for Pediatric Gastroenterology, Hepatology and Nutrition (ESPGHAN) recommended that an intestinal biopsy is not necessary to make the diagnosis of celiac disease in children who have all of the following clinical characteristics: symptoms suggestive of celiac disease, an IgA anti-TTG antibody level greater than 10 times the upper limit of normal, and a positive HLA haplotype (39). Nevertheless, asymptomatic children at high risk for celiac disease still need both positive serology and histological findings on duodenal biopsy to be properly diagnosed. Validation of ESPGHAN recommendations with prospective data in adults and children is lacking, and it is therefore unclear whether these guidelines proposed by ESPGHAN will be widely incorporated into the diagnostic scheme of celiac disease in Europe and North America. Patients with signs and symptoms that are suspicious for celiac disease (although markers for celiac disease may be negative) should also undergo intestinal biopsy, since approximately 10% of patients with celiac disease may have negative markers (31).

Scalloping of mucosal folds, absent or decreased duodenal folds, and fissures or a mosaic pattern of the mucosa are among the classic endoscopic findings in celiac patients (40). These manifestations are not always detected; therefore, the clinician should obtain biopsies if there is strong clinical suspicion that celiac disease is present (41). Conversely, the endoscopic findings related to celiac disease may also be detected in patients with other diseases (42).

Partial or total villous atrophy, elongation of crypts, a decreased villous-to-crypt ratio, and elevated intraepithelial lymphocytes are among the histological changes typical in patients with celiac disease. Poorly oriented biopsy specimens may appear like villous atrophy, which results in a high likelihood of a false-positive diagnosis, whereas false-negative determinations may result when there is a lack of adequate biopsies. However, villous atrophy is not unique to celiac disease (see Box 10.2), and diagnosis cannot be confirmed until the patient favorably responds to a gluten-free diet.

BOX 10.2   Differential Diagnoses of Villous Atrophy

- Celiac disease
- Giardiasis
- Collagenous sprue
- Common-variable immunodeficiency
- Autoimmune enteropathy
- Radiation enteritis
- Whipple's disease
- Tuberculosis
- Tropical sprue

- Eosinophilic gastroenteritis
- Human immunodeficiency virus enteropathy
- Intestinal lymphoma
- Zollinger-Ellison syndrome
- Crohn's disease
- Intolerance of foods other than gluten (eg, milk, soy, chicken, tuna)

Genetic Testing

As noted previously, among patients with celiac disease, 95% are HLA-DQ2 positive and most of the remaining 5% are HLA-DQ8 positive (8). Because virtually all patients diagnosed with celiac disease will have one of these two alleles, diagnosis is effectively excluded when these alleles are not present. For that reason, when other tests cannot confirm diagnosis, HLA testing could be a useful diagnostic tool. It may also be useful in testing patients who are already following a gluten-free diet, since the presence or absence of the haplotypes does not depend on gluten exposure.

It is important to note that approximately 40% of the US population is positive for either of these haplotypes. Therefore, genetic testing would generate many false-positive results and is not indicated in most initial evaluations of celiac disease (27).

Complications

Malignancy

Compared with the general population, patients with celiac disease have a substantially higher rate of malignancy(43,44) including non-Hodgkin's intestinal or extra-intestinal lymphomas (both B- and T-cell); esophageal adenocarcinoma; and cancers of the small intestine, colon, hepatobiliary system, and pancreas (43,45). If a patient with celiac disease has sudden onset of clinical relapse of symptoms after many successful years following a gluten-free diet, enteropathy-associated T-cell lymphoma may be the cause.

Refractory Celiac Disease

Refractory celiac disease is defined by the presence of symptoms—namely, diarrhea, weight loss, malabsorption, abdominal pain, bleeding, or anemia—in a patient with definitive celiac disease diagnosis who has been strictly following the gluten-free diet. Corticosteroids or other immunosuppressive medications may be necessary to induce clinical remission.

Treatment

Elimination of Gluten from Diet

The mainstay of treatment for celiac disease is lifelong elimination of the following:

- Wheat (including all types, such as spelt, einkorn, emmer, kamut, and durum)
- Rye
- Barley
- Triticale (a hybrid grain made from wheat and rye)
- Ingredients derived from the grains included in this list unless they have been processed to remove gluten

Oats do not naturally contain gluten, but they may be contaminated with gluten-containing grains. Therefore, patients are usually advised to avoid consuming oats unless they are labeled gluten-free (46,47).

Clinical improvement in patients with celiac disease is possible within days to weeks of initiating the gluten-free diet. In the case of repairing histological manifestations, however, it could take months to years to see any change. Even with stringent adherence to a gluten-free diet, some patients may achieve incomplete mucosal recovery (48).

No improvement in clinical or histological manifestations of celiac disease is possible in as many as 7% to 30% of patients who follow a gluten-free diet. The first step in this scenario is to reassess the initial diagnosis. As noted previously in this chapter, absence of the DQ2 and DQ8 alleles essentially rules out celiac disease diagnosis, so HLA-typing could be a beneficial assessment in this situation. The second step would be to consult the patient to determine the true level of dietary compliance. If a patient following the gluten-free diet for more than a year has persistent endomysial or tissue transglutaminase antibodies, this finding indicates exposure to gluten. Figure 10.3 shows diagnoses to consider if there is clinical certainty that a diagnosis of celiac disease is correct and the patient has not been ingesting gluten.

Screening for Bone Disease

Because of its high prevalence in the celiac disease patient population, patients should be screened for osteoporosis during the initial evaluation (49).

Treatment of Nutritional Deficiencies

Malabsorption of iron, folate, calcium, fat-soluble vitamins (A, D, E, and K), vitamins B-12 and B-6, zinc, and copper is linked to untreated celiac disease (50–52). Therefore, when the patient receives an initial diagnosis of celiac disease, he or she should be assessed for nutritional deficiencies.

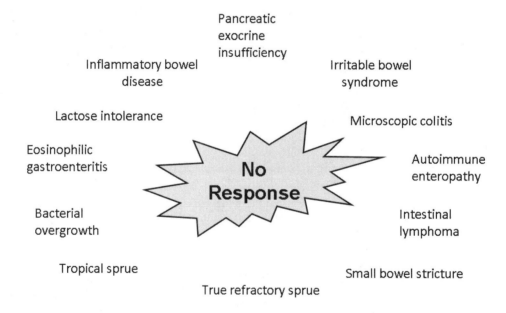

FIGURE 10.3   Nonresponders to the gluten-free diet. Differential diagnoses are wide for nonresponders to a gluten-free diet and include small intestine bacterial overgrowth, lactose intolerance, microscopic colitis, pancreatic insufficiency, inflammatory bowel disease, ulcerative jejunoileitis, collagenous sprue, and T-cell lymphoma, among others. These conditions must be excluded prior to making a diagnosis of refractory sprue in a celiac patient who presents with refractory symptoms despite a strict gluten-free diet.

Nutritional deficiencies can also be related to the gluten-free diet itself (see Table 10.2), because thiamin, riboflavin, niacin, folate, and iron are not found in many of the gluten-free grains (see Table 10.3) (53). Some patients on the gluten-free diet may require supplementation with a gluten-free multivitamin.

The Role of the Registered Dietitian

In 2010, the American Dietetic Association (now called the Academy of Nutrition and Dietetics) published the Celiac Disease Evidence-Based Nutrition Practice Guideline (54), which emphasizes the integral role of the registered dietitian (RD) in the care of patients with celiac disease. Refer to Box 10.3 for the recommendations in these guidelines. Resources that may help RDs apply the guidelines in practice include the companion *Celiac Disease Toolkit* (55) and the *Pocket Guide to Gluten-Free Strategies for Clients with Multiple Diet Restrictions* (53).

TABLE 10.2 Potential Nutritional Consequences of a Gluten-free Diet

Potential Consequence	*Contributing Factors*
↑ Fat	Decreased intake of grain food servings Foods high in fat are substituted for grain foods Gluten-free grain foods are often higher in fat compared to similar gluten-containing products (manufacturers may add "extra" fat to improve texture and mouth feel of food)
↓ Carbohydrate	Decreased intake of grain food servings Historically, poor palatability of grain foods, especially some bread products Gluten-free grain foods can be expensive
↓ Fiber	Low overall intake of carbohydrates, especially whole grain carbohydrates Overuse of refined grains and starches by manufacturers of gluten-free grain foods, such as breakfast cereal, pasta, and bread products
↓ Calcium	Decreased intake of milk-based products due to secondary lactose intolerance (usually a temporary condition that resolves as the intestine heals)
↓ Iron	Low overall intake of grain foods Low intake of gluten-free whole grains Lack of iron enrichment and fortification of gluten-free grain foods, such as bread products, pastas, and breakfast cereals
↓ Folate	Low overall intake of grain foods Low intake of gluten-free whole grains Lack of folic acid enrichment and fortification of gluten-free grain foods, such as bread products, pastas, and breakfast cereals
↓ Niacin	Low overall intake of grain foods Low intake of gluten-free whole grains Lack of niacin enrichment and fortification of gluten-free grain foods, such as bread products, pastas, and breakfast cereals
↓ Vitamin B-12	Decreased intake of milk-based products due to secondary lactose intolerance Lack of vitamin and mineral fortification (including vitamin B-12) of most gluten-free breakfast cereals
↓ Phosphorus	Decreased intake of milk-based products due to secondary lactose intolerance
↓ Zinc	Low overall intake of grain foods Low intake of gluten-free whole grains

Key: ↑: increased dietary intake of particular nutrient; ↓: decreased dietary intake of particular nutrient.
Source: Reprinted with permission from reference 53: Thompson T. *ADA Pocket Guide to Gluten-Free Strategies for Clients with Multiple Diet Restrictions.* Chicago, IL: American Dietetic Association; 2011.

TABLE 10.3 Nutrient Content of Selected Gluten-Free Grains

Grain	Fiber, g/oz	Iron, mg/oz	Thiamin, mg/oz	Riboflavin, mg/oz	Niacin, mg/oz	Folate, DFE/oz	Zinc, mg/oz
Amaranth	1.9	2.16	0.03	0.06	0.26	23	0.81
Brown rice	1.0	0.42	0.11	0.03	1.44	6	0.57
Buckwheat groats	2.9	0.70	0.06	0.08	1.46	12	0.69
Millet	2.4	0.85	0.12	0.08	1.34	24	0.48
Oats	3.0	1.34	0.22	0.04	0.27	16	1.13
Quinoa	2.0	1.30	0.10	0.09	0.43	52	0.88
Teff	2.3	2.16	0.11	0.08	0.95	n/a	1.03
White rice	0.4	0.23	0.02	0.01	0.45	2	0.31
White rice, enriched	0.4	0.81–1.63	0.13–0.25	0.08–0.15	1.00–2.00	110	0.31
Wild rice	1.8	0.56	0.03	0.07	1.91	27	1.69

Source: Reprinted with permission from reference 53: Thompson T. *ADA Pocket Guide to Gluten-Free Strategies for Clients with Multiple Diet Restrictions*. Chicago, IL: American Dietetic Association; 2011.

Selected Topics for Nutrition Education

When faced with the need to eliminate gluten from their diets, patients may be encouraged to learn there are many foods that they *can* eat. RDs should emphasize the variety of gluten-free choices available and assist patients in learning label-reading skills that will allow them to avoid gluten while selecting nutritious foods.

Alternatives to Gluten-Containing Ingredients

Grains that are permissible in the gluten-free diet include the following:

- Buckwheat
- Corn
- Millet
- Montina
- Oats (if labeled gluten-free)
- Quinoa
- Rice
- Sorghum
- Teff
- Wild rice

Additional sources of gluten-free starches that are useful as alternatives to flour include the following:

- Tubers: arrowroot, jicama, taro, potato, tapioca (cassava, manioc, yucca)
- Legumes: chickpeas, lentils, kidney beans, navy beans, pea beans, peanuts, soybeans
- Nuts: almonds, walnuts, chestnuts, hazelnuts, cashews
- Seeds: sunflower, flax, pumpkin

When teaching patients about these foods, RDs may wish to emphasize choices that are higher in fiber and/or enriched or fortified (53).

BOX 10.3   Recommendations from the Celiac Disease Evidence-Based Nutrition Practice Guideline

Screening and Referral

Medical Nutrition Therapy. Medical nutrition therapy (MNT) provided by a registered dietitian (RD) is strongly recommended for individuals with celiac disease. Consultation with an RD as part of a team-based approach results in improved self-management. (Consensus. Imperative.)

Nutrition Assessment

1. *Assessment of Food/Nutrition-Related History.* The RD should assess the food and nutrition-related history of individuals with celiac disease, including (but not limited to) the following:
   - Food and nutrient intake (eg, diet history, diet experience and macronutrient or micronutrient intake, specifically calcium, iron, vitamin B complex and vitamin D)
   - Medication and herbal supplement use
   - Knowledge, beliefs or attitudes (eg, readiness to change nutrition-related behaviors)
   - Behavior (eg, social network)
   - Factors affecting access to food and food and nutrition-related supplies (eg, safe food and meal availability)

   Assessment of the above factors is needed to effectively determine nutrition diagnoses and plan the nutrition intervention. Intake of gluten results may result in gastrointestinal symptoms, malabsorption and villous atrophy. (Strong. Imperative.)

2. *Assess Biochemical Data and Results of Medical Procedures.* The RD should assess the biochemical data and review the results of medical procedures in individuals with celiac disease, regardless of presentation and clinical symptoms, including (but not limited to) the following:
   - Gastrointestinal profile [eg, intestinal biopsy (or skin biopsy in the case of dermatitis herpetiformis) and celiac antibodies]
   - Nutritional anemia profile (eg, folate, ferritin and vitamin B-12)
   - Vitamin profile (eg, thiamin, vitamin B-6 and 25-hydroxy vitamin D)
   - Mineral profile (eg, copper and zinc)
   - Lipid profile
   - Electrolyte and renal profile

   Untreated celiac disease results in villous atrophy and malabsorption. The use of effective techniques to assess nutritional status is essential to prevention and treatment of malnutrition and the presence of iron deficiency anemia. (Strong. Imperative.)

3. *Bone Density Screening.* The RD should recommend bone density screening for adults with celiac disease within the first year. Clinical trials and cross-sectional studies have reported reduced bone mineral content and bone mineral density in untreated adults with celiac disease. (Strong. Conditional.)

4. *Assess Factors Affecting Quality of Life.* The RD should assess the factors affecting the quality of life of individuals with celiac disease when completing a comprehensive client history, which includes a medical history (eg, gastrointestinal, immune, neurological and psychological) and social history (eg, socioeconomic factors, religion, social and medical support and daily stress level). Individuals with celiac disease may not attain the same level of quality of life as the general population, due to social inconveniences of following a gluten-free dietary pattern. (Strong. Imperative.)

Continues

BOX 10.3   Recommendations from the Celiac Disease Evidence-Based Nutrition Practice Guideline (Continued)

5. *Assess Gastrointestinal Symptoms.* The RD should assess gastrointestinal symptoms (such as type, frequency and volume of bowel function; abdominal pain and bloating; nausea or vomiting; reduced gut motility and delayed gastric emptying) in individuals with celiac disease. Several studies have reported that people with celiac disease (treated and untreated) are more likely to experience gastrointestinal symptoms than are healthy control subjects. (Strong. Imperative.)

6. *Assessment of Other Disease States.* The RD should assess for the presence of other disease states, such as thyroid conditions, other autoimmune and endocrinologic disorders and diabetes, when implementing MNT. Identification of all nutritional issues is optimal to integrate MNT for individuals with celiac disease into overall disease management. (Consensus. Imperative.)

Nutrition Intervention

1. *Gluten-Free Dietary Pattern.* The RD should advise and educate individuals with celiac disease to be compliant with a gluten-free dietary pattern. Research on individuals with celiac disease reports that long-term compliance with a gluten-free dietary pattern improves outcomes related to bone density, iron deficiency anemia, villous atrophy, gastrointestinal and neurological symptoms, pregnancy outcomes and quality of life. (Strong. Imperative.)

2. *Consumption of Whole/Enriched Gluten-Free Grains and Products.* The RD should advise individuals with celiac disease to consume whole or enriched gluten-free grains and products such as brown rice, wild rice, buckwheat, quinoa, amaranth, millet, sorghum, teff, etc. Research reports that adherence to the gluten-free dietary pattern may result in a diet that is low in carbohydrates, iron, folate, niacin, zinc and fiber. (Strong. Imperative.)

3. *Addition of Multivitamin and Mineral Supplement.* If usual food intake shows nutritional inadequacies that cannot be alleviated through improved eating habits, the RD should advise individuals with celiac disease to consume a daily gluten-free age- and sex-specific multivitamin and mineral supplement. Research reports that adherence to the gluten-free dietary pattern may result in a diet that is low in iron, folate, niacin, vitamin B-12, calcium, phosphorus and zinc. (Strong. Conditional.)

4. *Inclusion of Gluten-Free Oats as Tolerated.* The RD should advise individuals with celiac disease who enjoy and can tolerate gluten-free oats to gradually include them in their gluten-free dietary pattern. Research on individuals with celiac disease reports that incorporating oats uncontaminated with wheat, barley or rye at intake levels of approximately 50 g dry oats per day is generally safe and improves compliance with the gluten-free dietary pattern. (Fair. Conditional.)

5. *Calcium/Vitamin D for Reduced Bone Density.* For adults with reduced bone density or reduced serum levels of 25-hydroxyvitamin D, the RD should advise the consumption of additional calcium and vitamin D through food or gluten-free supplements. Studies in adults with untreated celiac disease have shown that a gluten-free dietary pattern improves, but may not normalize bone mineral density. (Strong. Conditional.)

6. *Iron Supplementation for Iron Deficiency Anemia.* For individuals with iron deficiency anemia and celiac disease, the RD should advise the consumption of a daily gluten-free multivitamin with iron or additional individualized therapeutic doses of iron. Studies report that iron supplementation may be necessary to achieve normal values of hematological parameters. (Strong. Conditional.)

Continues

BOX 10.3   Recommendations from the Celiac Disease Evidence-Based Nutrition Practice Guideline *(Continued)*

7. *Provide Resources and Education on Label Reading.* The RD should provide resources and educate individuals with celiac disease about reviewing the ingredients on labels of food and supplements, using current publications, including those from the US Food and Drug Administration, for identification and avoidance of sources of gluten, namely wheat, rye, barley, malt and oats (unless oats are gluten-free). Education about the disease is optimal to integrate MNT for individuals with celiac disease into overall disease management. (Consensus. Imperative.)

8. *Coordination of Care.* The RD should implement MNT and coordinate nutrition care with a team of clinical professionals. Depending on the coexisting conditions of the individual with celiac disease, consultation with gastroenterologists, endocrinologists, allergists, dermatologists, hepatologists, pharmacists, social workers, etc., may be warranted. An interdisciplinary team approach is optimal to integrate MNT for individuals with celiac disease into overall disease management. (Consensus. Imperative.)

9. *Education on Food Cross-Contamination.* The RD should educate individuals with celiac disease regarding cross-contamination in gluten-free food preparation within manufacturing plants, restaurants and home kitchens. Education about the disease is optimal to integrate MNT for individuals with celiac disease into overall disease management. (Consensus. Imperative).

Nutrition Monitoring and Evaluation

1. *Monitoring and Evaluation of Dietary Compliance.* The RD should monitor the following to evaluate dietary compliance: (Strong. Imperative.)
   - Gluten-free dietary pattern
   - Antibody levels
   - Potential exposure to cross-contamination
   - Hidden sources of gluten in foods, medications and supplements.
   - Intake of gluten may result in gastrointestinal symptoms, malabsorption and villous atrophy.

2. *Monitoring and Evaluation of Factors Affecting Quality of Life.* The RD, at every encounter, should monitor and evaluate the factors affecting the quality of life of individuals with celiac disease, reviewing changes in client status, which includes medical status (eg, gastrointestinal, immune, neurological and psychological) and social status (eg, socioeconomic factors, religion, social and medical support and daily stress level). Individuals with celiac disease may not attain the same level of quality of life as the general population, due to social inconveniences of following a gluten-free dietary pattern. (Strong. Imperative.)

3. *Monitoring and Evaluation of Gastrointestinal Symptoms.* The RD, after ruling out gluten exposure, should monitor and evaluate persistent gastrointestinal symptoms in individuals with celiac disease, such as bloating, gas, constipation and diarrhea, as there may be other potential causes, such as leaky gut, lactose, fructose and carbohydrate intolerances, bacterial overgrowth, refractory sprue, related cancers, and other gastrointestinal diseases and conditions. Several studies have reported that people with celiac disease (treated and untreated) are more likely to experience gastrointestinal symptoms than healthy controls; compliance with a gluten-free diet reduces but may not eliminate these symptoms. (Fair. Imperative.)

Source: Adapted with permission from reference 54: Celiac Disease Evidence-Based Nutrition Practice Guideline. Academy of Nutrition and Dietetics Evidence Analysis Library. 2010. http://and evidencelibrary.com.

Label Reading

To improve the nutritional adequacy of their gluten-free diet, patients may benefit from general education about using the Nutrition Facts panel in making food choices. In addition, the RD should focus on teaching patients label-reading skills that help them avoid gluten-containing ingredients (55).

FOOD ALLERGEN LABELING

Wheat is considered a major food allergen under the Food Allergen Labeling and Consumer Protection Act of 2004 (FALCPA). When any ingredient in a food contains protein from wheat, the manufacturer is obligated to clearly indicate this fact on the label, either by including wheat in the ingredients list or by providing a "Contains" statement that lists wheat (and any of the other eight major food allergens). Therefore, if a product's ingredients list includes wheat, the patient can know to avoid that food (53,55,56).

However, patients also need to understand that the omission of the word "wheat" does *not* guarantee that the food is gluten-free (53,56).

- Barley and rye are not included as major food allergens covered by FALCPA.
- FALCPA regulates ingredients only; foods could contain wheat through cross contact without this being noted on the ingredients list or "Contains" statement.
- FALCPA is mandatory for only those foods regulated by the US Food and Drug Administration (FDA). Most manufacturers of foods regulated by the US Department of Agriculture (eg, meat products, poultry products, and eggs) comply, but their compliance is not mandatory. The Alcohol and Tobacco Tax and Trade Bureau has proposed rules for the *voluntary* labeling of major allergens in spirits, wine, and malt beverages (57).

GLUTEN-FREE LABELING

In August 2013, the FDA passed a final rule regarding the use of the phrases "gluten-free," "without gluten," "free of gluten," or "no gluten" on food product labels. The rule dictates that any foods listed as "gluten-free" must limit the unavoidable presence of gluten to less than 20 parts per million (ppm). Foods that are labeled gluten-free *cannot* contain any of the following (58):

- An ingredient that is any type of wheat, rye, barley, or crossbreeds of these grains
- An ingredient derived from these grains that has not been processed to remove gluten
- An ingredient derived from these grains that has been processed to remove gluten, if it results in the food containing 20 or more parts per million (ppm) gluten

Avoiding Cross-Contamination

RDs can assist patients by teaching them techniques to avoid cross-contamination of gluten-free foods when grocery shopping, storing and preparing foods, and eating out.

Conclusion

Occurring in nearly 1% of most countries' population, celiac disease is an autoimmune disease incited by gluten, a naturally occurring protein in wheat, rye, and barley. When a patient with celiac disease ingests gluten, it provokes a range of immunological responses in the small intestinal mucosa, which ultimately lead to villous atrophy and crypt hyperplasia, which are typically observed in this patient population.

Treatment for celiac disease is rooted in strict compliance with a lifelong gluten-free diet, and the RD can greatly assist patients in learning about and adhering to this diet.

References

1. West J, Logan RF, Hill PG, et al. Seroprevalence, correlates, and characteristics of undetected coeliac disease in England. *Gut.* 2003;52:960–965.
2. Mäki M, Mustalahti K, Kokkonen J, et al. Prevalence of celiac disease among children in Finland. *N Engl J Med.* 2003;348:2517–2524.
3. Fasano A, Berti I, Gerarduzzi T, et al. Prevalence of celiac disease in at-risk and not-at-risk groups in the United States: a large multicenter study. *Arch Intern Med.* 2003;163:286–292.
4. Bingley PJ, Williams AJ, Norcross AJ, et al. Undiagnosed coeliac disease at age seven: population based prospective birth cohort study. *BMJ.* 2004;328:322–323.
5. Tommasini A, Not T, Kiren V, et al. Mass screening for coeliac disease using antihuman transglutaminase antibody assay. *Arch Dis Child.* 2004;89:512–515.
6. Green PH, Stavropoulos SN, Panagi SG, et al. Characteristics of adult celiac disease in the USA: results of a national survey. *Am J Gastroenterol.* 2001;96:126–131.
7. Logan RF. Screening for celiac disease: has the time come for mass screening? *Acta Paediatra.* 1996;412(Suppl):S15–S19.
8. Green PH, Jabri B. Celiac disease. *Lancet.* 2003;362:383–391.
9. Greco L, et al. The first large population-based twin study of celiac disease. *Gut.* 2002;50:624–628.
10. Green PH, Jabri B. Celiac disease. *Annu Rev Med.* 2006;57:207–221.
11. Green PH, Cellier C. Celiac disease. *N Engl J Med.* 2007;357:1731–1743.
12. Persson LA, Ivarsson A, Hernell O. Breastfeeding protects against celiac disease in childhood: epidemiological evidence. *Adv Exp Med Biol.* 2002;503:115–123.
13. Norris JM, Barriga K, Hoffenberg EJ, et al. Risk of celiac disease autoimmunity and timing of gluten introduction in the diet of infants at increased risk of disease. *JAMA.* 2005;293:2343–2351.
14. Rampertab SD, Pooran N, Brar P, Singh P, Green PH. Trends in the presentation of celiac disease. *Am J Med.* 2006;119(4):e9–e14.
15. Fine KD. The prevalence of occult gastrointestinal bleeding in celiac sprue. *N Engl J Med.* 1996;334:1163–1167.
16. Dahele A, Ghosh S. Vitamin B12 deficiency in untreated celiac disease. *Am J Gastroenterol.* 2001;96:745–750.
17. Karpati S. Dermatitis herpetiformis: close to unraveling a disease. *J Dermatol Sci.* 2004;34:83–90.
18. Chin RL, Sander HW, Brannagan TH, et al. Celiac neuropathy. *Neurology.* 2003;60:1581–1585.
19. Hadjivassiliou M, Gibson A, Davies-Jones GA, et al. Does cryptic gluten sensitivity play a part in neurological illness? *Lancet.* 1996;347:369–371.
20. Abdo A, Meddings J, Swain M. Liver abnormalities in celiac disease. *Clin Gastroenterol Hepatol.* 2004;2:107–112.
21. Moreno ML, Vazquez H, Mazure R, et al. Stratification of bone fracture risk in patients with celiac disease. *Clin Gastroenterol Hepatol.* 2004;2:127–134.
22. Collin P, Kaukinen K, Valimaki M, Salmi J. Endocrinological disorders and celiac disease. *Endocr Rev.* 2004;23:464–483.
23. Ciacci C, Cirillo M, Auriemma G, et al. Celiac disease and pregnancy outcome. *Am J Gastroenterol.* 1996;91:718–722.
24. Gasbarrini A, Sanz Torre E, Trivellini C, et al. Recurrent spontaneous abortion and intrauterine fetal growth retardation as symptoms of celiac disease. *Lancet.* 2000;256:399–400.
25. Tata LJ, Card TR, Logan RF, et al. Fertility and pregnancy-related events in women with celiac disease: a population based cohort study. *Gastroenterology.* 2005;128:849–855.

26. Fasano A, Catassi C. Celiac disease. *N Engl J Med.* 2012;367(25):2419–2426.

27. Rostom A, Murry JA, Kagnoff MF. American Gastroenterological Association (AGA) Institute technical review on the diagnosis and management of celiac disease. *Gastroenterology.* 2006;131(6):1981–2002.

28. Lebwohl B, Rubio-Tapia A, Assiri A, Newland C, Guandalini S. Diagnosis of celiac disease. *Gastrointest Endosc Clin N Am.* 2012;22(4):661–677.

29. Rostom A, Dubé C, Cranney A, et al. The diagnostic accuracy of serologic tests for celiac disease: a systematic review. *Gastroenterology.* 2005;128(Suppl 1):S38–S46.

30. Hill ID. What are the sensitivity and specificity of serologic tests for celiac disease? Do sensitivity and specificity vary in different populations? *Gastroenterology.* 2005;128(4 Suppl 1):S25–S32.

31. Leffler DA, Schuppan D. Update on serological testing in celiac disease. *Am J Gastroenterol.* 2010;105(12):2520–25244.

32. Rostami K, Kerckhaert J, Tiemessen R, von Blomberg BM, Meijer JW, Mulder CJ. Sensitivity of antiendomysium and antigliadin antibodies in untreated celiac disease: disappointing in clinical practice. *Am J Gastroenterol.* 1999;94(4):888–894.

33. Dahlbom I, Olsson M, Forooz NK, Sjöholm AG, Truedsson L, Hansson T. Immunoglobulin G (IgG) anti-tissue transglutaminase antibodies used as markers for IgA-deficient celiac disease patients. *Clin Diagn Lab Immunol.* 2005;12(2):254–258.

34. Rubio-Tapia A, Hill ID, Kelly CP, et al. ACG clinical guidelines: diagnosis and management of celiac disease. *Am J Gastroenterol.* 2013;108:656–676.

35. Bonamico M, Mariani P, Thanasi E, et al. Patchy villous atrophy of the duodenum in childhood celiac disease. *J Pediatr Gastroenterol Nutr.* 2004;38:204–207.

36. Ravelli A, Bolognini S, Gambarotti M, Villanacci V. Variability of histologic lesions in relation to biopsy site in gluten sensitive enteropathy. *Am J Gastroenterol.* 2005;100:177–185.

37. Evans KE, Aziz I, Cross SS, et al. A prospective study of duodenal bulb biopsy in newly diagnosed and established adult celiac disease. *Am J Gastroenterol.* 2011;106(10):1837–1842.

38. Gonzalez S, Gupta A, Chang J, et al. Prospective study of the role of duodenal bulb biopsies in the diagnosis of celiac disease. *Gastrointest Endosc.* 2010;72(4):758–765.

39. Husby S, Koletzko S, Korponay-Szabó IR, et al. European Society for Pediatric Gastroenterology, Hepatology, and Nutrition guidelines for the diagnosis of coeliac disease. *J Pediatr Gastroenterol Nutr.* 2012;54(1):136–160.

40. Lee SK, Green PH. Endoscopy in celiac disease. *Curr Opin Gastroenterol.* 2005;21:589–594.

41. Oxentenko AS, Grisolano SW, Murray JA, et al. The insensitivity of endoscopic markers in celiac disease. *Am J Gastroenterol.* 2002;97:933–938.

42. Shah VH, Rotterdam H, Kotler DP, Fasano A, Green PH. All that scallops is not celiac disease. *Gastrointest Endosc.* 2000;51:6:717–720.

43. Askling J, Linet M, Gridley G, et al. Cancer incidence in a population-based cohort of individuals hospitalized with celiac disease or dermatitis herpetiformis. *Gastroenterology.* 2002;123:1428–1435.

44. Rampertab SD, Forde KA, Green PH. Small bowel neoplasia in coeliac disease. *Gut.* 2003;52:1211–1214.

45. Smedby KE, Akerman M, Hildebrand H, et al. Malignant lymphomas in coeliac disease: evidence of increased risks for lymphoma types other than enteropathy-type T cell lymphoma. *Gut.* 2005;54:54–59.

46. Thompson T. Oats and the gluten-free diet. *J Am Diet Assoc.* 2003;103:376–379.

47. Peräaho M, Kaukinen K, Mustalahti K, et al. Effect of an oats-containing gluten-free diet on symptoms and quality of life in coeliac disease: a randomized study. *Scand J Gastroenterol.* 2004;39:27–31.

48. Haines ML, Anderson RP, Gibson PR. Systematic review: the evidence base for long-term management of celiac disease. *Aliment Pharmacol Ther.* 2008;28(9):1042–1066.

49. Barton SH, Kelly DG, Murray JA. Nutritional deficiencies in celiac disease. *Gastroenterol Clin N Am.* 2007;36(1):93–108.

50. Reinken L, Zieglauer H. Vitamin B6 absorption in children with acute celiac disease and in control subjects. *J Nutr.* 1978;108(10):1562–1565.

51. Meyer D, Stavropoulos S, Diamond B, et al. Osteoporosis in a North American adult population with celiac disease. *Am J Gastroenterol.* 2001;96:112–119.

52. Lee SK, Lo W, Memeo L, Rotterdam H, Green PH. Duodenal histology in patients with celiac disease after treatment with a gluten-free diet. *Gastrointest Endosc.* 2003;57:187–191.

53. Thompson T. *ADA Pocket Guide to Gluten-Free Strategies for Clients with Multiple Diet Restrictions.* Chicago, IL: American Dietetic Association; 2011.

54. Celiac Disease Evidence-Based Nutrition Practice Guideline. Academy of Nutrition and Dietetics Evidence Analysis Library. 2010. http://andevidencelibrary.com/topic.cfm?cat=3677. Accessed April 3, 2014.

55. Academy of Nutrition and Dietetics. *Celiac Disease Evidence-Based Practice Toolkit.* Chicago, IL: Academy of Nutrition and Dietetics; 2011.

56. US Food and Drug Administration. Food Allergen Labeling And Consumer Protection Act of 2004 Questions and Answers. December 12, 2005; updated July 18, 2006. www.fda.gov/food/guidanceregulation/guidance documentsregulatoryinformation/allergens/ucm106890.htm. Accessed April 3, 2014.

57. US Department of Treasury Alcohol and Tobacco Tax and Trade Bureau. Major Food Allergen Labeling for Wines, Distilled Spirits, and Malt Beverages. www.ttb.gov/labeling/major_food_allergen_labeling.shtml. Accessed April 4, 2014.

58. US Food and Drug Administration. What Is Gluten? FDA Has an Answer. www.fda.gov/ForConsumers /ConsumerUpdates/ucm363069.htm. Accessed April 4, 2014.

PART III

Nutrition and Liver and Exocrine Disorders

CHAPTER 11

Liver Disease

Dawn McDowell Torres, MD, and
Gerard E. Mullin, MD, CNSP, FACN, AGAF

In 2004, NHANES data indicated that chronic liver disease (CLD) was the 12th leading cause of death in the United States (1). The prevalence of CLD varied between 15% and 30% for different ethnicities, with higher rates seen in Hispanic and nonwhite populations (1). However, Asrani et al have recently suggested that these data underestimate liver-related mortality, and US rates may actually be much higher (2).

The management of patients with CLD will depend on the underlying etiology. In particular, treatment for patients with nonalcoholic fatty liver disease (NAFLD) is distinct from treatment of all other CLDs. Patients with cirrhosis, liver transplantation, or acute liver failure require specific types of nutrition care.

Nutrition Assessment of CLD Patients

When assessing nutritional status in patients with CLD disease, keep in mind the following points (3,4):

- Due to interference from fluid overload, body mass index (BMI) and weight may not be helpful indicators of nutritional status.
- Plasma protein and prealbumin data can be misleading due to edema, but these data can reflect that inadequate liver synthesis is causing malnutrition.
- Anthropometric measurements, such as mid-arm muscle circumference, can be misleading if the patient has edema.
- Handgrip strength is relatively easy to assess and correlates well with outcomes.

Nonalcoholic Fatty Liver Disease

The most common cause of CLD in Western nations is hepatic steatosis; its prevalence in the United States is estimated to be at least 25% (5). Risk factors for NAFLD include obesity, metabolic syndrome, and insulin resistance (IR).

The progressive form of NAFLD is nonalcoholic steatohepatitis (NASH), which affects approximately 25% of all patients with NAFLD (6). These patients are at risk of developing cirrhosis and hepatocellular carcinoma.

Management

Lifestyle modifications, including diet and exercise, seem to be important in management of NAFLD, although an optimal approach has not been established (7,8). Slow gradual weight loss along with increased physical activity seems to be beneficial (9).

Roux-en-Y and laparoscopic banding can also benefit individuals with NAFLD, but these procedures have inherent risks, such as surgical complications, malabsorption, and malnutrition (10). See Chapter 14 for more information on bariatric procedures.

Diabetes medications, including thiazolidinediones, metformin, and incretin mimetics, may be used to treat patients with NAFLD (10). See Table 11.1 for information about the effects of these medications.

Nutrition Care

Nutrition considerations in the management of NAFLD include the following (11):

- Saturated fatty acids (SFAs): Limit SFAs to less than 10% of total energy intake (but maintain some minimal intake).
- Monounsaturated fatty acids (MUFAs): MUFAs such as olive oil, nuts, and avocadoes may be beneficial if they replace carbohydrates and SFAs (11–13).
- Polyunsaturated fatty acids (PUFAs): Replacing omega-6 fatty acids with omega-3 fatty acids as found in fish oil and walnuts improves international normalized ratio (INR), liver enzymes, and hepatic steatosis (14–16).
- Sucrose and fructose: Intake of refined sugars and sweetened drinks lead to de novo synthesis of fatty acids and should be limited in NAFLD patients (17).
- Protein: It is unclear whether high levels of protein intake are beneficial, but moderate amounts of lean protein that are high in omega-3 fatty acids (such as wild salmon) seem to be helpful. Intake of red meat that is high is saturated fat should be limited (18,19).
- Vitamin E: 400 to 800 IU of vitamin E daily seems to be promising for controlling the liver inflammation in NAFLD. The use of long-term, high-dose vitamin E in people without NAFLD has been associated with increased mortality, but the four major studies to date using vitamin E in NASH demonstrate histological improvement with therapy (20).

Cirrhosis and Liver Transplantation

Nutrition-Related Problems

Nutrition-related problems observed in patients with cirrhosis include protein-energy malnutrition, vitamin deficiencies, and osteoporosis. Nutritional deficiencies can affect liver transplant outcomes, morbidity, and mortality. Aggressive management of nutritional status in the pre- and posttransplant populations is imperative.

TABLE 11.1 Diabetes Medications Used to Treat Nonalcoholic Fatty Liver Disease (NAFLD)

Type of Medication	Comments	Adverse Effects
Thiazolidinediones	• Most studied type of diabetes medication used for NAFLD • Show biochemical and histological benefit in NAFLD	• Weight gain • Decreased bone mineral density • Increased triglycerides (rosiglitazone) • Increased rates of cardiovascular events (rosiglitazone) • Complications and exacerbation of congestive heart failure
Metformin	• Biochemical but no histological benefit as monotherapy • Cannot use if creatinine >1.5 mg/dL	• Diarrhea • Lactic acidosis (rarely)
Incretin mimetics	• Studies ongoing but no proven histological benefit	• Nausea • Delayed gastric emptying

MALNUTRITION

Between 20% and 80% of patients with cirrhosis experience malnutrition (21). Factors that contribute to undernutrition in this patient population include the following:

• Nausea and early satiety
• Hypermetabolic state
• Reduced glucose storage (in alcohol-induced cirrhosis)
• Insufficient intake of protein and energy

In prospective studies, 53% of patients awaiting orthotopic liver transplantation (OLT) for CLD were malnourished. Presence of malnutrition was the only independent risk factor associated with length of stay in intensive care and total number of days in hospital (22,23).

OSTEOPOROSIS

The pathophysiology of osteoporosis in CLD is not well understood, but the prevalence of osteoporosis in patients with cirrhosis is between 12% and 55% (24). Risk factors for osteoporosis in patients with cirrhosis include the following:

• Vitamin K deficiency
• Vitamin D deficiency (found in two-thirds of patients with cirrhosis) (24)
• Excess alcohol intake
• Hypogonadism/reduced serum testosterone levels
• Corticosteroids

The prevalence of osteoporosis in patients after liver transplantation is 15% to 27%. Osteoporosis will typically be seen in the first 2 years after transplant, and its risk is related to corticosteroid use (24).

Osteoporosis is also seen in patients with noncirrhotic biliary disease (primary sclerosing cholangitis [PSC] and primary biliary cirrhosis [PBC]), hemochromatosis, and excessive alcohol intake in the absence of cirrhosis (25).

Guidelines for the treatment for osteoporosis in patients with CLD include the following (25,26):

- One gram of calcium plus 800 IU vitamin D daily (To prevent osteoporosis, the optimal serum level for 25-OH vitamin D in all individuals is 50 ng/mL.)
- Bisphosphonates
- Physical activity
- Vitamin K (if deficient)
- Second-line treatments, such as hormone replacement therapy (raloxifene, testosterone, calcitonin)
- Biannual bone density tests, regardless of whether patient is treated for osteoporosis

MICRONUTRIENT DEFICIENCIES

Deficiency of certain micronutrients can occur in patients with cirrhosis. Table 11.2 identifies selected trace elements that should be monitored in this patient population (25–28).

OTHER NUTRITION-RELATED PROBLEMS FOR CIRRHOSIS PATIENTS

Additional nutrition-related problems for patients with cirrhosis may include edema and ascites, hypoglycemia related to the inability to maintain glycogen stores in the liver, and septicemia caused by *Vibrio vulnificus*. The following points are therefore part of the optimal diet plan for this patient population:

- If the patient has edema/ascites, limit sodium to 2 g/d or 88 mmol/d.
- To maintain stable blood glucose levels, the patient should eat frequent small meals.
- The patient should avoid raw seafood because it may be contaminated with *Vibrio vulnificus*.

Obesity and Liver Transplantation

Outcomes of liver transplant surgery tend to be less favorable for severely/morbidly obese patients than for those with normal BMI. Nair et al have concluded that patients with severe obesity (defined as BMI >32.3 for women and >31.1 for men) who undergo OLT are likely to have higher morbidity, mortality, and costs, and a lower long-term survival rate (29). Patients with BMI more than 40 are not considered transplant candidates at most centers.

Medical Complications and Nutritional Implications of Chronic Liver Disease

Pancreatic Insufficiency

If CLD patients experience pancreatic insufficiency, the goal of steatorrhea treatment is to limit malabsorption of long-chain fatty acids while increasing absorption of short- and medium-chain fatty acids. Pancreatic enzyme supplementation is used.

TABLE 11.2 Micronutrient Deficiencies Associated with Cirrhosis

Potential Deficiency	Notes
Zinc	• Signs and symptoms of deficiency include dysgeusia, dermatitis, testicular atrophy, loss of body hair, night-blindness, poor wound-healing, and decreased neurocognitive performances. • Replacement may be helpful in managing hepatic encephalopathy as well as night-blindness that is not responsive to vitamin A replacement.
Selenium	• Signs and symptoms include cardiomyopathy.
Magnesium	• Signs and symptoms include neuromuscular and cardiac arrhythmias.
Water-soluble vitamins (B complex, vitamin C, thiamin)	• Deficiency is particularly common in alcoholic liver disease.
Fat-soluble vitamins	• Deficiency occurs particularly in cholestatic liver disease such as primary biliary cirrhosis.
Vitamin A (retinol)	• Signs and symptoms of deficiency include night-blindness. • Deficiency of vitamin A is a risk factor for hepatocellular carcinoma and fulminant hepatic failure (ie, ito cell hyperplasia).
Vitamin D	• Deficiency leads to increased bone resorption and decreased bone formation. • Low vitamin D levels occur in two-thirds of patients with cirrhosis and 96% of patients awaiting liver transplant. • Mechanism of deficiency: 25 hydroxylation in liver is impaired in severe chronic liver disease; impaired synthesis of bile acids that are required for micelle formation leads to malabsorption of 25-hydroxy-vitamin D; reduced exposure to ultraviolet light due to inactivity due to chronic disease; dietary insufficiency (anorexia and impaired energy intake are common in CLD); impaired cutaneous synthesis of vitamin D. • Treatment: usually, give 800 IU in conjunction with 1 g calcium daily.
Vitamin E	• Deficiency occurs particularly in cholestatic and alcoholic liver disease. • Signs and symptoms of deficiency include hemolytic anemia. • Deficiency can lead to the following neurological deficits: spinocerebellar ataxia with loss of deep tendon reflexes; truncal and limb ataxia; loss of vibration and position senses; ophthalmoplegia; muscle weakness; ptosis; dysarthria.
Vitamin K	• Monitoring requires direct measurement, using vitamin K levels or PIVKA II (protein-induced by vitamin K absence or antagonist II) levels. • Relying on the international normalized ratio (INR) is not best practice for preventing subclinical deficiency. • Easy to replace (10 mg orally × 3 days).

Source: Data are from references 25–28.

Hepatic Encephalopathy

CLD patients have increased protein requirements (30). Therefore, patients with cirrhosis who do not have encephalopathy do not need to restrict protein. In the setting of hepatic encephalopathy, daily protein intake should be limited to 0.8 g per kilogram of body weight. Oral supplementation with branched-chain amino acids (BCAAs, ie, leucine, isoleucine, and valine) may be beneficial. However, specific recommendations about the supplementation regimen are not well established. (See Table 11.3, on page 134, for more information.) Probiotics may eventually prove useful in treating hepatic encephalopathy, but the efficacy has not yet been fully established. In a review of relevant studies, Sheth and Garcia-Tsao found that not all probiotics proved to be equally efficacious (31).

Alcoholic Hepatitis

In the absence of infection, corticosteroids are indicated for patients with alcoholic hepatitis whose Maddrey Discriminant score for alcoholic hepatitis is more than 32. Nutritional status is a prognostic variable for alcoholic hepatitis, and nutrition is a primary treatment modality (32). The optimal nutrition intervention has not been established, but general daily guidelines are 1.2 to 1.5 g protein per kilogram of body weight and 35 to 40 kcal/kg (33).

Acute Liver Failure

Due to the loss of hepatic gluconeogenic and glycogen capacity, patients with acute liver failure may initially experience hypoglycemia and require an intravenous glucose infusion (34). In later stages of the disease, patients may experience hyperglycemia, which is often secondary to infection. Strict blood glucose control (between 70 and 100 mg/dL) should be a priority.

Patients with acute liver failure often have vitamin deficiencies. Deficiencies of vitamin B-1 and vitamin B-6 are particularly common, and patients undergoing renal replacement therapy are at risk of deficiencies for all water-soluble vitamins.

Patients may benefit from early initiation of enteral nutrition to help decrease protein catabolism. Their metabolic requirements are 20% to 30% higher than those of healthy control subjects (35). Initial feedings should provide 20 to 25 kcal/kg/d. Energy goals during the recovery phase are 30 kcal/kg/d (36).

Dietary Supplements in Management of Liver Disease

As mentioned previously, BCAAs and probiotics have been considered for use in the management of hepatic encephalopathy. Table 11.3 summarizes indications and evidence for the use of BCAAs as well as selected other supplements in treating liver disease.

TABLE 11.3   Selected Dietary Supplements Used in Treatment of Liver Disease

Supplement	Indications	Level of Evidence	Comments
Branched-chain amino acids	Hepatic encephalopathy	No controlled studies in intensive care patients. Mixed results for use of oral supplementation in less critically ill patients.	Expensive, bad taste, overprescribed
S-adenosylmethionine (SAMe)	Alcoholic liver disease; gestational cholestasis	In one randomized controlled trial, patients with alcoholic liver disease showed benefit with SAMe use. In patients with gestational cholestasis, SAMe use was associated with less pruritis and decreased bilirubin.	Expensive; shown to help alcoholic hepatitis and depression
Polyenylphosphatidyl-choline (lecithin)	Prevention of alcoholic cirrhosis	Animal models only.	Inexpensive

Conclusion

CLD is a leading cause of morbidity and mortality worldwide. Nutrition-related disorders are common in CLD, and patients benefit from appropriate dietary management. Deficiencies in fat-soluble vitamins and other micronutrients require evaluation in the setting of CLD. Osteoporosis is an overlooked complication of CLD that requires ongoing monitoring and frequent treatment. Patients with CLD have elevated protein and energy requirements, but they tend to be underfed due to fears of protein intoxication. In CLD, protein restriction is only warranted in patients with hepatic encephalopathy or gastrointestinal bleeding. The use of BCAAs for the nutrition management of CLD is passé. BCAAs may benefit patients with hepatic encephalopathy but should otherwise be avoided because of their expense and poor palatability.

Acute liver failure is a catabolic state with a heightened metabolic demand for energy, protein, glucose, thiamin, and pyridoxine. Alcoholic hepatitis is a condition with an appreciable mortality whereby nutritional status is a prognostic indicator and dietary therapy plays a key role is disease management. NAFLD responds to calorie restriction, weight loss, and vitamin E supplementation.

References

1. Flores YN, Yee HF, Leng M, et al. Risk factors for chronic liver disease in blacks, Mexican Americans, and whites in the United States: Results from NHANES IV, 1999–2004. *Am J Gastroenterol.* 2008;103:2231–2238.
2. Asrani SK, Larson JJ, Yawn B, Therneau TM, Kim WR. Underestimation of liver-related mortality in the United States. *Gastroenterology.* 2013;145(2):375–382.
3. Sasidharan M, Nistala S, Narendhran RT, et al. Nutritional status and prognosis in cirrhotic patients. *Trop Gastroenterol.* 2012;33(4):257–264.
4. Taylor RM, Dhawan A. Assessing nutritional status in children with chronic liver disease. *J Gastroenterol Hepatol.* 2005;20(12):1817–1824.
5. Lazo M, Hernaez R, Eberhardt MS, et al. Prevalence of nonalcoholic fatty liver disease in the United States: The Third National Health and Nutrition Examination Survey, 1988–1994. *Am J Epidemiol.* 2013;178:38–45.
6. Clark JM, Brancati FL, Diehl AM. The prevalence and etiology of elevated aminotransferase levels in the United States. *Am J Gastroenterol.* 2003;98:960–967.
7. Nobili V, Alisi A, Raponi M. Pediatric non-alcoholic fatty liver disease: preventive and therapeutic value of lifestyle intervention. *World J Gastroenterol.* 2009;15(48):6017–6022.
8. Fu JH, Sun HS, Wang Y, et al. The effects of a fat- and sugar-enriched diet and chronic stress on nonalcoholic fatty liver disease in male wistar rats. *Dig Dis Sci.* 2010;55(8):2227–2236.
9. Hickman IJ, Jonsson JR, Prins JB, et al. Modest weight loss and physical activity in overweight patients with chronic liver disease results in sustained improvements in alanine aminotransferase, fasting insulin, and quality of life. *Gut.* 2004;53:413–419.
10. Torres DM, Harrison SA. Diagnosis and therapy of nonalcoholic steatohepatitis. *Gastroenterology.* 2008;134(6):682–698.
11. Perito ER, Rodriguez LA, Lustig RH. Dietary treatment of nonalcoholic steatohepatitis. *Curr Opin Gastroenterol.* 2013;29(2):170–176.
12. Ryan MC, Itsiopoulos C, Thodis T, et al. The Mediterranean diet improves hepatic steatosis and insulin sensitivity in individuals with non-alcoholic fatty liver disease. *J Hepatol.* 2013;59(1):138–143.
13. Hanke D, Zahradka P, Mohankumar SK, Clark JL, Taylor CG. A diet high in α-linolenic acid and monounsaturated fatty acids attenuates hepatic steatosis and alters hepatic phospholipid fatty acid profile in diet-induced obese rats. *Prostaglandins Leukot Essent Fatty Acids.* 2013;89(6):391–401.
14. Capanni M, Calella F, Biagini MR, et al. Prolonged n-3 polyunsaturated fatty acid supplementation ameliorates hepatic steatosis in patients with non-alcoholic fatty liver disease: a pilot study. *Aliment Pharmacol Ther.* 2006;23:1143–1151.

15. Leclercq IA, Horsmans Y. Nonalcoholic fatty liver disease: the potential role of nutritional management. *Curr Opin Clin Nutr Metab Care.* 2008;11:766–773.

16. Spadaro L, Magliocco O, Spampinato D, et al. 738 omega-3 polyunsaturated fatty acids: a pilot trial in non-alcoholic fatty liver disease. *J Hepatol.* 2006;44(Suppl):S264.

17. Collison KS, Saleh SM, Bakheet RH, et al. Diabetes of the liver: the link between nonalcoholic fatty liver disease and HFCS-55. *Obesity.* 2009;17(11):2003–2013.

18. Gentile CL, Pagliassotti MJ. The role of fatty acids in the development and progression of nonalcoholic fatty liver disease. *J Nutr Biochem.* 2008;19(9):567–576.

19. Zivkovic AM, German JB, Sanyal AJ. Comparative review of diets for the metabolic syndrome: implications for nonalcoholic fatty liver disease. *Am J Clin Nutr.* 2007;86:285–300.

20. Pacana T, Sanyal AJ. Vitamin E and nonalcoholic fatty liver disease. *Curr Opin Clin Nutr Metab Care.* 2012;15(6):641–648.

21. O'Brien A, Williams R. Nutrition in end-stage liver disease: principles and practice. *Gastroenterology.* 2008;134:1729–1740.

22. Ferreira LG, Anastácio LR, Lima AS, Correia MI. Malnutrition and inadequate food intake of patients on the waiting list for liver transplant. *Rev Assoc Med Bras.* 2009;55(4):389–393.

23. Merli M, Giusto M, Gentili F, et al. Nutritional status: its influence on the outcome of patients undergoing liver transplantation. *Liver Int.* 2010;30(2):208–214.

24. Collier J. Bone disorders in chronic liver disease. *Hepatology.* 2007;46:1271–1278.

25. Collier JD, Ninkovic M, Compston JE. Guidelines on the management of osteoporosis associated with chronic liver disease. *Gut.* 2002;50:i1–i9.

26. Roux C, Bischoff-Ferrari HA, Papapoulos SE, et al. New insights into the role of vitamin D and calcium in osteoporosis management: an expert roundtable discussion. *Curr Med Res Opin.* 2008;24(5):1363–1370.

27. Ioannis Stamoulis I, Kouraklis G, Theocharis S. Zinc and the liver: an active interaction. *Dig Dis Sci.* 2007;52:1595–1612.

28. Takahashi S, Kudo M, Chung H, Inoue T, et al. PIVKA-II is the best prognostic predictor in patients with hepatocellular carcinoma after radiofrequency ablation therapy. *Oncology.* 2008;75(Suppl 1):91–98.

29. Nair S, Cohen DB, Cohen MP et al. Postoperative mortality, costs, and long term survival in severely obese patients undergoing orthotopic liver transplantation. *Am J Gastroenterol.* 2001;96:842–845.

30. Cordoba J, Lopez-Hellin J, Planas M, et al. Normal protein diet for episodic hepatic encephalopathy: results of a randomized study. *J Hepatol.* 2004;41:38–43.

31. Sheth AA, Garcia-Tsao G. Probiotics and liver disease. *J Clin Gastroenterol.* 2008;42(Supp 2):S80–S84.

32. Bergheim I, McClain CJ, Artell GE. Treatment of alcoholic liver disease. *Dig Dis Sci.* 2005;23–24:275–284.

33. McCullough AJ, O'Connor JF. Alcoholic liver disease: proposed recommendations for the American College of Gastroenterology. *Am J Gastroenterol.* 1998;93:2022–2036.

34. Bernal W, Auzinger G, Sizer E, Wendon J. Intensive care management of acute liver failure. *Semin Liver Dis.* 2008;28:188–200.

35. Schneeweiss B, Pammer J, Ratheiser K, et al. Energy metabolism in acute hepatic failure. *Gastroenterology,* 1993;105:1515–1521.

36. Plauth M, Cabre E, Riggio O, et al. ESPEN guidelines on enteral nutrition: liver disease. *Clin Nutr.* 2006;25:285–294.

CHAPTER 12

Pancreatic Disease

Arlene Stein, MS, RD, CDN, CNSD,

Sunita Sidhu-Buonocore, MD, and James H. Grendell, MD

The pancreas is the master digestive gland of the body, secreting about 1 liter of protein- and bicarbonate-rich clear fluid into the duodenum each day. The pancreas is responsible for the following:

- Producing and secreting the digestive enzymes necessary for the digestion of macronutrients into forms that can be either absorbed directly by enterocytes or acted upon further by enterocyte brush border enzymes
- Producing and secreting the bicarbonate that is necessary for the optimal environment in the small intestine for the activity of pancreatic digestive enzymes and bile salts
- Producing and secreting the hormones insulin and glucagon, which are essential for glucose homeostasis

This chapter focuses on nutritional considerations for patients with acute pancreatitis or pancreatic insufficiency. Pancreatic insufficiency in cystic fibrosis is covered in Chapter 5, and pancreatic cancer is addressed in Chapter 13.

Effects of Nutrition on the Pancreas

The pancreas depends on the overall nutritional state of the body for its growth and function. The pancreas grows in parallel to general body growth and atrophies in the absence of food (1). Feeding increases the rate of synthesis and secretion of digestive enzymes. The content and secretion of major digestive enzymes change in proportion to the dietary content of their respective substrates (carbohydrate, fat, and protein) over 5 to 7 days, primarily because of changes in the mRNA levels for these enzymes. Ingestion of large amounts of amino acids or proteins stimulates pancreatic growth (2,3).

Hormones (eg, cholecystokinin, secretin, gastrin, insulin, insulin-like growth factor-1) and neurotransmitters mediate trophic effects of feeding, whereas neuropeptide Y and somatostatin inhibit pancreatic growth. In response to injury or surgical resection, dietary protein, cholecystokinin, insulin, and insulin-like growth factor-1 seem to be of primary importance in pancreatic regeneration (4). See Box 12.1 for a list of the potential effects of nutrition on the pancreas.

BOX 12.1   Effects of Nutrition on the Pancreas

- Pancreas atrophies in the absence of food.
- Ingestion of large amounts of amino acids or proteins stimulates pancreatic growth.
- Feeding increases rate of synthesis and secretion of digestive enzymes.
- Content and secretion of digestive enzymes change in response to composition of diet.
- Dietary protein, cholecystokinin, insulin, and insulin-like growth factor-1 are of primary importance in pancreatic repair and regeneration after injury or surgery.

Nutrition Issues in Acute Pancreatitis

For patients with acute pancreatitis, the two primary concerns are to reduce the metabolic work of the pancreas and to meet the nutritional needs of the patient. Because the presence of gastric acid, fats, amino acids, and peptides in the proximal duodenum stimulates the pancreas to synthesize and secrete digestive enzymes, thus increasing the metabolic work of an already inflamed gland, oral intake is initially prohibited (5,6).

Patients with mild acute pancreatitis can usually resume oral feeding within a few days of onset of symptoms. Therefore, they are usually managed with intravenous hydration and electrolytes. Oral feeding can resume once patients experience a substantial improvement in symptoms (eg, abdominal pain and nausea) and serum amylase and/or lipase levels trend toward normal. Oral feeding can be initiated with a low-fat solid diet rather than with clear liquids, which may shorten the length of hospitalization (5,6).

Patients with severe acute pancreatitis often have a prolonged course involving organ failure and other complications leading to extended stays in an intensive care unit. Nutrition support may be required for these patients. See Box 12.2 for a summary of nutrition care considerations in severe acute pancreatitis. The following sections elaborate on some of the main issues.

Nutrition Support

Historically, the treatments for acute pancreatitis included *complete* bowel rest and, therefore, total parenteral nutrition (TPN). However, enteral feeding into the jejunum provides minimal stimulation of pancreatic secretion because the hormonal and neural factors resulting in meal-related stimulation of the pancreas are primarily located in the proximal duodenum. Prospective, randomized studies have demonstrated no improvement in survival in patients receiving TPN compared to those receiving enteral nutrition (EN) through a nasojejunal feeding tube. Patients receiving EN had fewer complications, particularly line sepsis, and EN was significantly less costly than PN (7–9).

Because EN is more physiologic and may decrease the translocation of bacteria from the gastrointestinal (GI) tract into areas of pancreatic necrosis, institution of EN within 24 to 48 hours of hospital admission has been advocated with the goals of modulating the acute stress response, promoting more rapid resolution of the disease process, and maintaining the integrity of the intestinal mucosa (10). TPN should be reserved for those patients who do not tolerate EN (eg, due to severe ileus), when an enteral feeding tube cannot be placed, or when nutrition goals cannot be met within a few days of initiating EN.

JEJUNAL AND GASTRIC FEEDINGS

If an operation is being performed for a major complication of acute pancreatitis, placement of a jejunal feeding tube is often beneficial because the duration of time until oral feeding can be resumed is

---

BOX 12.2   Nutrition Care Considerations in Severe Acute Pancreatitis

- Enteral feeding is as effective as total parenteral nutrition, is associated with fewer complications, and is less expensive.
- Enteral feeding should be initiated within 24 to 48 hours of hospital admission.
- Jejunal feeding is preferred to gastric or duodenal feeding (although conflicting data exist).
- For jejunal feeding, elemental/semi-elemental feeding offers no greater benefits than polymeric formulas.
- Oral feeding should be initiated once complications are successfully treated and the patient is free of significant pain and nausea.
- There is no benefit associated with the use of probiotics or immunonutrition.

---

often difficult to predict. Because nasojejunal feeding tubes are more difficult to place than nasogastric tubes and more likely to migrate, studies have been done to determine whether the same results could be obtained with nasogastric feeding as with jejunal feeding. Although some studies have shown no difference (11,12), one report described a significant increase in pulmonary and total complications in the nasogastric-fed group (13). Further studies need to be done before accepting nasogastric feeding as an acceptable alternative to nasojejunal feeding.

ELEMENTAL/SEMI-ELEMENTAL VS POLYMERIC FEEDING SOLUTIONS
A meta-analysis involving up to 20 randomized controlled studies did not demonstrate a difference in feeding intolerance, infectious complications, or death for patients fed lower-cost polymeric formulas compared to patients fed elemental or semi-elemental formulas (14).

RESUMPTION OF ORAL FEEDING
Oral feeding should be initiated once complications have been successfully treated and the patient is no longer experiencing significant pain or nausea. If oral feeding is not initially tolerated, it should be suspended for 1 to 2 days and then retried. If it is still not tolerated, it should again be suspended and a search initiated for potential problems (eg, walled-off pancreatic necrosis, pseudocyst) that may be preventing the patient from eating.

Probiotics and Immunonutrition

Probiotics have been studied as a way to reduce the incidence of infectious complications for patients with acute pancreatitis. However, one large randomized controlled study of a multispecies probiotic product demonstrated that patients treated with the probiotic had increased mortality due to bowel ischemia (15). More studies with probiotics using other species of organisms may be needed. Until there is more evidence, the use of probiotics in patients with acute pancreatitis cannot be recommended.

Immunomodulating diets (IMDs) are nutritional formulations supplemented with increased amounts of nutrients that have been shown to modulate inflammation and improve immune function. These nutrients include arginine, glutamine, omega-3 fatty acids (as fish oil), and antioxidants. The use of IMDs in critically ill patients is controversial (5). These feeding formulas may seem theoretically appealing for the treatment of patients with acute pancreatitis, but a meta-analysis concluded that IMDs did not reduce infectious complications, mortality, or length of hospital stay (16). Because immunonutrition formulas are substantially more expensive than standard enteral formulas, there is no reason to recommend their use.

Nutrient Needs

The nutrient needs of the patient with acute pancreatitis depend on the severity of the pancreatitis and other comorbidities. See Box 12.3 for a summary of nutrient needs for patients with acute pancreatitis.

ENERGY
The patient's resting energy expenditure is significantly increased if there is sepsis or multiorgan failure. General guidelines for enteral or parenteral feeding are 25 to 35 kcal per kg of body weight per day. Certainly, overfeeding and underfeeding should be avoided, and indirect calorimetry, when available, can help assess needs more accurately.

PROTEIN
Protein needs generally are between 1.2 and 1.5 g per kg body weight per day. However, individual needs may approach 2 g per kg body weight per day, depending on the clinical situation. On the other hand, less protein may be beneficial for patients with renal or hepatic failure (17).

LIPIDS
Intravenous lipid does not stimulate pancreatic secretion and can be given to patients with acute pancreatitis as long as serum triglyceride concentrations are maintained below 400 mg/dL (18). In general, less than 2 g fat per kg body weight per day, or no more than 20% to 30% of the daily energy load from lipid, is recommended (6,19).

CARBOHYDRATES
Carbohydrates can be provided at levels of 3 to 6 g per kg body weight per day or 50% to 60% of the daily energy load to maintain blood glucose levels less than 180 to 200 mg/dL (6,19). Tighter glucose control may be desirable, depending on the clinical situation. Insulin may be helpful in attaining this goal.

Pancreatic Insufficiency

A patient's pancreatic insufficiency is clinically significant when the patient consumes a diet with 100 g fat per day and there is more than 15 g of fat per day in the stool (20). Steatorrhea and weight loss are manifestations of pancreatic exocrine insufficiency with malabsorption due to maldigestion. Steatorrhea requires the loss of 90% or more of the capacity of the pancreas to secrete digestive enzymes (17,21).

Etiology

Causes of pancreatic insufficiency include chronic pancreatitis, pancreatic cancer, cystic fibrosis, surgery of the pancreas or GI tract, Zollinger-Ellison syndrome, lipase/colipase deficiency, Shwachman-Diamond syndrome, celiac disease, and type 1 diabetes mellitus. There are also two very rare causes in children: Pearson syndrome and Johanson-Blizzard syndrome (20).

BOX 12.3   Nutrient Needs for Patients with Acute Pancreatitis

- Total energy: 25–35 kcal per kg body weight per day
- Protein: 1.2–1.5 g per kg body weight per day (may approach 2g/kg in some cases)
- Fat: <2 g per kg body weight per day, comprising 20% to 30% of daily energy intake (maintain serum triglycerides <400 mg/dL)
- Carbohydrate: 3–6 g per kg body weight per day, comprising 50%–60% of daily energy intake (maintain blood glucose levels <180–200 mg/dL, or achieve tighter glucose control, depending on the clinical situation)

Diagnosis

Historically, quantitative determination of fecal fat excretion in a 72-hour stool collection has been the "gold standard" for diagnosing pancreatic insufficiency. Because this is a cumbersome and unpopular test for patients, other simpler tests have been developed. The best of these in current practice is measurement in a random stool sample of fecal elastase concentration. Elastase is a pancreatic enzyme that is relatively resistant to degradation as it passes through the intestine; therefore, its concentration in stool is a reliable indicator of pancreatic exocrine secretory function. The normal value is more than 200 mcg elastase per gram of stool. Values between 100 and 200 mcg/g are considered to indicate mild-to-moderate insufficiency. A value less than 100 mcg/g demonstrates severe pancreatic insufficiency.

Dietary Management

Dietary management of pancreatic insufficiency includes abstinence from alcohol, if it is thought to be a contributing factor to the underlying disease process (eg, chronic pancreatitis) causing the pancreatic insufficiency. If serum values indicate a deficiency of fat-soluble vitamins (A, D, E, and K), supplementation is recommended (17). Small, frequent meals that are low in fiber are also recommended because fiber may inhibit pancreatic lipase activity (17,20).

Although strict fat restriction had been recommended in the past, experimental studies in dogs with pancreatic insufficiency found that fat absorption was actually improved when a high-fat diet was ingested along with effective pancreatic enzyme replacement therapy (PERT) (22). Therefore, fat restriction is probably not necessary for patients using effective pancreatic enzyme supplements at appropriate doses.

Medium-chain triglycerides (MCT) can be used by patients who are unable to maintain or gain weight despite appropriate PERT. MCT are absorbed directly across the enterocyte brush border and pass into the bloodstream without the need for pancreatic enzymes.

Pancreatic Enzyme Replacement Therapy

Currently available pancreatic enzyme supplements are derived from porcine pancreas and are the primary treatment for pancreatic insufficiency. Although pancreatic enzyme supplements contain all the enzymes secreted by the pancreas (approximately 20), dosing is based on the amount of lipase units contained in a given supplement. When the appropriate dose is administered, PERT can substantially reduce steatorrhea and help the patient maintain or gain weight (23,24).

Pancreatic enzyme supplements work best if given during and right after a meal. Enzyme supplements given before a meal may leave the stomach prior to the food and be degraded in the small intestine.

Because pancreatic enzymes are inactivated or denatured at acidic pHs, most are enteric-coated (ie, encapsulated in microspheres or microtablets that release their contents at a pH > 5.5, a situation normally encountered in the proximal small intestine) (25). Non-enteric-coated enzyme supplements require concomitant use of an H_2-receptor antagonist or one of the proton pump inhibitors (PPIs) to prevent inactivation of the enzymes in the stomach (25). Even some patients taking enteric-coated enzyme preparations may benefit from acid suppression because decreased bicarbonate secretion by the pancreas may lead to a pH in the proximal small intestine low enough to prevent appropriate release of the digestive enzymes in the supplement. Overall, using non-enteric-coated enzymes along with PPIs is not advisable due to the long-term adverse consequences of PPI use (21,26).

A patient's baseline weight should be obtained just before he or she starts PERT because weight stabilization is usually the goal of therapy. Subsequent weights are then assessed to determine whether the patient is benefitting from the treatment.

TREATMENT OF PANCREATIC EXOCRINE INSUFFICIENCY IN CYSTIC FIBROSIS

For children with cystic fibrosis, pancreatic enzyme supplementation is crucial to growth and development because malabsorption leads to malnutrition and growth retardation as well as to an increased risk of pulmonary complications (23,27). Pancreatic enzyme replacement therapy leads to a better quality of life for patients with cystic fibrosis.

In the past, fibrosing colonopathy presenting with bloody diarrhea, symptoms of GI obstruction, or chylous ascites was observed in children treated with very large daily doses of pancreatic lipase (>24,000 lipase units per kg body weight per day). This treatment used enzyme supplement capsules or tablets with much higher lipase contents than is provided by currently available supplements. With the current enzyme supplements and dosing guidelines, this complication of enzyme replacement no longer occurs (28). For additional information on cystic fibrosis and PERT, refer to Chapter 5.

REGULATION OF PANCREATIC ENZYME SUPPLEMENTS

The use of pancreatic enzyme supplements antedated the creation of the US Food and Drug Administration (FDA). Consequently, studies to assess the safety, efficacy, stability, or bioavailability of these products prior to marketing were not required until recently. However, the FDA now requires that manufacturers complete the standard new drug application process for any pancreatic enzyme supplement to be prescribed in the United States. All pancreatic enzyme supplements currently available in the United States have passed the FDA approval requirements (28,29).

Conclusion

The pancreas is a complex organ with both endocrine and exocrine functions. Nutritional status and diet affect the function of the pancreas, and diseases of the pancreas generally require dietary interventions for symptom management.

References

1. Baumier MD, Koopann MC, Thomas DD, et al. Intravenous or luminal amino acids are insufficient to maintain pancreatic growth and digestive enzyme expression in the absence of intact dietary protein. *Am J Physiol Gastrointest Liver Physiol.* 2010;299:G338–G347.

2. Crozier SJ, D'Alecy LG, Ernst SA, et al. Molecular mechanisms of pancreatic dysfunction induced by protein malnutrition. *Gastroenterology.* 2009;137:1093–1101.

3. Corring T. The adaptation of digestive enzymes to the diet: its physiological significance. *Reprod Nutr Dev.* 1980;20:1217–1235.

4. Pap A. Effects of insulin and glucose metabolism on pancreatic exocrine function. *Int J Diabetes Metabol.* 2004;12:30–34.

5. Marik P. What is the best way to feed patients with pancreatitis? *Curr Opin Crit Care.* 2009;15:131–138.

6. Meier R, Beglinger C, Layer P, et al. ESPEN guidelines on nutrition in acute pancreatitis. *Clin Nutr.* 2002;21:173–183.

7. McClave SA, Green LM, Snider HL, et al. Comparison of the safety of early enteral vs. parenteral nutrition in mild acute pancreatitis. *JPEN J Parenter Enteral Nutr.* 1997;21:14–20.

8. Kalfarentzos F, Kehagias J, Mead N, et al. Enteral nutrition is superior to parenteral nutrition in severe acute pancreatitis: results of a randomized prospective trial. *Br J Surg.* 1997;84:1665–1669.

9. Marik PE, Zaloga GP. Meta-analysis of parenteral nutrition versus enteral nutrition in patients with acute pancreatitis. *BMJ.* 2004;328:1407–1410.

10. McClave SA, Chang WK, Dhaliwal R, et al. Nutrition support in acute pancreatitis: a systematic review of the literature. *JPEN J Parenter Enteral Nutr.* 2006;30:143–156.

11. Eatock FC, Chong P, Menezes N, et al. A randomized study of early nasogastric versus nasojejunal feeding in severe acute pancreatitis. *Am J Gastroenterol.* 2005;100:432–439.

12. Kumar A, Singh N, Prakash S, et al. Early enteral nutrition in severe acute pancreatitis: a prospective randomized controlled trial comparing nasojejunal and nasogastric routes. *J Clin Gastroenterol.* 2006;40:431–434.

13. Eckerwall GE, Axelsson JB, Andersson RG. Early nasogastric feeding in predicted severe acute pancreatitis. A clinical, randomized study. *Ann Surg.* 2006;244:959–967.

14. Petrov MS, Loveday BP, Pylpchuk RD, et al. Systematic review and meta-analysis of enteral nutrition formulations in acute pancreatitis. *Br J Surg.* 2009;96:1243–1252.

15. Besselink MGH, Van Santvoort HC, Buskens E, et al. Probiotic prophylaxis in predicted severe acute pancreatitis: a randomized, double-blind, placebo-controlled trial. *Lancet.* 2008;371:651–659.

16. Petrov MS, Atduev VA, Zagainov VE. Advanced enteral therapy in acute pancreatitis: is there room for immunonutrition? A meta-analysis. *Int J Surg.* 2008;6:119–124.

17. Meier RF, Beglinger C. Nutrition in pancreatic diseases. *Best Pract Res Clin Gastroenterol.* 2006;20:507–529.

18. Klein S, Kinney J, Jeejeebhoy K, et al. Nutrition support in clinical practice: review of published data and recommendations for future research directions. *JPEN J Parenter Enteral Nutr.* 1997;21:133–156.

19. McIsaac C, Helton WS. Intravenous nutrition in patients with acute pancreatitis. In: Rombeau JL, Roandelli RH, ed. *Clinical Nutrition Parenteral Nutrition.* 3rd ed. Philadelphia, PA: WB Saunders; 2001:230–257.

20. Dominguez-Munoz JE. Pancreatic enzyme therapy for pancreatic exocrine insufficiency. *Curr Gastroenterol Rep.* 2007; 9:116–122.

21. Krishnamurty DK, Jagannath SB, Andersen DK. Delayed release pancrelipase for treatment of pancreatic exocrine insufficiency associated with chronic pancreatitis. *Ther Clin Risk Manag.* 2009;5:507–520.

22. Suzuki A, Mizumoto A, Rerknimitr R, et al. Effect of bacterial or porcine lipase with low- or high-fat diets on nutrient absorption in pancreatic insufficient dogs. *Gastroenterology.* 1999;116:431–437.

23. Baker SS. Delayed release pancrelipase for the treatment of pancreatic exocrine insufficiency associated with cystic fibrosis. *Ther Clin Risk Manag.* 2008;4:1079–1084.

24. Layer P, Groger G. Fate of pancreatic enzymes in the human intestinal lumen in health and pancreatic insufficiency. *Digestion.* 1993;54(Suppl 2):10–14.

25. Friedman SL, McQuaid KR, Grendell JH. *Current Diagnosis and Treatment in Gastroenterology.* 2nd ed. New York, NY: Lange Medical Books; 2003:503–504.

26. Dimagno EP, Malagelada JR, Go VL, et al. Fate of orally ingested enzymes in pancreatic insufficiency. Comparison of two dosage schedules. *N Engl J Med.* 1977;296:1318–1322.

27. Borowitz DS, Grand RJ, Durie PR. Consensus Committee. Use of pancreatic enzyme supplements for patients with cystic fibrosis in the context of fibrosing colonopathy. *J Pediatr*. 1995;127:681–684.
28. Taylor JR, Gardner TB, Waljee AK, et al. Systematic review: efficacy and safety of pancreatic enzyme supplements for exocrine pancreatic insufficiency. *Aliment Pharmacol Ther*. 2010;31:57–72.
29. Nakajima K, Oshida H, Muneyuki T, Kakei M. Pancrelipase: an evidence-based review of its use for treating pancreatic insufficiency. *Core Evid*. 2012;7:77–91.

PART IV

Gastrointestinal Oncology and Surgery

CHAPTER 13

Gastrointestinal Oncology

Mary J. Marian, MS, RD, CSO

The incidence of new cancers in the United States is a little more than 1.4 million cases annually (excluding basal and squamous cell skin cancers), with cancer accounting for 1 in every 4 deaths (1). When deaths are aggregated by age, cancer surpasses heart disease as the leading cause of death for individuals younger than 85 years (2). The National Cancer Institute estimates that approximately 11.1 million adults in the United States have a history of a cancer diagnosis and the overall costs related to cancer diagnoses are approximately $228 billion per year (1). Gastrointestinal (GI) cancers, including cancers of the esophagus, stomach, small bowel, large bowel, rectum, liver, gallbladder, and pancreas, account for approximately 20% of all newly diagnosed cancers annually (see Table 13.1 on page 148) (3).

Approximately one-third of cancer deaths are related to excess body fat, sedentary lifestyle, and poor diet, all of which are largely modifiable contributors (4). Chronic inflammation is thought to play a key role in carcinogenesis, although scientists do not know the precise mechanism(s) (5). Increased cell proliferation and oxidative stress resulting in dysplasia are key aspects of inflammation that are thought to contribute to carcinogenesis. Increased amounts of reactive oxygen and nitrogen species and DNA damage due to oxidative stress are also thought to be key contributors (5).

Cancer Prevention

The role that lifestyle and diet play in cancer risk is increasingly clearer, and it is now estimated that 50% of cancers are preventable (6). Observational and epidemiologic studies reflect significant differences in cancer rates among countries. Migration patterns exhibit the importance of environmental influences; the incidence of cancer increases among populations that migrate from developing countries to more Westernized societies (4). Tobacco and alcohol have also been found to play a significant role in the development of many GI cancers. Table 13.2 (page 148) provides an overview of the lifestyle risk factors associated with GI cancer risk (1,2,7,8).

Carcinogenesis is a multistep process with three critical steps: initiation, promotion, and progression. Chemoprevention involves preventing, suppressing, or reversing a premalignancy so it does not progress into cancerous cells. Epidemiologic evidence provides support that natural dietary bioactive compounds can modify this response (7,9,10). A number of studies have shown that individuals in the lower quartiles for intake of fruits and vegetables have about twice the risk for cancers when compared with individuals

TABLE 13.1 Adult Gastrointestinal Cancers in the United States

Cancer	New Diagnoses per Year	Estimated Deaths per Year[a]	Comments
Esophageal	16,470	14,530	Adenocarcinoma rates are increasing.
Gastric	21,130	10,620	More common in people older than 70 years.
Small bowel	6,230	1,110	Median age at diagnosis is 67 years.
Colon	106,100	9,920[b]	3rd most common cancer, but incidence is decreasing.
Rectal	40,870	Not available[b]	
Pancreatic	42,470	35,240	Incidence is stable in men and increasing in women; early detection can be difficult.
Hepatocellular	22,620	18,160	

[a]Based on 2009 estimates.
[b]Rectal cancer deaths and colon cancer deaths are typically combined as colorectal cancer mortality statistics.
Source: Data are from reference 3.

TABLE 13.2 Risk Factors for Gastrointestinal Cancers

Type of Cancer	Factors Associated with Increased Risk	Factors Associated with Decreased Risk
Mouth/oral	Alcohol	Nonstarchy vegetables, fruits, carotenoids
Esophageal	Abdominal fatness, alcohol, smoked foods, long-standing gastroesophageal reflux disease	Nonstarchy/cruciferous vegetables, vitamin C, carotenoids
Gastric	Salt, salted foods, smoking, *H. pylori* infection	Nonstarchy/allium vegetables, vitamin C, whole grains, carotenoids, green tea
Large bowel	Red meat, processed meats, alcohol, body fatness, adult-attained height	Fruits, vegetables, high-fiber foods, garlic, calcium, physical activity
Liver	Aflatoxins, alcohol, body fatness	Fruits
Pancreas	Red meat, body fatness, high vitamin D levels, smoking, chronic pancreatitis, diabetes, family history	Fruits, carotenoids, high-folate foods, physical activity

Source: Data are from references 1, 2, 7, and 8.

in the upper quartiles (11). Although the nutrient profile varies among these foodstuffs, plant foods are typically rich sources of many natural constituents associated with a reduced risk for cancers: fiber, vitamins, minerals, flavonoids, sulforaphane, resveratrol, and organosulfur compounds. Rich food sources of chemopreventive phytochemicals include cruciferous vegetables, carrots, celery, tomatoes, peppers, flaxseed, grapes, soybeans, parsley, garlic, onions, turmeric, and ginger.

The chemopreventive benefits that may be provided by specific phytonutrients are reviewed in Table 13.3 (7,9,10). Possible effects include the following (8):

- Antioxidant and anti-inflammatory properties
- Induction of phase II enzymes, anti-cell growth signaling pathways
- Induction of cellular defense systems resulting in apoptosis and/or cell cycle arrest

Additional chemopreventive advantages may include insulin-sensitizing effects that increase adiponectin levels or enhance adiponectin signaling (8).

TABLE 13.3 Phytochemicals and Cancer Prevention

Phytochemical	Food Source(s)	Clinical Significance
Allylic sulfides	Garlic, onion, shallots, chives, leeks	Anti-cancer activity; may decrease risk for colon and stomach cancers; decreases lipid peroxidation
α-Linoleic acid	Flaxseed, soy, walnuts	Reduces inflammation; may protect against breast cancer; enhances immunity
Anthocyanins	Blackberries, blueberries, strawberries, other berries	Antioxidants; inhibit HMG-CoA reductase
Ascorbic acid	Green and yellow vegetables; fruits	Antioxidant
β-carotene	Green and yellow fruits and vegetables	Reduces risk of lung and breast cancers; enhances immunity (in the elderly)
Capsaicin	Chili peppers	Antioxidant; reduces risk for colon, gastric, and rectal cancers
Catechin (flavonoid): theaflavins, thearubigins	Green and black tea, berries	Reduces risk of gastric cancer; antioxidant; increases immune function
Coumarin	Parsley, carrots, citrus	Reduces risk of cancers
Curcumin (plant phenol)	Turmeric, curry, cumin	Anti-inflammatory properties; reduces risk of skin cancer
Cynarin	Artichoke	Decreases cholesterol levels
Ellagic acid (polyphenol)	Wine, grapes, currants, nuts (pecans), berries (strawberries, blackberries, raspberries), seeds	Reduces cancer risk
Flavonoids and polyphenolic acids; other phenolic compounds (caffeic, ferulic acids; sesame; vanillin)	Parsley, carrots, citrus fruits, broccoli, cabbage, cucumbers, squash, yams, tomatoes, eggplant, peppers, soy products, berries, potatoes, broad beans, pea pods, colored onions, radishes, horseradish, tea, onions, apples, red wine, grape juice	Extend activity of vitamin C; act as antioxidants; anticarcinogenic activity
Genistein (phytoestrogen/ isoflavone)	Soybeans	Reduces risk of hormone-dependent cancers
Indoles	Cabbage, broccoli, brussels sprouts, spinach, watercress, cauliflower, turnip, kohlrabi, kale, rutabaga, horseradish, mustard greens	Reduce risk of hormone-related cancers; may "inactivate" estrogen
Isoflavones and saponins	Soybeans and soybean products	Decrease risks of certain cancers
Isothiocyanates, such as sulforaphane (released during chewing of cruciferous vegetables)	Cabbage, cauliflower, broccoli and broccoli sprouts, brussels sprouts, mustard greens, horseradish, radish	Reduce risk of tobacco-induced tumors; stimulate glutathione S-transferases (GST) activity
Lignans (phytoestrogen)	High-fiber foods, especially seeds; flax	Reduce cancer risk (colon); bind to estrogen receptor sites and may reduce risk of estrogen-stimulated breast cancer

Continues

TABLE 13.3 Phytochemicals and Cancer Prevention *(Continued)*

Phytochemical	Food Source(s)	Clinical Significance
Lignin	Soybean products, flaxseed	May reduce risk of certain types of cancers, including breast and prostate
Lycopene (carotenoid)	Tomato sauce, ketchup, red grapefruit, guava, dried apricots, watermelon	Antioxidant; reduces risk of prostate cancer; may reduce cardiovascular disease
d-Limonene	Citrus, citrus oils	Antioxidant; reduces cancer risk
Monoterpenes	Parsley, carrots, celery, broccoli, cabbage, cauliflower, cucumbers, squash, yams, tomatoes, eggplant, peppers, mint, basil, caraway seed oil	Anti-cancer activity
Organosulfur compounds (allylic acid)	Garlic, onion, watercress, cruciferous vegetables, leeks	Decrease lipid peroxidation; reduce risk of gastric cancer
Phenolic acid	Cruciferous vegetables, eggplant, peppers, tomatoes, celery, parsley, soy, licorice root, flaxseed, citrus, whole grains, berries	Inhibits cancer through inhibition of nitrosamine formation; reduces risk for lung and skin cancers
Plant sterols	Broccoli, cabbage, cucumbers, squash, yams, tomatoes, eggplant, peppers, soy products, whole grains	May decrease risk for colon, rectal, stomach, lung and breast cancers; decrease cardiovascular disease
Polyacetylene	Parsley, carrots, celery	Decreases risk for tobacco-induced tumors; alters prostaglandin formation
Retinol	Green and yellow vegetables, fruits	Potentially decreases risk for certain cancers
Selenium	Seafood, garlic	Antioxidant
Tocopherol (vitamin E)	Nuts, wheat germ, oils	Antioxidant

Source: Data are from references 7, 9, and 10.

Nutritional Implications of Cancer and Cancer Therapies

Available anticancer therapies include surgery, chemotherapy, radiation, and immunotherapy. Both the disease itself and treatment-related toxicities can contribute to deteriorations in nutritional status, including significant weight loss and malnutrition. In fact, malnutrition is often the ultimate cause of death in cancer patients (12,13).

Weight Loss and Cancer Cachexia

The prevalence of weight loss among cancer patients seems to be influenced by the type of tumor or cancer. For example, 30% to 80% individuals with gastric or pancreatic cancers have significant weight loss. Breast cancer, lymphomas, leukemias, and sarcomas are associated with the lowest incidence of weight loss (14).

The following factors may be associated with weight loss:

- Decreased nutritional intake
- Acute metabolic stress and increased nutrient demands associated with surgery, radiotherapy, or chemotherapy
- An increase in nutrient demands resulting from the systemic effect of the tumor, which competes with the host for nutrients, resulting in metabolic derangements leading to anorexia, increased basal metabolic rate, and abnormal metabolism of nutrients (15)
- Tumor phenotype or host genotype (although weight loss is not universal in all patients with similar tumor types) (16)

The wasting syndrome known as cancer anorexia-cachexia syndrome (CACS) can cause malnutrition (15,17). In addition to profound losses in lean body mass and fat stores, CACS is often characterized by the following:

- Weight loss
- Anorexia, early satiety, dysgeusia, nausea, constipation, fatigue, anemia, and edema
- Other inflammatory conditions, such as cardiac failure, rheumatoid arthritis, and chronic obstructive pulmonary disease

A marked loss of lean body mass leads to significant reductions in mobility and quality of life for cancer survivors, and cachexia has been estimated to be the primary cause of death in up to 33% of patients with cancer (18). Weight loss prior to cancer diagnosis is an important prognosticator in terms of morbidity and mortality. Weight loss (as little as 6%) predicted response to therapy, reduced overall survival, and correlated with performance status and quality of life, all of which decreased concurrently with weight (15). Approximately 80% of patients lose weight before they are diagnosed with cancer.

MECHANISMS OF CACS

Although CACS is not well understood, a variety of mechanisms that likely contribute to nutritional deterioration and ultimately cancer cachexia have been implicated. They include cytokines (tumor necrosis factor alpha [TNF-α], interleukin-1 [IL-1], interleukin-6 [IL-6], and interferon gamma [IFN γ]), which are protein mediators secreted by a wide variety of cell types, including macrophages, monocytes, lymphocytes, and endothelial and epithelial cells in response to malignancy, trauma, or sepsis (14). Other mediators that may play a role in the development of cancer cachexia include PIF, a glycoprotein proteolysis-inducing factor that has been isolated from the urine of weight-losing cancer patients but not in those losing weight from other causes (14).

Several neurotransmitter systems within the hypothalamus have also been implicated in cancer cachexia, particularly with regard to anorexia (15). Hypothalamic melanocortin (α-MSH) has been strongly implicated in the control of normal food intake (15). α-MSH facilitates anorexia by activating two melanocortin receptors expressed in the hypothalamus and other regions of the brain (15). In animal studies, inhibiting these pathways has resulted in increased food intake and body weight (19).

TREATMENTS FOR CANCER CACHEXIA

Curing the cancer is the most effective way to treat cancer cachexia, although a cure is not always possible in the advanced stages of cancer. Increasing nutrient intake would seem to be a logical way to reverse weight loss and promote nutritional repletion; however, this strategy is not always successful (20).

Recent investigations have revealed that a multimodal approach targeting the various mechanisms associated with inflammation, anorexia, and cachectic mediators or signaling pathways is likely to be more effective than the use of single agents (21). Pharmacologic agents (eg, megestrol acetate, a synthetic progestin) are used to stimulate appetite. Although high-dose progestin therapy results in statistical improvements in both appetite and weight, body composition analysis studies found that the weight gain was primarily due to an increase in body fat over lean tissue mass (22).

Eicosapentaenoic acid (EPA) is an omega-3 fatty acid that has been evaluated for its ability to attenuate weight loss. EPA's benefits are thought to be related to its ability to inhibit activation of NFκB by proteolysis inducing factor (PIF) through preventing signaling pathways upstream—potentially by inhibiting the release of arachidonic acid from phospholipids (23). EPA also seems to downregulate zinc-alpha2-glycoprotein (ZAG) expression by interfering with glucocorticoid signaling, which may in turn preserve adipose tissue (24). The results of clinical studies investigating the benefits of EPA regarding weight loss have been mixed, and the strength of the evidence is limited by poor compliance, poor study design, and short study duration. Barber et al reported that increases in plasma levels of EPA were associated with increases in weight and lean body mass (25). Well-designed placebo-controlled trials are needed to continue investigating the anticachetic activity of EPA. Further information about EPA is provided later in this chapter, in the Selected Nutrition Interventions section.

β-Hydroxy-β methyl butyrate (HMB) has been shown to downregulate PIF-induced muscle protein degradation by reducing the expression of and activity of the ubiquitin-proteasome pathway (26). In placebo-controlled clinical trials, HMB together with L-glutamine and L-arginine resulted in increased body weight and lean tissue mass with no changes in fat mass in study participants with advanced cancers (27).

Malnutrition Related to Antineoplastic Treatments

Antineoplastic therapies, including surgery, chemotherapy, and radiation, are known contributors to malnutrition (see Table 13.4). Surgically induced malnutrition results from a reduced GI absorptive capacity for nutrients or postoperatively increased metabolic demands for tissue repair in the face of inadequate nutrition intake. Chemotherapy can result in a number of treatment-related side effects, as described in Table 13.4. Radiation therapy, as outlined in Table 13.4, also augments deterioration in nutritional status when the radiotherapy field involves regions that are associated with the mechanics of eating or nutrient absorption. Treatment-related toxicities should be aggressively treated to prevent or reduce the likelihood of malnutrition associated with these therapies. Table 13.5 provides nutrition intervention strategies for combating these treatment-related issues (14,16,28).

Nutrition Screening, Nutrition Assessment, and Planning the Nutrition Intervention

Ideally, a nutrition screening and surveillance program should be in place in all types of oncology settings. However, most patients with cancer are likely to receive therapy in an outpatient setting, where nutrition screening and intervention protocols are less likely to be implemented than in acute care.

The use of nutrition protocols and/or algorithms for nutrition referral can result in optimized nutrition care. Patients who are newly diagnosed with cancer may have a variety of symptoms/nutrition problems, including the following (15):

- Abdominal fullness (60%)
- Constipation (58%)

- Taste changes (46%)
- Mouth dryness (40%)
- Nausea (39%)
- Vomiting (27%) prior to initiation of oncologic treatment

Malnutrition can be insidious from the onset of cancer. Therefore, early detection and intervention are essential to correct existing nutritional deficiencies or to promote maintenance of optimal nutritional status. Severe malnutrition has been defined in the literature in two ways:

- Functional definition (increased risk of morbidity and/or mortality)
- Definition by degree of weight loss, where any of the following indicates malnutrition (29):
  ○ Weight loss >2% of body weight per week
  ○ Weight loss >5% per month
  ○ Weight loss >7.5% per 3 months
  ○ Weight loss >10% per 6 months

The National Cancer Institute Grading System for weight loss is as follows (30):

- Grade 0: <5.0%
- Grade 1: 5.0%–9.9%
- Grade 2: 10.0%–19.9%
- Grade 3: >20.0%
- Grade 4 (life-threatening) is not specifically defined.

Unfortunately, this grading system does not take into account the baseline deficit or the length of time that has elapsed. Attention to weight loss at early time points can successfully prevent deterioration of weight, body composition, and performance status. CACS should be suspected when an involuntary weight loss of 5% within 6 months is detected, especially when muscle wasting is manifested (31).

TABLE 13.4 Anticancer Modalities That Affect Nutritional Status

Treatment	Potential Adverse Effects
Cytotoxic chemotherapy	Nausea, vomiting, anorexia, diarrhea, myelosuppression, fatigue, mucositis, dysgeusia, renal/hepatic side effects, peripheral neuropathies
Hormonal: glucocorticoids, anti-androgens/estrogens, gonadotropin-releasing hormone analogs	Nausea, vomiting, mucositis, bone loss, bone pain, hot flashes, neuropathy, fatigue, fever, hypercalcemia, myelosuppression, edema
Radiation to oropharyngeal region	Anorexia, dysphagia, mucositis, odynophagia, early satiety, fatigue
Radiation to thorax region	Esophagitis, dysphagia, nausea, anorexia, fatigue, odynophagia
Radiation to abdominal/pelvic region	Nausea, vomiting, diarrhea, abdominal cramping/bloating/gas, lactose intolerance, malabsorption, chronic colitis, enteritis
Surgery	Reduced surface area for digestion/absorption, increased nutrient needs, delayed wound healing, chyle leak, dumping syndrome, diarrhea, abdominal gas and bloating, gastroparesis, lactose intolerance, fluid and electrolyte imbalance

TABLE 13.5 Strategies for the Management of Treatment-Related Nutrition Impact Symptoms

Symptom	Etiology	Recommendation
Anorexia	Pain, depression, cytokine oncological therapies	Small, frequent, nutrient-dense meals; avoid fluids with meals; avoid low-calorie filler foods; increase physical activity; appetite stimulants
Constipation	Anticancer treatments, pain medication	High-fiber diet/use of fiber supplements, adequate hydration, physical activity
Diarrhea	Antineoplastic therapies	Low-fat, lactose-free diet; increase soluble fiber; avoid spicy foods; caffeine and alcohol; drink more fluids; probiotics
Dysgeusia	Anticancer treatments	Strong flavored foods (spicy, tart), zinc supplements
Dysphagia	Tumor burden, anticancer treatment	Thickened, moist, soft/blenderized/ground/pureed foods; nutrition support when risk of aspiration is too great for oral intake
Early satiety	Anticancer treatment, tumor burden	Small, frequent, nutrient-dense meals; no fluids with meals
Fatigue	Tumor burden, anticancer therapies, anemia, dehydration, chronic pain, medications, stress, depression, poor nutrition, poor sleep	Small, frequent, nutrient-dense meals; physical activity; assistance with meal planning/shopping/preparation; stress management; treat depression; improve sleep hygiene; maintain adequate hydration
Nausea and vomiting	Anticancer therapies, malignant gastroparesis	Small, frequent, low-fat and low-fiber meals; avoid spicy foods and caffeine; avoid eating 1–2 hours before treatment; ginger supplements; antiemetics; hypnosis; acupuncture; music therapy
Stomatitis/mucositis	Anticancer therapies	Soft nonirritating and nutrient-dense foods, liquids/nutritional supplements, "miracle mouth"/viscous lidocaine swishes, lemon/glycerin swabs, analgesics
Weight gain	Anticancer therapies, edema, steroids	Avoid excess energy intake, increase physical activity, assess fluid status
Weight loss	Tumor burden, cachexia, anticancer therapies	Small, frequent, nutrient-dense meals and snacks; liquid/powder nutritional supplements; appetite stimulants; omega-3 fatty acids
Xerostomia	Tumor burden, anticancer treatment	Drink/swallow small amounts of food at one time, sip water/fluid after each bite, try sweet or tart foods, soft/pureed foods, suck on hard candies, artificial saliva, acupuncture

Source: Data are from references 14, 16, and 28.

Patients identified to be at nutritional risk should receive a comprehensive nutrition assessment, which evaluates the following:

- Anthropometric measurements (including weight-for-height, weight history, BMI, waist-to-hip ratio)
- Nutrition history

- Physical examination findings that can indicate potential nutritional deficiencies
- Laboratory data (eg, electrolytes; data related to renal function; glucose; serum albumin and prealbumin; and hemoglobin/hematocrit together with mean corpuscular volume [MCV] or mean corpuscular hemoglobin concentration [MCHC])
- Performance status and quality of life

Following the assessment, an *individualized* nutrition plan that includes goals for clinical outcomes should be developed. Strategies on how to meet nutritional requirements, as well as strategies to combat treatment-related toxicities, should be reviewed with cancer survivors. Nutrition care plans should coincide with not only the medical team's desires but also with the patient and/or caregiver's wishes. Reassessment should also occur at regular time points. The patient-generated Subjective Global Assessment described in Chapter 3 is an assessment tool that can be used (32).

Nutrition outcome goals can include the following:

- Maintaining or improving nutritional status
- Avoiding or improving treatment-related toxicities
- Avoiding nutrition-related interruptions in treatment
- Decreasing morbidity related to disease/treatment
- Maintaining or improving functional ability
- Maintaining or improving quality of life

As noted previously, nutrition management strategies for patients struggling to consume adequate oral intake or facing other short-term and long-term issues, such as diarrhea, xerostomia, or mucositis, are found in Table 13.5.

Nutritional Requirements of Individuals with Cancer

Adequate intake of energy, protein, and micronutrients can improve nutritional status for most patients with cancer (28). The nutrition principles outlined by the American Cancer Society's guidelines on diet, nutrition, and cancer prevention should be used for the basis of a healthy diet for all patients with cancer, including those who are well nourished, during and after treatment (1).

Energy

The impact of cancer on energy needs is inconsistent. Resting energy expenditure (REE) has been found unchanged, increased, or decreased in comparison to predicted needs (28). The European Society for Parenteral and Enteral Nutrition (ESPEN) has generally recommended the following energy estimates when REE cannot be measured directly, although ESPEN states that these recommendations are less accurate for individuals who are underweight (33):

- 30 to 35 kcal/kg body weight per day for ambulatory patients
- 20 to 25 kcal/kg body weight per day for bedridden patients

Protein

Protein metabolism is altered with cancer, and protein needs typically increase with treatment because of the stress and cellular damage that commonly occur with therapies, particularly radiation. In general, protein requirements for nonstressed cancer patients are thought to be 1 to 1.5 g/kg/d, and individuals with elevated protein needs due to hypermetabolism or protein-losing enteropathy should receive 1.5 to 2.5 g/kg/d (34).

Micronutrients

Individuals with cancer may be at risk of micronutrient deficiencies due to poor intake, increased requirements, and increased nutrient losses. Unfortunately, specific guidelines are not available. The Tolerable Upper Intake Levels (ULs) of the Dietary Reference Intakes should not be exceeded unless some objective data indicate a need for a greater intake to facilitate repletion.

Selected Nutrition Interventions

Immune-Enhancing Formulas

Several investigators have assessed the preoperative and perioperative impact on clinical outcomes of immune-enhancing formulas (arginine, omega-3 fatty acids, and nucleotides) vs standard formulas (35–40). Compared with standard care, the preoperative and perioperative use of the specialty formulas was associated with a significant reduction in postoperative infections. The mean length of hospitalization was also significantly shorter for patients receiving both the pre- and perioperative immune-enhancing formulas, and inflammatory markers such as C-reactive protein and interleukin-6 have been reduced with the use of these products. In a prospective, randomized double-blind clinical trial, perioperative consumption of immunonutrition reportedly reduced infectious complications in well-nourished patients with colorectal, stomach, or pancreatic cancer (40).

Clinical practice guidelines by both the American Society for Parenteral and Enteral Nutrition (A.S.P.E.N.) (41) and ESPEN (33) recommend the *perioperative* use of such formulations for patients undergoing elective surgeries (including for cancer) and critically ill patients to achieve favorable clinical outcomes (Grade A from both societies). However, further study is warranted before the use of immune-enhancing formulas can be recommended on a more global basis.

Nutritional Supplements

The strategies for maintaining adequate oral intake depend on the challenges experienced by the individual (see Table 13.5, earlier in this chapter). Aggressive management of symptoms has been found to not only improve/maintain nutritional status but also enhance quality of life and social interactions (42–44). The use of commercially prepared nutritional supplements has resulted in increased weight gain and reduced incidence of postoperative complications in patients undergoing surgery for GI cancers (45).

The omega-3 fatty acid EPA has been associated with an anti-inflammatory response, including downregulation of both proinflammatory cytokine synthesis and the acute phase response in both healthy individuals and patients with cancer. In some clinical trials (35,46,47), nutritional supplements enriched with EPA have been found to reverse weight loss, increase lean body mass, and improve quality of life and survival. For example, in the Fearon et al study, patients with GI cancers who received EPA experienced a significant increase in body weight compared to participants who received a placebo (47). However, other studies (34,48,49) have found no improvements associated with use of EPA. A.S.P.E.N.'s clinical practice guidelines for nutrition support during adult anticancer treatment give a Grade B recommendation to the use of omega-3 fatty acid supplements in cancer patients consuming oral diets and exhibiting continued unintentional weight loss (50). It seems that consumption of 2 g of EPA per day is necessary to obtain any benefit from supplementation; higher doses do not seem to confer additional benefits.

Nutrition Support

Nutrition support should be considered when oral nutritional intake is insufficient to maintain nutritional status or is contraindicated. The time at which nutrition support should be instituted for patients with cancer is controversial. Few studies have found any statistically significant difference in clinical endpoints (postoperative complications or mortality rates) between patients receiving nutrition support (PN or enteral tube feeding) and those who did not (50).

According to the A.S.P.E.N. clinical guidelines for nutrition support during anticancer treatment, current available evidence does not show that the routine use of any nutrition support therapy for all patients undergoing major surgery for cancer improves clinical outcomes. There have been no documented benefits associated with routine use in terms of reductions in morbidity and mortality (50). A.S.P.E.N. clinical guidelines recommend that specialized nutrition support should be initiated for patients with an inadequate oral intake for 7 to 14 days or in patients in whom inadequate oral intake is expected for a 7- to 14-day period (41).

ENTERAL NUTRITION

Enteral nutrition (EN) should be considered for patients unable to consume adequate oral nutrition when the GI tract can be safely used. When specialized nutrition support is warranted and the GI tract is functional and available, EN is clearly preferred over parenteral nutrition (PN). A meta-analysis of 27 prospective randomized controlled studies investigating the use of early enteral nutrition in hospitalized patients with a variety of medical conditions, including surgical oncology patients, found a significant reduction in hospital length of stay and infectious complications with early EN (51).

EN is also associated with positive clinical measures such as earlier reduction in inflammatory markers such as C-reactive protein levels, and shorter duration of nutrition support (52–54). Clinical practice guidelines recommend that EN should be initiated within 24 to 48 hours after injury or hospital admission to gain these positive clinical outcomes (41).

PARENTERAL NUTRITION

The A.S.P.E.N. clinical guidelines for nutrition support during adult anticancer treatment support the perioperative use of PN for severely malnourished patients with cancer (50). Parenteral nutrition for patients receiving chemotherapy with or without radiation can result in increased weight and body fat mass, correction of vitamin and mineral deficiencies, and improved hydration (50). The A.S.P.E.N. guidelines suggest that PN should not be routinely used in all patients (41,50). In summary:

- PN should not be routinely administered to cancer patients undergoing chemotherapy, radiation, or surgery (50).
- PN should be considered only in patients who are moderately to severely malnourished and unable to tolerate EN or oral diet for at least 1 week.
- Perioperative PN may be indicated for moderately to severely malnourished patients in whom surgery may safely be delayed 7 to 14 days and when EN is not possible (41,50).
- Lastly, PN is recommended for individuals with severe mucositis, ileus, or intractable vomiting following hematopoietic stem cell transplantation (50).

NUTRITION SUPPORT IN ALTERNATIVE CARE SITES AND HOME CARE

Nutrition support, especially EN, is widely used in long-term care, hospice, and other alternative care sites (52). The A.S.P.E.N. guidelines for the provision of home nutrition support stress the importance of in-depth nutrition assessment; assessment of the patient's home environment; evaluation of his or her medical suitability for EN or PN, education level, and rehabilitative potential; and the need for close evaluation of reimbursement sources prior to making a decision about home nutrition support (41,55). PN or EN should be terminated when the patient no longer benefits from the therapy or the burden exceeds the benefit (44,50). PN may prolong survival for patients with cancer (primarily ovarian and gastric) but at the expense of greater incidence of overall and infectious complications (56). For additional information on home enteral and parenteral nutrition, refer to Chapter 22.

Nutrition and Specific GI Cancers

Head and Neck Cancer

Malnutrition plays a key role in the morbidity of head and neck cancer patients receiving surgery, chemotherapy, radiotherapy, or combined modality therapy. Weight loss prior to diagnosis of head and neck cancer is common (57). Following diagnosis, an additional 10% of pretherapy body weight may be lost during radiotherapy or combined-modality treatment (57). A reduction of more than 20% of total body weight results in an increase in toxicity and mortality (14). Severe treatment-related toxicities can result in prolonged treatment times because of poor nutritional status, and prolonged treatment time has been implicated in poor clinical outcome. Swallowing function is also commonly adversely affected by treatment. Severe mucositis and neutropenia are also common sequelae of chemoradiation.

Individualized nutrition counseling has been shown to effectively increase dietary intake, maintain or improve nutritional and functional status, and improve quality of life in patients undergoing radiotherapy with a variety of head and neck cancers (58).

Gastrostomy (G-tubes) or percutaneous endoscopic gastrostomy (PEG) tubes are frequently used for the provision of nutrition (57). Estimates of the percentage of patients who must depend on enteral nutrition support for 6 to 12 months following surgical, radiotherapy, and/or chemotherapy interventions vary from 6% to 64% (59,60). At long-term (≥1 year) follow-up after chemoradiation, patients without recurrence of cancer typically had at least some oral intake, but one-third still required supplemental enteral support due to chronic dysphagia.

Esophageal Cancer

Although esophageal cancer is relatively uncommon compared to other types of cancer (approximately 16,470 new cases in 2009), incidence of adenocarcinoma of the esophagus is increasing, with these tumors primarily being located in the distal esophagus (61). Unfortunately, the prognosis for individuals with esophageal cancer is poor, with a 5-year survival rate ranging from 10% to 13% (61). According to the National Cancer Institute, routine screening for esophageal cancers would not decrease mortality associated with esophageal cancer in the United States (61).

Esophageal cancer affects men more than women, and white people are at increased risk compared with other racial groups. Risk factors for esophageal cancer include the following:

- Tobacco and alcohol use
- Obesity
- Barrett's esophagus (which is associated with persistent gastric acid reflux)
- Diet

Dietary factors that may increase risk include the following (62):

- Consuming foods high in N-nitroso compounds
- Ingestion of very hot foods and beverages
- Diets low in fruits and vegetables

Zinc deficiency has also been noted as a potential risk factor (63).

Diets high in cereal fiber, beta-carotene, vitamin C, folate, and vitamin B-6 have been cited as possible protective agents (62). Aspirin and other NSAIDS may provide protective benefits as well.

Patients with esophageal cancer should be screened for presence of malnutrition (32) and reassessed at established time points for re-evaluation. An estimated 57% to 69% of patients with esophageal cancer experience malnutrition (61).

Esophageal obstruction, dysphagia, anorexia, and the side effects of treatment modalities (such as severe mucositis and vomiting) often affect nutritional status in this patient population (28). Progressive dysphagia resulting in weight loss affects more than 10% of patients prior to diagnosis (64). Early signs of esophageal cancer can also include complaints of food "sticking" in the throat, retrosternal discomfort, or a burning sensation.

EN is often necessary for patients with esophageal cancer due to the frequency of severe dysphagia or luminal obstruction. In a study of 50 malnourished esophageal cancer patients, Bozzetti et al concluded that the body weight and serum proteins of the 29 patients who received EN stabilized, while 21 patients who received standard oral diets continued to experience deteriorations in both weight and serum proteins (65). A.S.P.E.N. recommends the use of perioperative nutrition support for moderately to severely malnourished patients, including patients with esophageal cancer, if administered for 7 to 14 days preoperatively (50).

Gastric Cancer

Gastric cancer is the 14th most commonly diagnosed cancer in the United States; more than 21,000 cases of gastric cancer are diagnosed annually, and approximately 10,000 deaths are caused each year by this type of cancer. Incidence in the United States is relatively low, but gastric cancer is the fourth leading cause of cancer deaths worldwide, with particularly high rates in Asia and South America (66). Individuals older than 65 years are the most likely to be diagnosed. The most common type of gastric cancer (>90% of cases) is adenocarcinoma.

Risk factors for gastric cancer include the following:

- Genetic factors (Asian descent) and environmental factors (smoking)
- Dietary factors, such as:
  - A diet high in salted, smoked foods; N-nitroso compounds; or processed and red meats; alcohol intake
  - Low intake of fruits and vegetables (66)
  - Low vitamin A intake (66)

Chronic superficial gastritis and gastric atrophy are thought to play a role in the progression to gastric cancer (66–68). Chronic gastritis caused by chronic *H. pylori* infection and pernicious anemia results in chronic atrophic gastritis and intestinal metaplasia (68). Metaplasia and dysplasia progress to gastric carcinoma in 21% to 57% of the cases (68). In the Japanese population, a higher prevalence of *H. pylori* correlates with a higher salt intake (69).

Signs and symptoms of gastric cancer include malnutrition (with anorexia reportedly experienced by approximately two-thirds of patients diagnosed), as well as abdominal pain, anemia, and nausea and vomiting (reported in 66%, 42%, and 32% of patients, respectively) (32).

Gastric resection is associated with an increased risk for morbidity, depending on the disease state and type of resection needed (67). The presence and type of disease dictates whether a small portion of the stomach must be removed vs a total gastrectomy. Whether a Billroth I (anastomosis of the esophagus or the remaining stomach to the duodenum) or a Billroth II (anastomosis of the esophagus or remaining stomach to the jejunum) is done, the patient's ability to consume adequate oral nutrition postoperatively is affected.

After gastric surgery, dumping syndrome is common, especially when the pylorus is either removed or bypassed. Dumping syndrome occurs when the food passes through the GI tract quickly without being significantly absorbed. It includes symptoms such as abdominal cramping, diarrhea, sweating, nausea, dizziness, and tachycardia (69). Symptoms usually appear within 30 to 60 minutes of eating or 2 to 3 hours after eating.

Dietary modifications to help combat these symptoms include the following:

- Eating small frequent bland and low-fat meals
- Avoiding spicy foods, alcohol, and sugar and sweets
- Avoiding very hot or cold foods
- Limiting fluids to 4 ounces during meals and instead drinking liquids 30 to 45 minutes before and after eating

Some nutrients, vitamins, and minerals may be poorly absorbed, with subsequent deficiencies in iron, calcium, folate, and vitamin B-12. To avoid or correct deficiencies, patients may need liquid or chewable multivitamin/multimineral supplements and vitamin B-12 shots.

Small Bowel Cancers

Small bowel cancers are extremely rare (slightly more than 6,000 cases diagnosed annually) (70). The most common type diagnosed is adenocarcinoma. Other types include sarcoma, carcinoid tumors, and lymphoma, which account for between 1% and 2% of all GI cancers (70). The 5-year survival rate varies between 20% for resectable adenocarcinomas and 50% for leiomyosarcoma tumors (70).

The treatment modalities for other types of GI cancers previously discussed are also used for the treatment of small bowel cancers. Surgery is the most common when resection of the tumor is possible.

Pancreatic Cancer

Pancreatic cancer is the fourth leading cause of cancer death in the United States, Canada, and Western Europe, with approximately 42,000 cases diagnosed annually in the United States and 35,000 US deaths (71). Pancreatic cancer is rare in individuals younger than the age of 45 years; however, rates increase sharply thereafter, with men affected more often than women. Compared with other racial groups, African Americans are at increased risk (71). Risk factors for pancreatic cancer also include the following:

- A first-degree relative with a history of the disease. Between 5% and 10% of pancreatic cancers are thought to occur in individuals with a first-degree relative who has had pancreatic cancer.
- Smoking.
- Hereditary chronic pancreatitis and other inherited cancer-susceptibility syndromes.

- Diabetes mellitus, alterations in glucose metabolism, and insulin resistance. In a meta-analysis by Everhart and Wright, the pooled relative risk (RR) for pancreatic cancer in individuals with diabetes (predominantly type 2) compared to patients without diabetes was estimated to be 2.1 (95% CI 1.6–2.8) (72).
- Excess body fat (body mass index [BMI] >30). In the Nurses' Health Study and the Health Professionals Follow-up Study, BMI >30 was significantly associated with a greater risk for pancreatic cancer when compared with BMI <23 (73).
- Tall height.
- Lower levels of physical activity.

Some, but not all, studies have found that increased risk of pancreatic cancer is associated with consumption of a Western-style diet that is high in fat and/or meat. Both coffee and alcohol exposure have been investigated as risk factors, and neither has been associated with increased risk (74). Lastly, the potential association between serum vitamin D levels and pancreatic cancer risk has been evaluated in case-control studies (75,76). However, more research is needed before public health recommendations about vitamin D can be made.

The most common treatment options for pancreatic cancer are chemotherapy and radiation. Tumor resection with curative intent is possible in only 10% to 15% of subjects, with many patients facing limited therapeutic options and a poor prognosis (71).

At diagnosis, many patients with pancreatic cancer present with significant weight loss (10% to 15% of pre-illness weight). A median loss of 25% of pre-illness weight by time of death has been reported (71). Such weight loss is associated with impairments in functional status and worse outcomes. Reduced intake is caused by a number of factors, including nausea, pain, anxiety, depression, and gastric outlet obstruction (77). Malabsorption and altered glucose tolerance further complicate nutritional status. Nutrition interventions are not likely to extend the survival of a patient with advanced, progressive pancreatic cancer but may have a role in palliative care and improvement in quality of life (77,78).

Malabsorption should be suspected in the face of continued weight loss and the presence of abdominal symptoms (eg, bloating, abdominal pain, greasy stools). Pancreatic enzymes should be prescribed when malabsorption is diagnosed. Enzymes are typically dosed based on lipase content (79). See Chapter 13 for more information on the use of pancreatic enzymes.

Malabsorption also typically leads to vitamin and mineral deficiencies. Absorption of vitamins A, D, E, and K is dependent on fat absorption; vitamin B-12 absorption relies on the presence of protease enzymes. Iron, calcium, vitamin B-12, and vitamin D deficiencies can occur when proton pump inhibitors are prescribed. Whipple procedures can result in deficiencies of calcium, zinc, and iron (80). Guidelines for providing vitamin and mineral supplements to patients with pancreatic cancer are lacking. Supplementation needs are likely to vary depending on the severity of malabsorption. Trace element deficiencies have been documented in patients with chronic pancreatitis and may occur in those with pancreatic cancer (79).

A multivitamin supplement with the fat-soluble vitamins provided as water-soluble components is recommended. The use of omega-3 fatty acid supplements has been investigated in this patient population with mixed results. The A.S.P.E.N. clinical practice guidelines recommend using omega-3 fatty acid supplements in the face of progressive unintentional weight loss (50).

Patient compliance with the nutrition prescription seems to improve outcomes in patients with unresectable pancreatic cancers (80). Nutrition support should be reserved for patients who are moderately to severely malnourished and when the benefits outweigh the harm.

Large Bowel Cancers

Colorectal cancers, the third most common type of cancer worldwide (accounting for approximately 9% of US cancer deaths annually), start primarily from adenomatous polyps, which may take a decade or more to become cancers (81). While large bowel cancers are influenced by genetic factors, colon cancer is more common in Westernized countries than in developing countries and is thought to be strongly influenced by lifestyle factors (81). In the United States, an estimated 70% of deaths resulting from colon cancers could be prevented by diet modifications. Commonly cited risk factors include the following (81):

- Family history (particularly of familial adenomatous polyposis and hereditary nonpolyposis colon cancer)
- Personal or family history of breast, ovarian, or endometrial cancers; adenomatous polyps
- Inflammatory bowel disease (chronic ulcerative colitis or Crohn's disease)
- Coronary heart disease
- Cholecystecotmy
- Ureterocolic anastomosis
- Obesity
- Systemic inflammation
- Diabetes and insulin resistance
- Age (colon cancer is rare before the age of 40 years)
- Sedentary lifestyle
- Smoking

The World Cancer Research Fund (WCRF) and the American Institute for Cancer Research (AICR) have concluded that red and processed meats, alcoholic drinks in men, body fatness, abdominal fatness, and adult-attained height are strong risk factors for colorectal cancer (74).

The role of the nutrition, particularly dietary fat, in chemoprevention for colon cancer has been examined by a number of investigators. A recent meta-analysis by Alexander et al found no statistically significant associations between animal fat intake and colorectal cancers (82). As described by the investigators, only data from the Nurses' Health Study showed that the risk for colon cancer increased as the intake of animal fat increased (83).

Epidemiologic studies have noted that fruit and vegetable intake is associated with a lower risk of colorectal cancer (84,85). However, the Nurses' Health Study and the Healthy Professionals Follow-up Study found no significant association between fruit and vegetable intake and colorectal cancer risk (86).

Risk can be decreased by increased physical activity and by increasing foods that contain fiber and calcium. Milk and garlic consumption are also associated with decreased risk (74).

Magnesium, vitamin D, folic acid, and selenium have been investigated for playing a potential role in colorectal cancer. Although magnesium and vitamin D may reduce the risk for colorectal cancer, the evidence has been inconsistent to date. According to the WCRF and AICR, there is limited evidence that foods containing folic acid protect against colorectal cancer (74). Furthermore, Mason (86) has concluded that supplemented folic acid may *promote* colon cancer in individuals with colon polyps.

O'Keefe and colleagues have hypothesized that modifying the interactions between diet and the colon microbiota can influence colorectal cancer risk, specifically through the regulation of butyrate (87). Butyrate has potent anti-inflammatory and antiproliferative properties that may confer antineoplastic benefits (88,89).

Postoperatively, most individuals advance to an oral diet fairly quickly and safely (90,91). EN or PN may be indicated for certain colon cancer patients with severe malnutrition and, in the latter case, inability to use the GI tract for nutrition support. Routine use of PN in patients with colon cancer has not been shown to be beneficial and is not recommended (92,93).

Conclusion

Cancer is expected to become the number 1 cause of death in the United States, and many malignancies are thought to be preventable. Multiple lifestyle factors, including tobacco and alcohol use, unhealthy diet, excess body weight, and lack of regular physical activity, have been identified as risk factors. Basic lifestyle changes can therefore have a significant impact on modifying one's risk.

Medical nutrition therapy plays an essential role in maintaining or improving the nutritional status of cancer survivors. Nutrition screening identifies patients at high risk for nutritional deterioration or who experience malnutrition. Many anticancer therapies are associated with a number of treatment-related toxicities that have a profound impact on nutritional status. Such treatment-related toxicities should be aggressively treated to maintain or improve nutritional status as well as quality of life. For additional information on medical nutrition therapy for cancer patients, readers are encouraged to review the Academy of Nutrition and Dietetics Oncology Nutrition Evidence-Based Nutrition Practice Guideline (http://andevidencelibrary.com).

References

1. American Cancer Society. www.cancer.org. Accessed January 16, 2010.
2. Jemal A, Murray T, Ward E, et al. Cancer statistics, 2005. *CA Cancer J Clin*. 2005;55:10–30.
3. American Cancer Society. *Cancer Facts & Figures 2009*. Atlanta, GA: American Cancer Society; 2009.
4. Khan N, Afaq F, Mukhtar H. Lifestyle as risk factor for cancer: evidence from human studies. *Cancer Letter*. 2010;293(2):133–143.
5. Kraus S, Arber N. Inflammation and colorectal cancer. *Curr Opin Pharmacol*. 2009;9:405–410.
6. Buc E, Kwiatkowski F, Alves A, Panis Y, Mantion G, Slim K. Tobacco smoking: a factor of early onset of colorectal cancer. *Dis Colon Rectum*. 2006;49:1893–1896.
7. Khan N, Afaq H, Hukhtar H. Cancer chemoprevention through dietary antioxidants: progress and promise. *Antioxid Redox Signal*. 2008;10:475–510.
8. Kim YS, Young MR, Bobe G, Colburn NH, Milner JA. Bioactive food components, inflammatory targets, and cancer prevention. *Cancer Prev Res*. 2009;2(3):200–208.
9. Surh YJ. Cancer chemoprevention with dietary phytochemical. *Nat Rev Cancer*. 2003;3:768–780.
10. Khan N, Adhami VM, Mukhtar H. Apoptosis by dietary agents for prevention and treatment of cancer. *Biochem Pharmacol*. 2008;76:1333–1339.
11. Vegetables, fruits, pulses (legumes), nuts, seeds, herbs, spices. In: World Cancer Research Fund/American Institute of Cancer Research. *Food, Nutrition, Physical Activity, and the Prevention of Cancer: A Global Perspective*. Washington, DC: AICR; 2007:75–115.
12. Warren S. The immediate cause of death in cancer. *Am J Med Sci*. 1932;185:610.
13. Copeland EM. Nutrition as an adjunct to cancer treatment in the adult. *Cancer Res*. 1977;37:2451–2456.
14. DeWys WD, Begg C, Llavin PT, et al. Prognostic effect of weight loss prior to chemotherapy in cancer patients. *Am J Med*. 1980;69:491–497.
15. Tisdale MJ. Mechanisms of cancer cachexia. *Physiol Rev*. 2009;89:381–410.
16. Monitto CL, Berkowitz D, Lee KM, et al. Differential gene expression in a murine model of cancer cachexia. *Am J Physiol Endocrinol Metab*. 2001;281:E289–E297.

17. Barber MD. The pathophysiology and treatment of cancer cachexia. *Nutr Clin Pract.* 2002;17:203–209.
18. Houten L, Reilly AA. An investigation of the cause of death from cancer. *J Surg Oncol.*1989;13:111–116.
19. Wisse BE, Schwartz MW. Role of melanocortins in control of obesity. *Lancet.* 2001;358(99285):857–859.
20. Bosaeus I. Nutritional support in multimodal therapy for cancer cachexia. *Support Care Cancer.* 2008;16:447–451.
21. Madeddu C, Mantovani G. An update on promising agents for the treatment of cancer cachexia. *Curr Opin Support Palliat Care.* 2009;3(4):258–262.
22. Loprinzi CL, Schaid DJ, Dose AM, Burnham NL, Jensen MD. Body-composition changes in patients who gain weight while receiving megestrol acetate. *J Clin Oncol.* 1993;11:152.
23. Whitehouse AS, Tisdale MJ. Increased expression of the ubiquitin-proteasome pathway in murine myotubes by proteolysis-inducing factor (PIF) is associated with activation of the transcription factor NF-$_K$B. *Br J Cancer.* 2003;89:1116–1122.
24. Russell ST, Tisdale MJ. Effect of eicosapentaenoic acid (EPA) on expression of a lipid mobilizing factor in adipose tissue in cancer cachexia. *Prostaglandins Leukot Essent Fatty Acids.* 2005;72:409–414.
25. Barber MD, Ross JA, Voss AC, Tisdale MJ, Fearon KCH. The effect of an oral nutritional supplement enriched with fish oil on weight-loss in patients with pancreatic cancer. *Br J Cancer.* 1999;81:80–86.
26. Smith HJ, Wyke SM, Tisdale MJ. Mechanism of the attenuation of proteolysis-inducing factor stimulated protein degradation in muscle by β-hydroxy-β-methylbutyrate. *Cancer Res.* 2004;64:8731–8735.
27. May PE, Barber A, D'Olimpio JT, Hourihane A, Abumrad NN. Reversal of cancer-related wasting using oral supplementation with a combination of β-hydroxy-β-methylbutyrate, arginine and glutamine. *Am J Surg.* 2002;183:471–479.
28. Brown J, Byers T, Thompson K, et al. Nutrition during and after cancer treatment: a guide for informed choices by cancer survivors. *CA Cancer J Clin.* 2001;51:153–181.
29. Blackburn GL, Bistrian BR, Maini BS, et al. Nutritional and metabolic assessment of the hospitalized patient. *JPEN J Parenter Enteral Nutr.* 1977;1(1):11–22.
30. National Cancer Institute. Common Toxicity Criteria. http://ctep.cancer.gov/protocoldevelopment/electronic _applications/docs/ctcv20_4-30-992.pdf. Accessed March 17, 2010.
31. Inui A. Cancer anorexia-cachexia syndrome: are neuropeptides the key? *Cancer Res.* 1999;59:4493–4501.
32. Langer CJ, Hoffman JP, Ottery FD. Clinical significance of weight loss in cancer patients: rationale for the use of anabolic agents in the treatment of cancer-related cachexia. *Nutrition.* 2001;17(1 Suppl):S1–S20.
33. European Society for Parenteral and Enteral Nutrition (ESPEN). Guidelines on Enteral Nutrition: Surgery Including Organ Transplantation. www.espen.org. Accessed December 4, 2009.
34. Hurst JD, Gallagher AI. Energy, macronutrient, micronutrient, and fluid requirements. In: Elliot L, Molseed LI, McCallum PD, ed. *The Clinical Guide to Oncology Nutrition.* 2nd ed. Chicago, IL: American Dietetic Association; 2006:54–71.
35. Ryan AM, Reynolds JV, Healy L, et al. Enteral nutrition enriched with eicosapentaenoic acid (EPA) preserves lean body mass following esophageal cancer surgery: results of a double-blinded randomized controlled trial. *Ann Surg.* 2009;249(3):355–363.
36. Giger U, Büchler M, Farhadi J, et al. Preoperative immunonutrition suppresses perioperative inflammatory response in patients with major abdominal surgery: a randomized controlled pilot study. *Ann Surg Oncol.* 2007;14(10):2798–2806.
37. Lobo DN, Williams RN, Welch NT, et al. Early postoperative jejunostomy feeding with an immune modulating diet in patients undergoing resectional surgery for upper gastrointestinal cancer: a prospective, randomized, controlled, double-blind study. *Clin Nutr.* 2006;25(5):716–726.
38. Wu GH, Liu ZH, Wu ZH, et al. Perioperative artificial nutrition in malnourished gastrointestinal cancer patients. *World J Gastroenterol.* 2006;12(15):2441–2444.
39. Braga M, Gianotti L, Nespoli L, et al. Nutritional approach in malnourished surgical patients: a prospective randomized study. *Arch Surg.* 2002;137:174–180.
40. Braga M, Gianotti L, Radaelli G, et al. Perioperative immunonutrition in patients undergoing cancer surgery: results of a randomized double-blind phase 3 trial. *Arch Surg.* 1999;134:428–433.

41. McClave SM, Martindale RG, Vanek VW, et al. Guidelines for the provision and assessment of nutrition support therapy in the adult critically ill patient: Society for Critical Care Medicine (SCCM) and American Society for Parenteral and Enteral Nutrition (A.S.P.E.N.). *JPEN J Parenter Enteral Nutr.* 2009;33(3):277–316.

42. Nitenberg G, Raynard B. Nutritional support of the cancer patient: issues and dilemmas. *Crit Rev Oncol Hematol.* 2000;34:137–168.

43. Clifford C, Kramer B. Diet as risk and therapy for cancer. *Med Clin N Am.* 1993;77:725–744.

44. Grindel CG, Whitmer K, Barsevick A. Quality of life and nutritional support in patients with cancer. *Cancer Pract.* 1996;4:81–87.

45. Keele AM, Bray MJ, Emery PW, et al. Two phase randomised controlled clinical trial of postoperative oral dietary supplements in surgical patients. *Gut.* 1997;40:393–399.

46. Barber MD, Ross JA, Preston T, et al. Fish oil-enriched nutritional supplement attenuates progression of the acute phase response in weight-losing patients with advanced pancreatic cancer. *J Nutr.* 1999;129:1120–1125.

47. Fearon KC, Barber MD, Moses AG, et al. Double-blind, placebo-controlled, randomized study of eicosapentaenoic acid diester in patients with cancer cachexia. *J Clin Oncol.* 2006;24:3401–3407.

48. Bruera E, Strasser F, Palmer JL, et al. Effect of fish oil on appetite and other symptoms in patients with advanced cancer and anorexia/cachexia: a double-blind, placebo-controlled study. *J Clin Oncol.* 2003;21(1):129–134.

49. Jatoi A, Towland K, Loprinzi CL, et al. An eicosapentaenoic acid supplement versus megestrol acetate versus both for patients with cancer-associated wasting: a North Central Cancer Treatment Group and National Cancer Institute of Canada collaborative effort. *J Clin Oncol.* 2004;22(12):2469–2476.

50. August DA, Huhmann MB. A.S.P.E.N. Clinical Guidelines: nutrition support therapy during adult anticancer treatment and in hematopoietic cell transplantation. American Society for Parenteral and Enteral Nutrition (A.S.P.E.N.) Board of Directors. *JPEN J Parenter Enteral Nutr.* 2009;33(5):472–500.

51. Marik PE, Zaloga GP. Early EN in acutely ill patients: a systematic review. *Crit Care Med.* 2001;29:2264–2270.

52. Wu GH, Zhang YW, Wu ZH. Modulation of postoperative immune and inflammatory response by immune-enhancing enteral diet in gastrointestinal cancer patients. *World J Gastroenterol.* 2001;7:357–362.

53. Magnotti LJ, Deitch EA. Burns, bacterial translocation, gut barrier function, and failure. *J Burn Care Rehabil.* 2005;26:383–391.

54. Abou-Assi S, Craig K, O'Keefe SJ. Hypocaloric jejunal feeding is better than total parenteral nutrition in acute pancreatitis. *Am J Gastroenterol.* 2002;97:2255–2262.

55. Kovacevich DS, Frederick A, Kelly D, et al. Standards for specialized nutrition support: home care patient. *Nutr Clin Pract.* 2005;20(5):579–590.

56. Chermesh I, Mashiach T, Amit A, et al. Home parenteral nutrition (HTPN) for incurable patients with cancer with gastrointestinal obstruction: do the benefits outweigh the risks? *Med Oncol.* 2011;28(1):83–88.

57. Capuano G, Gentile PC, Bianciardi F, et al. Prevalence and influence of malnutrition on quality of life and performance status in patients with locally advanced head and neck cancer before treatment. *Support Care Cancer.* 2010;18(4):433–437.

58. Isenring E, Capra S, Bauer J, Davies PS. The impact of nutrition support on body composition in cancer outpatients receiving radiotherapy. *Acta Diabetol.* 2003;40(Suppl 1):S162–S164.

59. Raykher A, Russo L, Schattner M, et al. Enteral nutrition support of head and neck cancer patients. *Nutr Clin Pract.* 2007;22:68–73.

60. Lawson JD, Gaultney J, Saba N, et al. Percutaneous feeding tubes in patients with head and neck cancer: rethinking prophylactic placement for patients undergoing chemoradiation. *Am J Otolaryngol.* 2009;30(4):244–249.

61. National Cancer Institute. Esophageal cancer. www.cancer.gov/cancertopics/types/esophageal. Accessed March 17, 2010.

62. Sampliner RD. Epidemiology, pathobiology, and clinical manifestations of esophageal cancer. www.uptodate.com. Accessed February 12, 2010.

63. Limburg PJ, Wei W, Ahnen DJ, et al. Randomized, placebo-controlled, esophageal squamous cell cancer chemoprevention trial of selenomethionine and celecoxib. *Gastroenterology*. 2005;129(2):863–873.

64. Ryan AM, Rowley SP, Healy LA, et al. Post-oesophagectomy early enteral nutrition via a needle catheter jejunostomy: 8-year experience at a specialist unit. *Clin Nutr*. 2006;25:386–393.

65. Bozzetti F, Cozzaglio L, Gavazzi C, et al. Nutritional support in patients with cancer of the esophagus: impact on nutritional status, patient compliance to therapy, and survival. *Tumori*. 1998;84:681–686.

66. National Cancer Institute. Stomach (Gastric) Cancer Screening (PDQ). www.cancer.gov. Accessed March 1, 2010.

67. Chan AOO, Wong BCY. Risk factors for gastric cancer. www.utdol.com/online/content/topic.do. Accessed February 28, 2010.

68. Ito M, Haruma K, Kamada T, et al. Helicobacter pylori eradication therapy improves atrophic gastritis and intestinal metaplasia: a 5-year prospective study of patients with atrophic gastritis. *Aliment Pharmacol Ther*. 2002;16(8):1449–1456.

69. Rugge M, Farinati F, Baffa R, et al. Gastric epithelial dysplasia in the natural history of gastric cancer: a multicenter prospective follow-up study. Interdisciplinary Group on Gastric Epithelial Dysplasia. *Gastroenterology*. 1994;107(5):1228–1296.

70. National Cancer Institute. Small Intestinal Cancer. www.cancer.gov/cancertopics/types/smallintestine. Accessed March 17, 2010.

71. National Cancer Institute. Pancreatic Cancer. www.cancer.gov/cancertopics/types/pancreatic. Accessed March 4, 2010.

72. Everhart J, Wright D. Diabetes mellitus as a risk factor for pancreatic cancer. A meta-analysis. *JAMA*. 1995;273(20):1605–1609.

73. Michaud DS, Giovannucci E, Willett WC, et al. Physical activity, obesity, height, and the risk of pancreatic cancer. *JAMA*. 2001;286(8):921–929.

74. Cancers—Pancreas. In: World Cancer Research Fund/American Institute for Cancer Research. *Food, Nutrition, Physical Activity, and the Prevention of Cancer: a Global Perspective*. Washington, DC: American Institute for Cancer Research, 2007:271–276.

75. Skinner HG, Michaud DS, Giovannucci E, et al. Vitamin D intake and the risk for pancreatic cancer in two cohort studies. *Cancer Epidemiol Biomark Prev*. 2006;15:1688–1695.

76. Stolzenberg-Solomon RZ, Vieth R, et al. A prospective nested case-control study of vitamin D status and pancreatic cancer risk in male smokers. *Cancer Res*. 2006;66:10213–10219.

77. Ellisom NM, Chevlen E, Still C, Dubagunta S. Supportive care for patients with pancreatic adenocarcinoma: symptom control and nutrition. *Hematol Oncol Clin N Am*. 2002;16:105–121.

78. Brennan MF, Pfisters PW, Posner M, Quesada O, Shike M. A prospective randomized trial of total parenteral nutrition after major pancreatic resection for malignancy. *Ann Surg*. 1994;220:436–441.

79. Ottery F. Supportive nutritional management of the patient with pancreatic cancer. *Oncology*. 1996;9(Suppl):26–32.

80. Bauer J, Capra S, Battistutta D, Davidson W, Ash S. Compliance with nutrition prescription improves outcomes in patients with unresectable pancreatic cancer. *Clin Nutr*. 2005;24(6):998–1004.

81. Ahnen DJ, Macrae FA. Colorectal cancer: epidemiology, risk factors, and protective factors. www.utdol.com/online/content/topic.do.

82. Alexander DD, Cushing CA, Lowe KA, Sceurman B, Roberts MA. Meta-analysis of animal fat or animal protein intake and colorectal cancer. *Am J Clin Nutr*. 2009;89:1402–1409.

83. Willett WC, Stampfer MJ, Colditz GA, Rosner BA, Speizer FE. Relation of meat, fat, and fiber intake to the risk of colon cancer in a prospective study among women. *N Engl J Med*. 1990;323:1664–1672.

84. Slattery ML, Boucher KM, Caan BJ, et al. Eating patterns and risk of colon cancer. *Am J Epidemiol*. 1999;150(8):869–877.

85. Michels KB, Giovannucci E, Joshipura KJ, et al. Prospective study of fruit and vegetable consumption and incidence of colon and rectal cancers. *J Natl Cancer Inst*. 2000;92(21):1740–1752.

86. Mason JB. Folate, cancer risk, and the Greek god, Proteus: a tale of two chameleons. *Nutr Rev.* 2009;67(4):206–212.

87. O'Keefe SJD, Ou J, Aufreiter S, et al. Products of the colonic microbiota mediate the effects of diet on colon cancer risk. *J Nutr.* 2009;139:2044–2048.

88. Kim YS, Milner JA. Dietary modulation of colon cancer risk. *J Nutr.* 2007;137(suppl):S2576–S2579.

89. Nguyen KA, Cao Y, Chen JR, Townsend CM Jr, Ko TC. Dietary fiber enhances a tumor suppressor signaling pathway in the gut. *Ann Surg.* 2006;243:619–627.

90. Bufo A, Feldman S, Daniels G, Lieberman R. Early postoperative feeding. *Dis Colon Rectum.* 1994;37:1260–1265.

91. Reissman P, Teoh T, Cohen S, et al. Is early oral feeding safe after elective colorectal surgery? A prospective randomized trial. *Ann Surg.* 1995;222:73–77.

92. Fasth S, Hulten L, Magnusson O, Nordgren S, Warnold I. Postoperative complications in colorectal surgery in relation to preoperative clinical and nutritional state and postoperative nutritional treatment. *Int J Colorec Dis.* 1987;2:87–92.

93. Vitello J. Nutritional assessment and the role of preoperative parenteral nutrition in the colon cancer patient. *Semin Surg Oncol.* 1994;10:183–194.

CHAPTER 14

Gastrointestinal Tract Surgery

Gail A. Cresci, PhD, RD, CNSC

The nutritional needs of surgery patients vary depending on several factors, including the patient's disease process, other comorbidities, and baseline nutritional status. This chapter reviews recommendations for preoperative nutrition care of undernourished patients prior to gastrointestinal (GI) tract surgeries as well as issues related to nutrition care after such surgeries.

Preoperative Nutrition

Patients undergoing surgery of the GI tract often have suboptimal preoperative nutritional status as a result of the disease process that precedes the surgery (eg, cancer, obstruction). The patient's disease process may also cause a hypermetabolic state, placing the patient at nutritional risk. Preoperative malnutrition is associated with altered immune function, poor wound healing, and increased morbidity and mortality.

Ideally, a malnourished patient should be nutritionally repleted 7 to 10 days prior to surgery for optimal postoperative outcomes (1). Unless the GI tract is nonfunctional, nutrition should be provided enterally rather than parenterally (1).

Energy

Adequate energy should be provided, with carbohydrates comprising the majority of the calories (50%–60%) to supply sufficient glucose for optimal glycogen storage and to prevent lean muscle and adipose tissue catabolism (2).

Protein

Most surgical patients do not require extra protein before surgery, but their needs should be assessed individually. Patients who are nutritionally depleted have slightly elevated protein requirements and should be provided with adequate protein along with adequate total energy (2).

Micronutrients and Fluids

Any deficiency state, such as anemia, should be corrected. Electrolytes and fluids should be normalized and in balance; if the patient is dehydrated or has acidosis or alkalosis, these conditions should be resolved before surgery (2).

Postoperative Nutrition

The appropriate approach to postoperative nutrient provision will depend on the following factors:

- The surgical procedure performed and the anticipated time before the patient can resume oral intake
- Any complications of surgery and the patient's postoperative clinical status
- The patient's preoperative nutritional status

The well-nourished patient undergoing elective surgery will typically resume oral feeding by postoperative day 3 to 7. In this situation, nutrition therapy in the form of enteral or parenteral nutrition is not indicated.

If a malnourished patient is undergoing elective or emergent surgery and is not anticipated to meet his or her nutritional needs orally for 7 to 10 days, he or she should receive specialized nutrition support (1). If feasible, this nutrition therapy should be provided enterally rather than parenterally to minimize the incidence of complications. This nutrition therapy should be initiated within 24 to 48 hours after surgery, with advancement to goal amount of calories over the next 48 to 72 hours (1). The duration of the nutrition therapy will depend on the patient's clinical status and transition to adequate oral diet consumption and tolerance. See Chapters 19 and 20, respectively, for more information on enteral nutrition and parenteral nutrition.

In the immediate postoperative period, especially in the critically ill, the goal of nutrition therapy is to attempt to attenuate the metabolic response to stress, prevent oxidative cellular injury, and favorably modulate the immune response (1). Nutrition care includes providing appropriate macro- and micronutrients.

Energy

Energy requirements of surgical patients are generally higher postoperatively than preoperatively (see Table 14.1 on page 170) (2) and may be affected by complications such as infection, fever, sepsis, and wounds. These conditions alter metabolism and catabolism and thus elevate energy and protein requirements. If indirect calorimetry is not available to determine resting energy expenditure, predictive equations can be used for estimating energy requirements, but only a few have been validated (see Chapter 3 and 4). When it is not feasible to provide full energy requirements, efforts should be made to provide at least 50% to 65% of goal energy requirements to achieve the clinical benefits of nutrition therapy within the first week of surgery (1).

Protein

Postoperative patients have elevated protein requirements, particularly if they are critically ill (2). Reasons for increased requirements include increased catabolism and protein turnover and the need for tissue synthesis and wound healing. In critically ill patients, metabolic stress results in a loss of lean body mass,

TABLE 14.1 Energy and Protein Requirements in Surgical Patients

Patient Status	Energy, kcal/kg/d	Protein, g/kg/d
Adequately nourished preoperative patient	25	0.8–1.0
Adequately nourished postoperative patient	25	1.0–1.1
Adequately nourished, stressed postoperative patient	25–30	1.2–2.0
Nutritionally depleted, nonstressed preoperative patient	25	1.0–1.2
Nutritionally depleted, nonstressed postoperative patient	25	1.2–1.5
Nutritionally depleted, stressed patient	25–30	1.5–2.0

Source: Data are from reference 2.

which leads to elevated protein requirements for all age groups (see Chapter 4). Protein tolerance, as opposed to protein requirements, often determines the amount of protein provided. Patients with impaired renal or hepatic function may not be able to tolerate the standard recommended levels of protein.

Fluid

A variety of methods can be used to estimate normal body water requirements. The Food and Nutrition Board of the Institute of Medicine recommends 1 mL fluid per kcal of energy expenditure for adults with average energy expenditures who live in average environmental conditions (4). Fluid requirements increase with fever, high altitude, low humidity, profuse sweating, watery diarrhea, vomiting, hemorrhage, diuresis, surgical drains, and loss of skin integrity (eg, open wounds, burns) (3). Therefore, fluid status is of vital concern postoperatively. It is common for large volumes of fluids to be provided intraoperatively. Patients will typically diurese these volumes postoperatively; however, some patients may require diuretics.

To ensure fluid balance, surgical patients are typically provided with intravenous fluids until oral intake resumes and is tolerated. Daily weights can be monitored to assess fluid balance with 1 kg of body weight fluctuation roughly reflecting 1 liter of fluid gain or loss.

Vitamins and Minerals

Adequate vitamin and mineral nourishment is important for optimal postoperative recovery. Vitamins and minerals are involved with many metabolic processes in the body, many of which are altered as a result of surgery (Table 14.2). Surgical patients who experience excessive GI losses through nasogastric tube suctioning or surgical drains, diarrhea, and high ostomy or fistula outputs may be at risk for many vitamin and mineral deficiencies (5). If fluid losses exceed 800 mL/d, then micronutrient supplementation should be considered (2,6).

Nutrition Concerns Related to Specific Types of Surgery

The digestive tract is a metabolically active organ involved in digestion, absorption, and metabolism of many nutrients. Therefore, various surgical interventions involving the GI tract can result in malabsorption and maldigestion and lead to nutritional deficiencies. To appreciate the magnitude of the nutrient alterations that can occur as a result of surgery, one must be familiar with both the anatomy of the GI tract and sites of nutrient absorption (see Figure 14.1 on page 173).

TABLE 14.2 Selected Vitamins and Minerals of Concern in Surgical Patients

Nutrient	Biochemical Functions	Recommended Daily Intake
Vitamin A	• Retinol: reproduction • Retinaldehyde: vision • Retinoic acid: normal structure and function of epithelial cells	700–900 RE
Vitamin D	• Maintains serum calcium and phosphorus levels to support neuromuscular function, bone calcification, and other cellular processes; anti-inflammatory agent	5–15 mcg
Vitamin E	• Maintenance of membrane integrity in body cells via its role as antioxidant	15 mg α-tocopherol
Vitamin K	• Functions in the posttranslational gamma-carboxylation of clotting factors (II, VII, IX, X) and anticoagulant proteins (C and S) • May benefit bone health	75–120 mcg
Vitamin C	• Antioxidant; reacts with superoxide, hydroxyl radicals, and singlet oxygen • Provides reducing equivalents for a variety of reactions • Acts as a cofactor for reactions requiring a reduced metal • Required for synthesis of collagen, carnitine, and neurotransmitters • Enhances intestinal absorption of nonheme iron; cholesterol hydroxylation into bile acids; reduction of toxic transition metals; reductive protection of folic acid and vitamin E; and immune-mediated and antibacterial functions of white blood cells	65–90 mg
Vitamin B-12	• Involved in the metabolism of every cell of the body, especially affecting the DNA synthesis and regulation and fatty acid synthesis and energy production	2.4 mg
Folate (vitamin B-9)	• A coenzyme in the transfer of single-carbon fragments from one compound to another for amino acid metabolism and nucleic acid synthesis	400 mcg
Thiamin (vitamin B-1)	• Energy transformation • Synthesis of pentoses and NADPH • Membrane and nerve conduction • As thiamin pyrophosphate, serves as a magnesium-coordinated coenzyme for the oxidative decarboxylation of alpha-ketoacids involved in carbohydrate metabolism • Activity of transketolase in pentose phosphate pathway	1.0–1.2 mg
Zinc	• Catalyst for more than 200 enzymes • Structural function in metalloenzymes and zinc finger motif in proteins • Regulatory role in gene expression • Physiologic role in lipid peroxidation, apoptosis, cellular proliferation and differentiation, and immune function	8–11 mg
Copper	• Functions in oxidation-reduction and electron transfer reactions involving oxygen (copper enzymes: superoxide dismutase, ceruloplasmin, copper thioneins) • Ceruloplasmin is also responsible for manganese oxidation and oxidation of ferrous iron to ferric iron	700–900 mcg

Continues

TABLE 14.2 Selected Vitamins and Minerals of Concern in Surgical Patients *(continued)*

Nutrient	Biochemical Functions	Recommended Daily Intake
Copper *(continued)*	• Other copper-dependent enzymes include lysyl oxidase (forms cross linkages found in collagen and elastin); dopamine monooxygenase (necessary for conversion of dopamine to norepinepherine); peptidylglycine α-amidating monooxygenase (necessary for activation and deactivation of various peptide hormones); and other copper-containing enzymes used for formation of myelin • Copper is necessary for cholesterol and glucose metabolism and formation of melatonin pigment	
Iron	• Essential component of hemoglobin (oxygen transport), myoglobin (muscle iron storage), and cytochromes (oxidative production of cellular energy as ATP)	8–18 mg
Selenium	• Antioxidant • Thyroid hormone synthesis and metabolism	55 mcg

Abbreviations: ATP, adenosine triphosphate; NADPH, nicotinamide adenine dinucleotide phosphate.

Head and Neck Surgery

Preoperative patients with head and neck cancer are usually malnourished due to their disease state. Often the tumor inhibits the patient's ability to chew and swallow normally, which typically is what makes the patient seek medical attention. Also, preoperative treatment may involve radiation and/or chemotherapy to reduce tumor bulk. These therapies may diminish the patient's ability to swallow. Even if she or he can consume some liquids and soft foods, oral intake is often not enough to support nutritional needs. Furthermore, many patients have a long history of alcohol and tobacco use, which may also negatively affect nutrient intake (see Chapter 13 for more information on head and neck cancer).

Preoperative improvements in nutritional status are important for optimal postoperative recovery. Patients typically will require postoperative nutrition support, particularly if they receive chemotherapy and/or radiation therapy, which can further delay return of adequate oral nutrient consumption. A plan should be made preoperatively as to how nutrition therapy will be provided postoperatively to avoid the use of parenteral nutrition if feasible (see Chapter 20). If the tumor size permits, a percutaneous endoscopic gastrostomy (PEG) tube can be placed preoperatively to allow for perioperative enteral nutrition. A PEG, open gastrostomy, or nasoenteric feeding tube may also be placed intraoperatively to provide postoperative enteral nutrition.

Esophageal Surgery

Several medical conditions, such as corrosive injuries and perforation, achalasia, gastroesophageal reflux disease (GERD), and partial or full obstruction caused by cancer, strictures, or congenital abnormalities, affect the esophagus and inhibit the ability to swallow. When surgical intervention is required to correct the abnormality, it involves removal of a segment or the entire esophagus. The esophageal tract is then replaced with either the stomach (gastric pull-up) or the intestine (colonic/jejunal interposition) (see Figure 14.2 on page 174). A gastric pull-up procedure results in displacement of the stomach in the thoracic cavity (Figure 14.2A). This procedure results in a reduced stomach capacity, with potential delayed

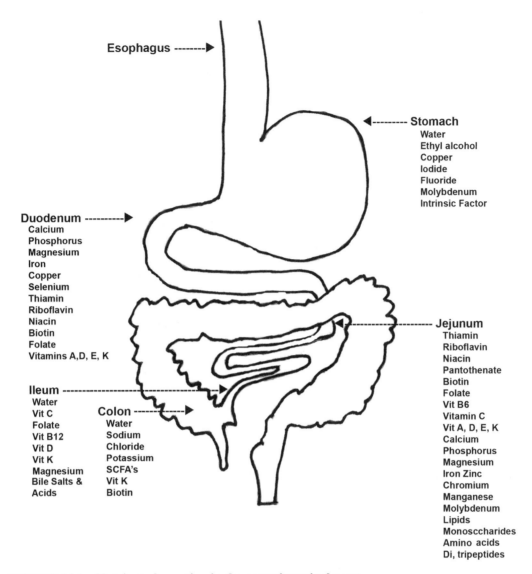

FIGURE 14.1   Nutrient absorption in the gastrointestinal tract.

gastric emptying and dumping syndrome (see Box 14.1 on page 174 for additional information on dumping syndrome). Another option for re-establishing esophageal continuity is by interposing a segment of colon (Figure 14.2B) or jejunum (Figure 14.2C) between the distal esophageal remnant and the stomach, or duodenum after subtotal gastrectomy. Complications following this procedure include dysphagia, strictures, and leakage at the anastomotic site.

Patients with dysphagia or strictures may be limited to a soft or liquid diet preoperatively. If the patient is unable to consume adequate nutrients orally, then a nasoenteric feeding tube may be placed, if feasible. A PEG tube is not indicated if a gastric pull-up procedure is planned because the stomach is used to make the esophageal conduit and a hole resulting from a gastrostomy tube would be contraindicated. Patients may require preoperative parenteral nutrition if the esophagus is obstructed. Intraoperatively, a jejunal feeding tube may be placed to allow for postoperative enteral nutrition therapy until adequate oral intake is achieved. If enteral access is not obtained intraoperatively, then parenteral nutrition is indicated because patients may not resume oral intake for 7 to 10 days (1).

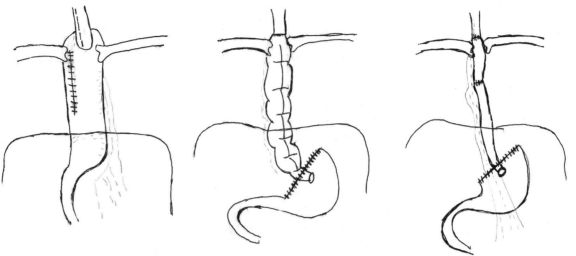

A. Gastric pull-up   B. Colonic interposition   C. Jejunal interposition

FIGURE 14.2   Options for surgical reconstruction after esophagectomy.

BOX 14.1   Dumping Syndrome

Dumping syndrome is a constellation of postprandial symptoms that result from rapid empty-ing of hyperosmolar gastric contents into the small intestine. The hypertonic load in the small intestine promotes reflux of vascular fluid into the bowel lumen. A rapid decrease in circulating blood volume results. Rapid symptoms include the following:
- Abdominal cramping
- Nausea
- Vomiting
- Palpitations
- Sweating
- Weakness
- Hypotension
- Tremors
- Osmotic diarrhea

Early symptoms begin 10 to 30 minutes postprandially. Late symptoms occur 1 to 4 hours after eating or drinking.

Dumping syndrome can result from insulin hypersecretion in response to carbohydrate loads dumped into the small intestine. Following carbohydrate absorption, the hyperinsu-linemia causes hypoglycemia, which results in vasomotor symptoms, such as diaphoresis, weakness, flushing, and palpitations.

A Nissen fundoplication procedure is the most common anti-reflux operation for patients with chronic GERD refractory to medical management. This procedure involves wrapping the stomach around the base of the esophagus (near the lower esophageal sphincter) to place pressure in this region and nar-row the lower esophageal opening in order to prevent reflux (Figure 14.3). Because esophageal swelling occurs postoperatively and produces a feeling of tightness and dysphagia, patients are typically placed on

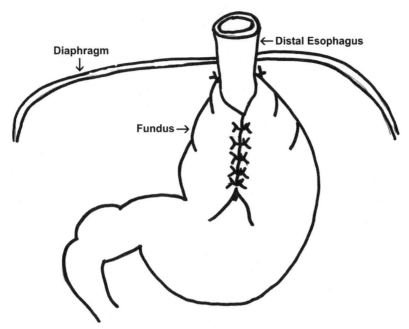

FIGURE 14.3   Nissen fundoplication.

BOX 14.2   Dietary Guidelines After a Nissen Fundoplication

- Eat pureed and moist foods for 2–4 weeks.
- Avoid nuts, seeds, fresh bread, rice, tough meats, foods with sharp edges (eg, chips, hard raw vegetables/fruits, pretzels, crackers).
- Consume small, frequent meals.
- Do not gulp fluids or food; chew and eat slowly.
- Avoid use of straws.
- Avoid gas-causing foods.
- Avoid carbonated beverages, onions, cabbage, beans.

---

a pureed diet for 2 to 4 weeks after this procedure until the swelling is reduced. Patients who undergo a Nissen fundoplication should subsequently avoid foods that can become lodged in the lower esophagus (eg, nuts, rice, and seeds). See Box 14.2 for other dietary guidelines.

Gastric Surgery

There are several indications for gastric surgery (see Box 14.3 on page 176). A vagotomy is often done to eliminate gastric acid secretion. Vagotomy at certain levels can alter the normal physiologic function of the stomach, small intestine, pancreas, and biliary system (Table 14.3 on page 176) (6). Vagotomy procedures are commonly accompanied by a drainage procedure (antrectomy or pyloroplasty) that aids with gastric emptying. Dumping syndrome, steatorrhea, and bacterial overgrowth may be associated with these procedures.

A total gastrectomy involves removal of the entire stomach, whereas only a portion of the stomach is removed with a subtotal gastrectomy. A gastrectomy is accompanied by a reconstructive procedure. A

BOX 14.3   Indications for Gastric Surgery

- Gastric tumor resection
- Ulcer disease
- Gastric perforation
- Gastric hemorrhage

- Zollinger-Ellison syndrome
- Gastric polyposis
- Menetrier's disease
- Pylorotomy for gastroparesis

TABLE 14.3 Potential Complications of Gastric Surgery

Procedure	Potential Complications
Vagotomy: total gastric and truncal vagotomy	• Impairs proximal and distal motor function of the stomach • Digestion and emptying of solids are retarded • Emptying of liquids is accelerated
Total gastrectomy	• Early satiety, nausea, vomiting • Weight loss • Inadequate bile acid and pancreatic enzyme availability due to anastomotic changes • Malabsorption • Protein-energy malnutrition • Anemia • Dumping syndrome • Bezoar[a] formation • Vitamin B-12 deficiency • Metabolic bone disease
Subtotal gastrectomy with vagotomy	• Early satiety • Delayed gastric emptying • Rapid emptying of hypertonic fluids

[a]*Bezoar* is retained concretions of indigestible foreign material that can accumulate in the stomach and cause a partial or complete blockage. *Phytobezoar* is bezoar consisting of nondigestible food material. *Pharmacobezoar* is bezoar consisting of medications. Precautions to prevent bezoar formation are to avoid nondigestible food ingredients and to crush medications or use liquid medications.
Source: Data are from reference 56.

Billroth I procedure (gastroduodenostomy) involves removal of the pylorus and/or antrum and an anastomosis of the proximal end of the duodenum to the distal end of the remnant stomach (Figure 14.4). A Billroth II procedure (gastrojejunostomy) involves removal of the stomach antrum and an anastomosis of the remnant stomach to the side of the jejunum, which creates a blind loop (Figure 14.5).

Patients who undergo any gastric surgical procedure are at risk for postoperative malnutrition (see Table 14.3). Dietary modifications are a key component of the medical therapy after these surgical procedures (see Box 14.4 on page 178) (2). Many patients only require an anti-dumping diet for several weeks after surgery, but some people may need to restrict their diet indefinitely.

When patients are malnourished preoperatively, a small bowel feeding tube may be placed intraoperatively so that low-rate enteral feedings can be initiated in the early postoperative phase. Enteral feedings can then be adjusted according to the patient's clinical progress and tolerance of an oral diet. It is not unusual to discharge patients to home care with tube feedings until their oral diet is optimal (see Chapter 22 for more information on enteral nutrition in the home setting). Oral supplements may be provided to

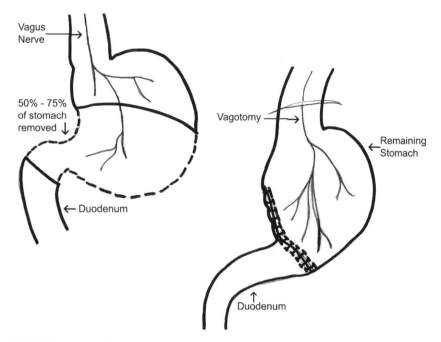

FIGURE 14.4   Gastroduodenostomy (Billroth I).

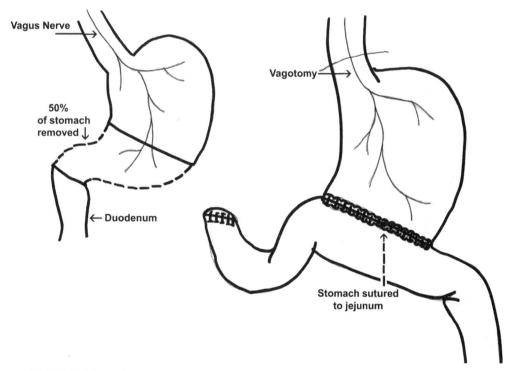

FIGURE 14.5   Gastrojejunostomy (Billroth II).

BOX 14.4   Postgastrectomy/Anti-dumping Diet

Principles of diet

Postoperatively, some discomfort (gas, bloating, cramping) and diarrhea may occur. To reduce the likelihood of these symptoms, a healthy, nutritionally complete diet should be followed. Each person may react to foods differently. Foods should be reintroduced into the diet slowly.

Diet guidelines

1. Eat small, frequent meals.
2. Limit fluids to 4 ounces (½ cup) at a meal, just enough to "wash" food down.
3. Drink remaining fluids at least 30 to 40 minutes before and after meals.
4. Eat slowly and chew foods thoroughly.
5. Avoid extreme temperatures of foods (very hot or very cold).
6. Use seasonings and spices as tolerated (may want to avoid pepper, hot sauce).
7. Remain upright while eating and for at least 30 minutes after eating.
8. Avoid simple sugars in foods and drinks. Examples: fruit juice, sport drinks, fruit-flavored drinks, sweet tea, sucrose, honey, jelly, corn syrup, cookies, pie, and doughnuts.
9. Complex carbohydrates, such as bread, pasta, rice, potatoes, and vegetables, do not need to limited.
10. Include a protein-containing food at each meal.
11. Limit fats (<30% of total energy). Avoid fried foods, gravies, fat-containing sauces, mayonnaise, fatty meats (sausage, hot dogs, ribs), chips, biscuits, and pancakes.
12. Lactose in milk and dairy products may not be tolerated. Introduce dairy foods slowly into the diet if they were tolerated preoperatively. Lactose-free milk or soy milk is suggested.
13. Avoid sugar alcohols (eg, sorbitol in beverages, candies, and medications).

Source: Data are from reference 2.

increase nutrient intake. However, to avoid dumping, these need to be isotonic and should not contain simple sugars (6). Unfortunately, many oral supplements contain simple sugars and are hyperosmolar, which means they are not well tolerated postoperatively. Parenteral nutrition is indicated only if enteral access is not available and the patient is malnourished and not able to tolerate adequate nutrients orally.

Anemia is a common consequence of gastric surgery. It may be a result of a deficiency or malabsorption of one or more nutrients, including iron, folate, and vitamin B-12 (see Table 14.4). Total gastrectomy and some subtotal gastrectomy patients require periodic intramuscular vitamin B-12 injections. Metabolic bone disease can also be a late complication of gastric surgery. In addition to consuming dietary calcium, patients require calcium and vitamin D supplementation (6).

Intestinal Surgery

If excessive lengths of intestine are removed, nutritional consequences can arise depending on the location resected (Table 14.5). Short bowel syndrome may occur if more than 50% of the small intestine is removed. This syndrome is characterized by severe diarrhea or steatorrhea, malabsorption, and malnutrition (see Chapter 8). Patients often require long-term parenteral nutrition to maintain nutritional status and fluid and electrolyte balance.

TABLE 14.4 Nutrient Deficiencies Associated with Gastric Surgery

Deficiency	Causes	Management

Microcytic anemia	• Iron malabsorption or deficiency.
	• Total and subtotal gastrectomy:
	  ◦ Achlorhydria leads to insufficient cleavage of iron from food sources.
	  ◦ Reduction and solubilization of ferric iron to the ferrous form.
	  ◦ Anemia is more common with Billroth II procedure than with Billroth I because Billroth II bypasses the primary sites of iron absorption.
	• Reduced intake of iron-rich foods due to intolerance and reduced gastric capacity.
		Supplementation with 325 mg ferrous sulfate twice daily and coadministration of vitamin C

Macrocytic anemia	• Folate or vitamin B-12 deficiency or anemia. • Achlorhydria leads to insufficient liberation of vitamin B-12 from protein food sources. • Decreased intrinsic factor leads to decreased binding of vitamin B-12. • Reduced intake of protein-rich foods due to intolerance and reduced gastric capacity.	Monthly intramuscular vitamin B-12 injections (1,500 mcg)
Metabolic bone disease	• Calcium deficiency or malabsorption. • Disease is more common with Billroth II than with Billroth I procedure because Billroth II bypasses the duodenum and proximal jejunum. • Rapid gastric emptying can reduce absorption. • Fat malabsorption can lead to insoluble calcium soap formation. • Vitamin D malabsorption may accompany fat malabsorption, which can impair calcium and phosphorus metabolism.	Daily supplementation with 1,500 mg calcium and 800 IU vitamin D

Source: Data are from reference 5.

TABLE 14.5 Nutritional Consequences of Intestinal Surgery

Location	Potential Consequences
Proximal small intestine Gastric bypass	• Malabsorption of calcium, magnesium, iron, vitamin A, and vitamin D • Protein-energy malnutrition from malabsorption due to dumping or unavailability of bile acids and pancreatic enzymes related to anastomotic changes • Bezoar formation
Distal small intestine	• Malabsorption of water-soluble vitamins (folate, vitamins B-12, B-1 [thiamin]), B-2 [riboflavin], B-6, and C) • Protein-energy malnutrition due to dumping • Fat malabsorption • Bacterial overgrowth if ileocecal valve is resected
Colon	• Fluid malabsorption • Electrolyte malabsorption (potassium, sodium, chloride)

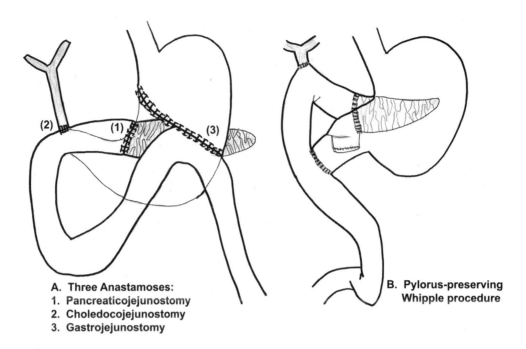

A. Three Anastamoses:
1. **Pancreaticojejunostomy**
2. **Choledocojejunostomy**
3. **Gastrojejunostomy**

B. Pylorus-preserving Whipple procedure

FIGURE 14.6   Pancreaticoduodenectomy (Whipple procedure).

Pancreaticoduodenectomy (Whipple Procedure)

In cases of ampullary, duodenal, and pancreatic malignancy, a pancreaticoduodenectomy may be performed. This procedure is one of the most technically difficult and challenging of GI surgeries and involves resecting the distal stomach, the distal common bile duct, the pancreatic head, and the duodenum. Three anastomoses must be done: pancreaticojejunostomy, choledocojejunostomy, and gastrojejunostomy (Billroth II). The pylorus-sparing pancreaticoduodenectomy (Whipple procedure) has become the preferred variation because it has fewer postoperative nutritional consequences (Figure 14.6).

Common complications after these procedures include delayed gastric emptying, dumping syndrome, weight loss, diabetes mellitus, and malabsorption due to pancreatic exocrine insufficiency. Nutrient guidelines after these procedures are similar to those following a gastrectomy.

Ileostomy and Colostomy

An ileostomy or colostomy may be required in the cases of intestinal lesions, obstruction, necrosis, or inflammatory bowel disease of the distal small intestine or colon or when diversion of fecal matter is necessary. These procedures involve the creation of an artificial anus on the abdominal wall by incision into the colon or ileum and bringing it out to the surface, forming a stoma. A pouch is placed externally over the stoma to collect the fecal matter.

In general, patients with ostomies should eat regular diets. Foods that are gas-forming or difficult to digest may be avoided to reduce adverse effects (Table 14.6). In the case of high-output ostomies (>800 mL/d), patients may need to avoid hypertonic, simple sugar–containing liquids and foods, fatty foods, and foods high in insoluble fiber.

TABLE 14.6 Foods of Interest for Patients with an Ostomy

Food Effect	Foods
Produce odor[a]	Asparagus, beans, brussels sprouts, cabbage, coffee, cucumber, eggs, fish, garlic, green peppers, milk, onions, prunes, radishes, turnips
Decrease odor	Buttermilk, cranberry juice, parsley, spinach, yogurt
Produce gas[b]	Apples (raw), asparagus, beans, broccoli, cabbage, carbonated beverages, cauliflower, corn, cucumber, dairy foods, eggs, melon, mushrooms, onions, peas, spicy foods, spinach
Thicken stools[c]	Applesauce, bananas (greener the better), breads, cheeses, marshmallows, milk, peanut butter (creamy), starches (rice, pasta, potatoes, tapioca), yogurt
Thin stools	Apple juice, chocolate, fresh fruits, fried foods, grape juice, green beans, highly seasoned foods, prune juice

[a]Vitamin supplements may also contribute to odor production.
[b]Chewing gum and use of straws (swallowing air) may also cause gas.
[c]Soluble fiber supplements may also help thicken stools.

Conclusion

Preoperative nutrition care of the malnourished patient can help improve postoperative outcomes. Postoperative nutrition care must focus on delivery of appropriate amounts of energy, fluids, and macro- and micronutrients. The nutritional needs of patients will depend in part on the type of GI tract surgery—the various types affect intake and absorption differently and may be associated with a variety of adverse nutritional consequences. Some patients will need long-term nutrition interventions, ranging from avoidance of certain foods to nutrient supplementation to enteral or parenteral nutrition in the home-care setting.

References

1. McClave SA, Martindale RG, Vanek VW, McCarthy M, Roberts P, Taylor B, Ochoa JB, Napolitano L, Cresci G. Guidelines for the provision and assessment of nutrition support therapy in the adult critically ill patient: Society of Critical Care Medicine (SCCM) and American Society for Parenteral and Enteral Nutrition (A.S.P.E.N.). *JPEN J Parenter Enteral Nutr.* 2009;33:277–316.
2. Cresci G, MacFadyen BV, Gregory JS, Marr AB, Warren J. Nutrition. In: Lawrence PF, ed. *Essentials of General Surgery.* 5th ed. Philadelphia, PA: Wolters Kluwer; 2013:57–75.
3. Langley G, Tajchman S. Fluids, electrolytes, and acid-base disorders. In: Mueller CM, ed. *The A.S.P.E.N. Adult Nutrition Support Core Curriculum.* 2nd ed. Silver Spring, MD: American Society for Parenteral and Enteral Nutrition; 2012:99–120.
4. Food and Nutrition Board, Institute of Medicine. Dietary Reference Intakes for Water, Potassium, Sodium, Chloride, and Sulfate. Washington, DC: National Academies Press; 2004.
5. Clark SF. Vitamins and trace elements. In: Mueller CM, ed. *The A.S.P.E.N. Adult Nutrition Support Core Curriculum.* 2nd ed. Silver Spring, MD: American Society for Parenteral and Enteral Nutrition; 2012:121–148.
6. Frantz D, Munroe C, Parrish CR, Krenitsky J, Willcutts K, Forturne A. Gastrointestinal disease. In: Mueller CM, ed. *The A.S.P.E.N. Adult Nutrition Support Core Curriculum.* 2nd ed. Silver Spring, MD: American Society for Parenteral and Enteral Nutrition; 2012:426–453.

CHAPTER 15

Bariatric Surgery

Karen M. Buzby, RD, LDN

Bariatric surgery is indicated for patients with a body mass index (BMI) ≥40, or for individuals with a BMI ≥35 who also suffer from serious obesity-related medical conditions (1,2). See Chapter 3 for additional information on interpreting BMI and Box 15.1 (3,4) for the formulas for calculating excess body weight and estimating weight loss. The impact of clinically severe obesity on overall health and life expectancy is dramatic. Obesity-related diseases contribute to increased morbidity and mortality (see Box 15.2). Weight loss surgery (WLS) helps the morbidly obese patient achieve sustainable weight reduction (averaging 61% of excess body weight), significantly improves or resolves many of the obesity-related comorbidities (see Table 15.1) (3), and increases life expectancy (5). Due to the complex factors inherent in this patient population, a multidisciplinary team approach is recommended to ensure comprehensive preoperative screening and patient education, as well as postoperative care and long-term follow-up.

BOX 15.1   Calculating Excess Body Weight and Estimating Weight Loss in Adults

Excess Weight = Preoperative Weight − Desirable Weight

Where: Desirable weight = Weight at body mass index of 25

Excess Weight Loss (%) = (Weight Loss/Excess Weight) × 100

Total Weight Loss (%) = (Weight Loss/Preoperative Weight) × 100

To estimate weight loss expected with each procedure:

Estimated Weight Loss = (Excess Weight × Average % of Excess Weight Loss for Procedure)/100

Where: The average % excess body weight loss is 61% for Roux-en-Y gastric bypass (3); 47.5% for adjustable gastric banding (3); and 61% for sleeve gastrectomy (4).

Weight Loss Goal = Preoperative Weight − Estimated Weight Loss

---

BOX 15.2 Obesity-Related Comorbidities

- **Cardiovascular**: Coronary artery disease; congestive heart failure; hypertension; peripheral vascular disease
- **Cancer**: Breast; colon; endometrial; prostate; renal cell
- **Endocrine**: Dyslipidemia; type 1 diabetes mellitus; type 2 diabetes mellitus; gestational diabetes mellitus; metabolic syndrome; polycystic ovary syndrome
- **Gastrointestinal**: Cholelithiasis; nonalcoholic steatohepatitis; gastroesophageal reflux disease; hiatal hernia
- **Genitourinary**: Female infertility; urinary incontinence
- **Musculoskeletal**: Degenerative joint disease; gout; osteoarthritis
- **Neurologic**: Pseudotumor cerebri
- **Psychological**: Depression; eating disorders
- **Pulmonary**: Obstructive sleep apnea; asthma; hypoventilation syndrome

---

TABLE 15.1 Resolution or Improvement of Obesity-Related Comorbidities After Bariatric Surgery[a]

| | Procedures | |
Comorbidity	*Gastric Bypass*	*Adjustable Gastric Banding*
Diabetes	Resolved: 83.7% Improvement: 93.2%	Resolved: 47.9% Improvement: 80.8%
Hyperlipidemia	Improvement: 96.9%	Improvement: 58.9%
Hypertension	Resolved: 67.5% Improvement: 87.2%	Resolved: 43.2% Improvement: 70.8%
Obstructive sleep apnea	Resolved: 80.4% Improvement: 94.8%	Resolved: 95.0% Improvement: 68.0%

[a]Percentages of patients as determined in a 2004 meta-analysis.
Source: Data are from reference 3.

Patient Screening and Selection

Potential candidates for bariatric surgery must be well informed about the types of surgeries and the risks involved, motivated to make diet and lifestyle changes, and have failed attempts at nonsurgical approaches to weight loss. Additional criteria for patient screening and selection are listed in Table 15.2 (page 184).

Preoperative Nutrition Management

The registered dietitian (RD) must play an integral role in the care of the WLS patient to ensure positive health outcomes and lasting weight loss (2,6,7). The nutrition management of the bariatric patient should follow the Academy of Nutrition and Dietetics Nutrition Care Process of nutrition assessment, nutrition diagnosis, nutrition intervention, and nutrition monitoring and evaluation (8), and current evidence-based practice recommendations, which are outlined in the Academy's position paper on weight management (9).

TABLE 15.2 Criteria for Weight-Loss Surgery Patient Screening and Selection

Characteristic or Issue	Criteria
Age	No universally accepted guidelines for age No minimum or maximum age identified
Clinically severe obesity	Body mass index (BMI) ≥40 *or* BMI >35 with obesity-related comorbidities
Previous weight loss	History of multiple weight loss attempts without successful weight maintenance
Medical/surgical clearance	Evaluate for diseases associated with increased risk for complications or mortality
Psychological evaluation	Absence of eating disorders, major depression or psychosis; no drug or alcohol abuse; ability to comprehend behavioral and lifestyle changes required
Other considerations	Cessation of smoking for at least 2 months prior to surgery; pregnancy not planned for at least 2 years after surgery; mobility and potential for physical activity; commitment to lifelong nutritional supplementation and medical monitoring after surgery

For many patients, the medical, psychological, and surgical evaluations required for WLS can take several months to complete. Insurance company requirements for physician-supervised diet and exercise programs can also extend the preoperative process. During this period, the RD should perform a nutrition assessment, make nutrition diagnoses, and work with the patient to improve his or her nutritional status. Nutrition intervention should also include initiating changes in the patient's diet, behavior, and lifestyle to set the stage for positive outcomes after surgery. In select patients, the use of a very–low-energy-diet may be indicated preoperatively to achieve rapid weight loss and reduce liver size, because an enlarged liver can increase surgical difficulty (10).

Types of Bariatric Surgical Procedures

Minimally invasive surgical techniques are often used in bariatric surgery. Laparoscopic procedures, using multiple small incisions, help speed patient recovery and return to normal activities as well as decrease operative morbidity and mortality.

When a laparoscopic approach is not an option, surgical access is obtained through an upper midline incision, which is referred to as an "open approach." Patients undergoing an open WLS procedure may have a longer hospital stay and higher incidence of some complications, such as infections, hernias, and wound dehiscence (11).

Bariatric surgical procedures (Figure 15.1) are classified as follows (12):

- Purely restrictive (adjustable gastric banding [AGB] and sleeve gastrectomy [SG])
- Restrictive with some malabsorption (Roux-en-Y gastric bypass [RYGB])
- Primarily malabsorptive with some restriction (biliopancreatic diversion with duodenal switch)

AGB and RYGB are the most common weight loss surgeries in the United States. SG is also gaining in popularity as a primary procedure. Selecting the most appropriate procedure for a patient requires surgical consultation and consideration of several variables including the patient's BMI, operative risk, and comorbidities.

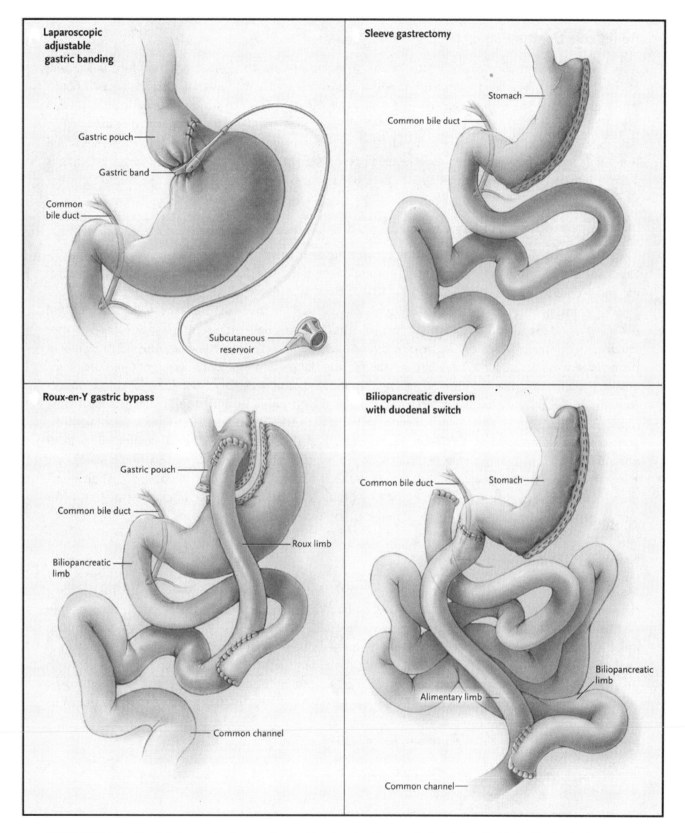

FIGURE 15.1 Bariatric surgical procedures. Reprinted with permission from: DeMaria EJ. Bariatric surgery for morbid obesity. *N Engl J Med.* 2007;356:2176–2183. Copyright 2007, Massachusetts Medical Society. All rights reserved.

Adjustable Gastric Banding

AGB is a gastric restrictive procedure that is used to create an early sense of satiety, limit food intake, and cause weight loss. The band is placed just below the gastroesophageal junction, creating a small pouch with a narrow opening to the larger lower stomach (see Figure 15.1). The size of the gastric pouch is less than 30 mL in volume. An access port, placed deep under the patient's skin, is connected to the band by tubing. Saline solution is used to add fluid to the interior lumen of the band, restricting the flow of food from the pouch to the lower stomach. The mean percentage of excess weight loss for gastric banding is 47.5%, with an observed range of 40.7% to 54.2% (3).

Roux-en-Y Gastric Bypass

The RYGB procedure restricts food intake by creating a small gastric pouch, causes malabsorption (ie, alters nutrient absorption) by bypassing a portion of the intestines, and impacts gastrointestinal neuronal and hormonal signals (see Figure 15.1) (13). The major feature of the RYGB is the proximal gastric pouch (30 mL in volume) made from the lesser curvature of the stomach. This part of the stomach will not distend and provides the restriction necessary for optimal long-term weight management. A gastrojejunostomy is made to connect the gastric pouch to the jejunum. This anastomosis, only 12 to 15 mm in diameter, limits the rate food flows through the pouch. The portion of jejunum brought up to the pouch creates the alimentary or Roux limb. The length of the Roux limb can vary from 75 to 150 cm. A longer Roux limb will increase the malabsorptive effects of the operation, resulting in greater weight loss. A longer Roux limb length may be indicated for patients with BMI more than 50. With the creation of the pouch and gastrojejunostomy, the larger distal stomach (or gastric remnant), the duodenum, and a small portion of the jejunum, referred to as the Y-limb or biliopancreatic limb, are bypassed. To permit gastric juices as well as bile and pancreatic secretions to mix with food, another anastomosis, a jejunojejunostomy, is created to connect the Y-limb to the Roux limb. The mean percentage of excess weight loss for gastric bypass is 61.6%, with an observed range of 56.7% to 66.3 % (3).

Sleeve Gastrectomy

SG is a bariatric procedure that restricts how much food the stomach can hold (see Figure15.1). During the surgery, a long, sleeve-shaped tube is created along the lesser curvature of the stomach using a 34 to 42 French bougie and 75% to 80% of the greater curvature is removed. The nutrients and calories in food are absorbed normally; however, food intake is limited due to gastric restriction and/or neurohumoral changes caused by the procedure. SG evolved from the first stage of the biliopancreatic diversion with duodenal switch (Figure 15.1), a malabsorptive WLS procedure for the superobese. It is now considered a primary operation to manage weight. However, a second operation (RYGB or duodenal switch) can be done if more weight loss is desired.

The following are medical indications for SG (14):

- BMI >60 with high risk for complications
- Inflammatory bowel disease
- Severe small bowel adhesions

- When weight loss is required before kidney transplant
- Use of immunosuppressant or anti-inflammatory medications

The percentage of excess body weight loss after sleeve gastrectomy has been observed to be 49% at 6 months postoperative, 59% at 1 year postoperative, and 61.5% at 2 years postoperative (15).

Postoperative Diet Stages

See Box 15.3 (page 188) for a summary of the five stages of a post–bariatric surgery diet (2,16). In the immediately following sections, management issues related to AGB, RYGB, and SG are discussed. More general principles and goals are covered later in the chapter.

Management of Adjustable Gastric Banding Patients

Early Postoperative Management

Standard intravenous (IV) fluids are administered while the patient is NPO. Consultation with RD is recommended. As noted in Box 15.3, patients usually advance to a bariatric clear liquid diet on post-op day 1 (2). Patients should be monitored for symptoms of postoperative stoma obstruction/gastric edema. After demonstrating tolerance to liquids, most patients are discharged within 24 hours of AGB surgery, depending on their medical status, pain control, and presence or absence of nausea. Diet is progressed to bariatric full liquids once the patient is at home, and is then advanced as outlined in Box 15.3.

Patients should be cautioned to strictly adhere to dietary guidelines to prevent vomiting in the early postop period. If persistent vomiting occurs before the stomach has healed, the lower stomach may prolapse above the band.

Patients may experience hunger approximately 1 week postoperatively. Encourage them to consume protein-containing food to increase satiety.

Diet-Related Complaints and Symptoms

DYSPHAGIA TO SOLID FOOD

Dysphagia can be caused by eating too quickly, taking too big a mouthful, not chewing food enough, eating food that is not easily masticated, or eating doughy foods. Some patients report dysphagia early in the day, with improvement over the course of the day. A liquid meal replacement or protein-containing beverage will help these patients maintain appropriate nutrition and decrease their feelings of anxiety associated with dysphagia.

OBSTRUCTION OF THE OUTLET OF THE POUCH

Severe pain and increased salivation can occur if the outlet of the pouch is obstructed. Vomiting or regurgitation may relieve the obstruction. If symptoms persist and liquid, including saliva, is not tolerated, all fluid in the band should be removed to permit the food bolus obstruction in the stoma to pass. If deflating the band does not work, endoscopy may be required to remove the obstruction.

BOX 15.3   Post–Bariatric Surgery Diet: Stages I to V

Stage I: Bariatric clear liquid diet
- **Indications**: The clear liquid diet is used to initiate oral intake after surgery and usually can be started 24 hours after any bariatric procedure (2).
- **Duration**: 1–2 days. If clear liquids are required for a longer period of time, a low-residue, high-protein nutritional supplement should be added and appropriate multivitamin and mineral supplements started, if not contraindicated (16).
- **Foods/fluids**: Noncarbonated, caffeine-free, sugar-free beverages and foods that are liquid at body temperature. Diet gelatin, broth, sugar-free popsicles, decaf/herbal teas, artificially sweetened beverages, and diluted 100% juice.
- **Other restrictions/considerations**: No straws are permitted; too much liquid and/or air may be ingested with use of straw.

Stage II: Bariatric full liquid diet
- **Indications**: A full liquid diet is indicated for the bariatric patient who has demonstrated tolerance to clear liquids for 2 meals or for patients being discharged from the hospital. The full liquid diet permits further healing and is an intermediate step in the progression from clear liquids to a pureed diet. This stage approximates the energy and protein equivalent of a very-low-calorie diet.
- **Duration**: 10–14 days; (Postop weeks 1 and 2).
- **Foods/fluids**: Low-fat milk products and milk alternatives; strained milk–based soups, vegetable juice, liquid low-calorie protein supplements. *Some programs permit thin refined/ hot cereals, low-fat/light yogurt and custards on the full liquid diet whereas other programs introduce these foods on the pureed diet.*
- **Vitamin and mineral supplementation**: Begin chewable or liquid supplements as per protocol.

Stage III: Bariatric pureed diet
- **Indications**: A pureed diet is indicated for the bariatric patient as an intermediate step in the progression from full liquids to a soft diet. Pureed foods gradually increase gastric residue and decrease the risk of obstruction due to improperly masticated foods.
- **Duration**:
  ○ AGB and RYGB: 2 weeks (postop weeks 3 and 4).
  ○ SG: may require 3–4 weeks on the pureed diet (postop weeks 3–6).
- **Foods/fluids**: Blended or liquefied foods low in sugar and fat. Scrambled eggs and egg substitutes; pureed meat and beans; flaked, water-packed tuna or salmon, and meat alternatives; yogurt, cottage cheese, soft cheeses; hot/cold cereal; pureed fruit or vegetables can be introduced but protein-containing foods and beverages should be consumed first in the meal. Continue liquid low-calorie protein supplements.
- **Vitamin and mineral supplementation**: Continue supplements as per protocol.

Stage IV: Bariatric soft diet
- **Indications**: A soft diet is indicated for the bariatric patient as an intermediate step in the progression from pureed foods to a regular diet. The diet focus is on foods "soft" in texture that decrease the risk of obstruction due to improperly masticated foods.

Continues

BOX 15.3   Post–Bariatric Surgery Diet: Stages I to V *(Continued)*

- **Duration**:
  - AGB: 14 days (postop weeks 5 and 6).
  - RYGB: ≥14 days (postop weeks 5 and 6). Patients often remain on a soft diet for a longer period of time).
  - SG: Progress as tolerated.
- **Foods/fluids**: Ground or chopped tender cuts of meat and poultry, fish, cooked beans/lentils, meat alternatives; low-fat dairy products; well-cooked vegetables and canned fruit; soft fresh fruit without peels or skins; toasted whole grain bread and crackers as tolerated.
- **Vitamin and mineral supplementation**: Continue supplements as per protocol.

Stage V: Bariatric regular diet (maintenance diet)
- **Indications**: Appropriate for bariatric surgery patients who are 2 months or more postop and able to tolerate foods of regular consistency.
- **Duration**: Initiated approximately 2 months after surgery or when tolerated.
- **Foods/fluids**: Solid foods, whole foods instead of processed; lean proteins; low-fat dairy; fresh fruits and vegetables; whole grain bread and cereals.
- **Food intolerances**: Patients are cautioned to avoid tough meats, doughy breads or starches, fibrous vegetable or fruits that cannot be chewed to pureed consistency. These foods do not easily digest through the narrow stoma or anastomosis and may not be tolerated for the first 6–12 months.
- **Vitamin and mineral supplementation**: Continue supplements as per protocol. Change to tablet or pill form (<11 mm in width and length) as tolerated.
- **Other dietary restrictions/considerations**: Alcohol consumption should be initially avoided. For all bariatric patients, intake should be limited because of caloric content of most alcoholic beverages. RYGB patients should be cautioned regarding the immediate absorption and intoxicating effects of alcohol. If alcohol is consumed, intake should be limited.

REFLUX

A patient may experience reflux if the band is too tight or has slipped or the stomach prolapses above the band. Treatment may include removing the fluid from the band or another surgery to reposition the band.

Band Adjustments

The process of incrementally adding fluid to the band is called an *adjustment* or *fill*. There are several bands approved for use in the United States. The type of band used will determine the total amount of fluid that can be added. Adjustment algorithms are available to guide how much fluid should be added during a fill (17).

If needed, the band can be adjusted at 6 weeks postoperatively. Multiple adjustments every 4 to 6 weeks may be needed in the first postoperative year for the patient to achieve optimal restriction and produce early satiety (2,17).

Patients should be frequently questioned about their appetites, portion sizes, eating behaviors, and weight loss. An adjustment may be needed if the patient reports the following:

- Hunger between meals
- Increased appetite
- Ability to eat larger portions
- Increased snacking
- Weight gain or weight plateau

Fluid may need to be removed from the band if the patient reports any of the following problems:

- Dysphagia
- Reflux or heartburn symptoms
- Developing a night cough
- Regurgitating food and liquids
- Maladaptive eating behaviors such as consuming soft foods and high-calorie liquids that digest easier through the tight band than do solid foods

Adjustments can be made in the physician's office with or without the use of fluoroscopy. Accessing the port under fluoroscopy permits visualization of the esophagus, stomach, band, and the outlet of the pouch, and helps to diagnosis complications.

After an adjustment of the band, a modified diet progression (see Box 15.4) is followed to give the patient the opportunity to slowly experience drinking and eating with more fluid in the band. Weight loss should be slow and steady (1 to 2 lb/wk in the first 24 to 36 months after surgery) (17).

Patient commitment to frequent follow-up can positively influence weight loss (17). Ongoing dietary and behavioral counseling, in addition to evaluating the need for an adjustment, are essential components of AGB outpatient monitoring.

Management of Roux-en-Y Gastric Bypass Patients

Early Postoperative Management

Postoperative dietary management includes NPO for the first 24 hours. Standard IV fluids are administered until the patient demonstrates tolerance to liquids. Consultation with registered dietitian is recommended.

Patients usually advance to a bariatric clear liquid diet on postop day 1 (2). Refer to the sections on initiating fluid and food intake in the postoperative patient, later in this chapter.

Patients are typically hospitalized for 2 to 3 days. After demonstrating tolerance to liquids, most patients are discharged, depending on their medical status, pain control, and presence or absence of nausea.

Diet is progressed to bariatric full liquids at home and is advanced as outlined in Box 15.3. Patients should be cautioned to strictly adhere to dietary guidelines to prevent dehydration and vomiting in the early postoperative period. Patients may not be hungry for weeks or months after surgery and need to be counseled on the importance of following diet instructions to develop positive eating behaviors and good dietary habits.

BOX 15.4   Adjustable Gastric Banding: Post–Adjustment Diet Progression

- **Indications**: To gradually introduce solid foods after the band is filled.
- **Duration**: Full liquids for 1–2 day(s), pureed/soft foods for 3 days, regular foods as tolerated by day 5.
- **Foods/fluids**: As described in Stages II-V. (See Box 15.3.)
- **Other restrictions/considerations**: Patients should be reminded to chew foods well to facilitate digestion through a tighter stoma and to decrease the likelihood of an obstruction.

Diet-Related Complaints and Symptoms

NAUSEA AND VOMITING

Nausea and vomiting may be related to specific food intolerance or due to eating/drinking too quickly, too much, or not chewing foods well enough.

EARLY-STAGE DUMPING SYNDROME

Early-stage dumping usually occurs 10 to 30 minutes after eating a food or drinking a beverage containing simple sugar (6). The hyperosmolar sugar particles rapidly empty into the jejunum, causing an influx of fluid into the intestine and producing symptoms that may include nausea, vomiting, abdominal cramping, diarrhea, dizziness, diaphoresis, and tachycardia. Often patients need to lie down until symptoms resolve. To prevent dumping, instruct patients to select food containing less than 15 g sugar per serving and to separate drinking and eating.

Ingesting foods that are high in fat may cause GI symptoms similar to those observed with dumping syndrome. Therefore, high-fat foods should be avoided because they are calorically dense and may cause abdominal discomfort.

LATE-STAGE DUMPING SYNDROME

Late-stage dumping (postprandial hyperinsulinemic hypoglycemia or reactive hypoglycemia) occurs 1 to 3 hours after eating. The symptoms are usually flushing, dizziness, palpitation, and lightheadedness. In severe cases, loss of consciousness may result from hypoglycemia due to an exaggerated release of insulin after a high-carbohydrate meal (18).

The onset of late-stage dumping is typically 1 to 2 years after RYGB. Symptoms are usually not observed in patients less than 1-year postop. The etiology is hypothesized to result from an increase in beta-cell mass or function and the decreased insulin resistance observed with weight loss. Treatment includes increasing protein content and lowering carbohydrate concentration of meals.

LACTOSE INTOLERANCE

Symptoms of lactose intolerance include flatulence, bloating, cramps, and diarrhea. It is caused by compromised ability to digest lactose and dumping syndrome. Consumption of milk, dairy products, and protein supplements containing whey protein concentrates may substantially increase after WLS secondary to the need to increase protein intake.

Patients should only use soy-based protein drinks or protein supplements that contain whey protein isolates (the lactose has been filtered out of the whey in these products). Lactose-free milk products or milk-alternatives are also recommended.

CONSTIPATION

Constipation may be due to decreased food and fluid intake. Recommend the use appropriate fiber supplements as well as dietary modifications to increase fluid and fiber consumption. Patients may use stool softeners and laxatives when indicated.

MICRONUTRIENT DEFICIENCIES

Micronutrient deficiencies have been reported after RYGB (16). Deficiencies of vitamin B-12, iron, and vitamin D are frequently reported. Changes in calcium metabolism are also common, and patients should therefore be monitored for long-term risk of metabolic bone disease.

Thiamin deficiency, while rare, can quickly arise in RYGB patients with persistent vomiting who are unable to consume the recommended supplements (16). Early diagnosis and treatment is essential to prevent serious health problems.

Patients must adhere to vitamin and mineral supplementation protocols. Routine monitoring of laboratory values is required to detect deficiencies before they progress to functional impairments.

STRICTURE OF THE GASTROJEJUNOSTOMY

A stricture may occur 1 to 3 months after surgery. Patients may complain of an inability to advance their diet or notice that they are only able to tolerate fluids.

Treatment for a stricture is endoscopic balloon dilatation of the anastomosis. Several dilatations may be required before the stricture resolves and the patient can tolerate diet advancement. During this time, provide patients with dietary guidance to ensure nutritional goals are met. Patients may also develop a fear of eating and require psychological or emotional support.

MARGINAL ULCERS OF THE POUCH

The incidence of ulcers is higher in patients who resume smoking or who use nonsteroidal analgesics. Symptoms include vomiting, epigastric pain, and gastrointestinal bleeding. Endoscopy is required for evaluation and treatment.

Ulcers may compromise the patient's ability to meet nutritional goals. They are treated with acid-suppression medications. Severe cases may require bowel rest and parenteral nutrition.

INTERNAL HERNIA OR BOWEL OBSTRUCTION

Hernia or bowel obstruction may occur in the immediate postoperative period or many years later. Patients may complain of intermittent or severe postprandial pain. Reoperation is necessary for hernia repair and to relieve the obstruction.

LEAK OF THE STAPLE LINE

Leaks of the staple line can be a life-threatening complication of RYGB if not diagnosed early. Reoperation is necessary, and patients may require nutrition support in the postoperative period.

Management of Sleeve Gastrectomy Patients

Early Postoperative Management

Postoperative dietary management includes NPO for the first 24 hours. Standard IV fluids are administered until the patient demonstrates tolerance to liquids. Patients should consult with a registered dietitian.

Patients usually advance to a bariatric clear liquid diet on postop day 1 (see Box 15.3) (2). Patients are typically hospitalized for 2 to 3 days. After demonstrating tolerance to liquids, most patients are discharged, depending on their medical status, pain control, and presence or absence of nausea.

Diet is progressed to bariatric full liquids at home and is advanced as outlined in Box 15.3. Patients should be cautioned to strictly adhere to dietary guidelines to prevent dehydration and vomiting in the early postoperative period. Patients may not be hungry for weeks or months after surgery and need to be counseled on the importance of following diet instructions to develop positive eating behaviors and good dietary habits.

Diet-Related Complaints and Symptoms

NAUSEA AND VOMITING

Nausea and vomiting may be related to specific food intolerances or due to eating and drinking too quickly, eating and drinking too much, or not chewing foods well enough. Pureed consistency foods may be necessary for 3 to 4 weeks after surgery, depending on patient tolerance.

GASTROESOPHAGEAL REFLUX

In the early postoperative period, many patients report symptoms of reflux. Over time, the incidence of reflux significantly decreases or completely resolves (4).

CONSTIPATION

Constipation may be due to decreased food and fluid intake. Recommend the use of appropriate fiber supplements as well as dietary modifications to increase fluid and fiber consumption. Patients may use stool softeners and laxatives when indicated.

Postoperative Diet Principles and Modifications

Prior to surgery patients must be instructed on the principles of the postoperative diet and the required nutritional supplements. Above all, understanding both *how* to eat and *what* to eat is essential for safe and successful weight loss. Take care to instruct patients in both the "how" and the "what."

The goals of the bariatric diet are as follows:

- To ensure adequate hydration
- To consume high-quality protein to decrease loss of lean body mass, promote wound-healing, and maintain visceral protein stores
- To facilitate/promote weight loss by focusing on low-calorie foods and beverages
- To use the recommended vitamin and mineral supplements to ensure that micronutrient needs are met
- To maximize food digestibility and tolerance with a gradual diet progression

Initiating Postoperative Fluid Intake

Patients must learn to sip liquids slowly, beginning with 1 oz over 15 minutes. Instruct patients to increase the rate of fluid intake as tolerated, progressing from 4 oz/h to 6 oz/h to 8 oz/h, and so on, eventually establishing a new "normal" pace of drinking. Drinking too quickly may cause patients to experience fluid stacking in their esophagus or foaming of saliva in the back of the throat; nausea and vomiting may also occur. Allowed fluids include the following:

- Sugar-free or low-calorie beverages (≤15 g sugar per serving).
- Decaffeinated beverages. (Caffeine intake is limited due to its mild diuretic effect, which can increase the risk of dehydration.)
- Noncarbonated beverages. (Carbonated beverages may cause cramping, bloating, nausea, and vomiting.)
- Protein-containing liquids, including low-fat and fat-free milk, lactose-free milk, soy milk, and liquid protein supplements meeting the dietary criteria. To improve tolerance to protein drinks, limit use of protein powder supplements to 20 to 30 g in 8 oz of fluid.

Fluid requirements are 48 to 64 oz of total fluid per day. Clears liquids should account for half of total fluids.

Initiating Postoperative Food Intake

Eating and drinking at the same time after WLS may cause rapid digestion of food, resulting in increased consumption. It may also cause dumping symptoms in the RYGB patient. Therefore, an important diet principle for all WLS patients is to separate eating and drinking. Patients should be instructed to do the following:

- Stop drinking 30 minutes before a meal.
- Refrain from drinking during a meal.
- Wait at least 30 to 45 minutes after eating to drink.

Patients must also be educated to limit their food volume appropriately. Food volume is initially limited to ¼ cup or 2 oz per meal. Over time, more food is tolerated at each meal.

Due to volume limitations, patients are encouraged to eat 3 to 6 small meals daily. The pace of eating is very important. Food should be consumed slowly over a 20- to 30-minute period. A bite, forkful, or spoonful of food should be very, very small. Using an infant spoon and small-pronged fork will help remind patients to take very small mouthfuls. Food must be chewed until it is of semi-liquid consistency.

Teach patients to recognize the signs of fullness, such as pressure, pain, and/or nausea, and to stop eating as soon as signs of fullness occur. Patients may feel like food is getting "stuck" if they eat too quickly. If the bolus of food cannot be digested, the body may expel the obstruction through vomiting or regurgitation. Slippage or prolapse of the stomach through the gastric band may occur if overeating causes frequent vomiting. If the obstruction persists, patients should be instructed to contact their physician.

Macronutrient Recommendations

PROTEIN

The recommended goal for protein intake may be 60 to 80 g/d or 1.0 to 1.5 g per kg of ideal body weight (IBW) (16). It may be difficult for patients to meet a goal of 1.5 g per kg IBW without excluding other macronutrients.

Commercially produced liquid or powder protein supplements of high biological value (whey, casein, soy protein, and egg albumin) are recommended until the patient is able to meet protein needs with food alone. Collagen-based products with added casein or another complete protein may not provide sufficient amounts of several indispensable amino acids (16). Therefore, collagen-based products should not be used as the sole protein source after weight loss surgery. Whey protein isolates are lactose-free; whey concentrates contain lactose in varying amounts. Patient compliance may be influenced by taste, texture, convenience, ease of mixing, and price. Prior to surgery, it is imperative patients find a protein supplement that they find palatable.

Patients should select foods containing high–biological value protein, such as lean meat, poultry, fish, low-fat dairy, and soy products and other meat alternatives. The development of food intolerance to meat, poultry, and/or dairy foods may compromise protein intake. At meals, patients are typically instructed to eat the protein-containing foods first.

FAT

The recommended minimum for fat intake is 20 g/d (19). Patients should be instructed to select low-fat foods to minimize caloric intake. Patients who have an RYGB should also understand that ingesting high-fat foods causes dumping-like symptoms. Encourage patients to choose healthy sources of essential fatty acids.

CARBOHYDRATES

The recommended minimum for carbohydrate intake is 130 g/d (19). Patients should select nutrient-dense complex carbohydrates and limit starchy carbohydrates. Patients should also avoid concentrated sweets because of their simple-sugar and calorie content.

Gastric bypass patients may experience dumping syndrome if food(s) with more than 15 g sugar are consumed. Dumping syndrome is more common in the early postoperative period, with symptoms decreasing in severity over time. The degree and severity of symptoms vary from patient to patient.

Sugar alcohols may have a laxative effect in sensitive individuals. Therefore, foods containing high concentrations of sugar alcohols should be avoided.

The fiber content of the postoperative diet is negligible. Powder fiber supplements may be added to liquids.

Vitamin and Mineral Requirements

Multivitamins with iron and trace minerals are recommended. Specific requirements vary depending on the WLS procedure:

- RYGB and SG: Two adult multivitamins/day
- AGB: One adult multivitamin/day

All supplements must be purchased prior to surgery and approved by the RD. Products should contain a minimum of 100% of daily value for at least two-thirds of nutrients (16). Patients should avoid products that are incomplete or lacking an essential vitamin or mineral. Check to ensure that the following nutrients are present and at 100% of the Dietary Reference Intake (DRI) (6):

- Iron
- Thiamin
- Vitamin B-12
- Folic acid
- Zinc
- Biotin
- Vitamin K

Bariatric vitamin brands are available and are formulated with more than 100% of the Daily Value for most nutrients. Chewable or liquid multivitamins should be started upon discharge from the hospital. Progression from a chewable or liquid vitamin to a vitamin tablet is as tolerated. Typically, tablets can be started by 3 months after surgery. Tablet size should be less than 11 mm in length/width to facilitate digestion.

Ensuring adequate folic acid intake for women of childbearing age is essential to prevent deficiency and fetal neural tube defects if pregnancy occurs. Two adult multivitamins will provide 800 mcg/d (200% DRI). Folic acid intake should be limited to less than 1,000 mcg/d, because excess folic acid can mask B-12 deficiency.

CALCIUM WITH VITAMIN D

Calcium requirements are 1,200 to 1,500 mg/d (2). A product containing calcium citrate with vitamin D should be recommended (16). Calcium citrate is better absorbed than calcium carbonate in a low-acid environment. Begin with a chewable, liquid, or crushed tablet.

Patients should begin taking calcium upon discharge from the hospital, taking it in divided doses of less than or equal to 500 to 600 mg to enhance calcium absorption. Advise patients to avoid taking calcium with supplements that contain iron. Ingestion of calcium and iron-containing supplements should be separated by at least 2 hours.

Vitamin D requirements are at least 3,000 IU/d and should be titrated to blood levels of >30 ng/mL 25-hydroxyvitamin D (2). An additional supplement may be required if the total vitamin D, from multivitamins and calcium, is less than the recommended intake.

VITAMIN B-12

Patients who undergo an RYGB or SG require more vitamin B-12 than is found in a multivitamin. Surgically bypassing or removing a portion of the stomach causes a decreased availability of intrinsic factor, which is needed for B-12 absorption in the terminal ileum. AGB patients may not need additional B-12 supplementation since the anatomy of the stomach is not changed. Patients should begin vitamin B-12 when discharged from the hospital, and one of the following routes of B-12 administration should be selected:

- Sublingual tablet or liquid drops: ≥500 mcg/d
- Oral tablet (crystalline form): ≥350 mcg/d
- Nasal spray: 500 mcg/wk
- Intramuscular injection: 1,000 mcg once a month

IRON

Total daily iron intake between 45 and 60 mg is recommended (2). Menstruating women and patients with a history of iron deficiency or a change in laboratory indices of iron status may require additional oral iron (ferrous sulfate, fumerate or gluconate) to provide 150 to 200 mg elemental iron daily (2). They should take iron with 250 mg vitamin C between meals to enhance iron absorption. They should not use enteric-coated or extended-release products. Additionally, they should not take iron supplements with calcium (ingestion of iron and calcium supplements should be separated by at least 2 hours).

OPTIONAL B COMPLEX

The daily recommended B-50 dosage is 1 tablet (16). B complex supplements are used as prophylaxis against B vitamin deficiencies in all WLS. They provide water-soluble vitamins that are absorbed in the proximal jejunum. They are required in patients with frequent vomiting or memory loss. When considering B complex supplements, remember that the combined total of folic acid should not exceed 1,000 mcg/d. Levels greater than 1,000 mcg could mask vitamin B-12 deficiency (16).

Diet Progression

Current clinical practice is to use a multistage diet progression after WLS (2,16). However, there is considerable variability in diet recommendations among bariatric programs. The RD, in collaboration with the bariatric team, should develop institution-specific protocols for diet advancement.

Patients are typically NPO for 24 hours after surgery, with intravenous fluids providing adequate hydration. Some surgeons/institution protocols require the patient to have a limited upper GI contrast study to evaluate the anastomosis and identify leaks prior to initiating liquids.

Fluids can be introduced starting with water. Instruct the patient to sip 1 oz over 15 minutes. If 4 oz are tolerated, the diet can be advanced to bariatric clear liquids.

As noted in Box 15.3, earlier in this chapter, the diet is advanced in stages. Tolerance and rate of progression will vary with each individual and type of surgery (see Box 15.4 on page 191 for information about progression after AGB).

Timeline for Outpatient Monitoring

To achieve optimal results after WLS, patients should seek regular follow-up, adhere to dietary recommendations, and commit to an active lifestyle. During the first 3 months after surgery, visits are suggested at 2 weeks, 1 month, 2 months, and 3 months to monitor diet tolerance and progression. Thereafter, quarterly visits are scheduled for the first year. Patients should make annual appointments or follow-up more frequently, if needed, for an adjustment or other medical or nutritional indication (16).

Evaluating Weight Changes

In the first 3 months after malabsorptive procedures, significant weight loss (ranging between 40 and 90 lb) may be observed (20). This translates into a loss of 0.5 to 1.0 lb per day (20). Weight loss is more gradual at 6 to 9 months, with the goal being 1 to 2 lb per week.

After RYGB, maximum weight loss is achieved within 12 to 18 months and averages 61% excess body weight (3). A more gradual weight loss is observed with AGB. Goal weight may be achieved after 2 to 3 years and averages 48% of excess body weight (3). Weight loss after SG can be achieved in 1 to 2 years after surgery and is similar to the weight loss observed with the RYGB (approximately 60%) (4,15).

Weight loss alone should not be the only parameter used to define success after bariatric surgery. Resolution or improvement in comorbid conditions and improved sense of well-being and quality of life are also important factors to consider when evaluating surgical outcomes.

Weight regain can occur after surgery. Sjostrom et al have reported that weight lost from baseline at 10 years after surgery is 25% for RYGB and 14% for AGB (SG patients were not included in this review) (5). If patients fail to lose weight or experience weight regain, assess to determine the cause. Potential reasons include maladaptive eating behaviors, psychological issues, and inadequately adjusted bands.

Reviewing Diet and Ability to Meet Nutrition Goals

Patients should be instructed to keep daily diet diaries for self-monitoring and for review by the RD. In this review, the RD should do the following:

- Assess fluid and protein intake, portion size, food texture and tolerance, frequency of eating, and overall dietary quality.
- Evaluate compliance with diet principles and progression and readiness to advance diet.
- Evaluate frequency of protein supplementation and daily use of vitamin and mineral supplements.
- Assess hunger/satiety.
- Review of symptoms of obstruction (reflux, vomiting, or pain) or other complications.

Evaluating Laboratory Markers of Nutritional Status

Box 15.5 presents nutrition-related laboratory data that should be periodically assessed in WLS patients (2). Monitor at 3 months, 6 months, 9 months, and then annually or as needed. Treat deficiencies per established protocols.

Assessing and Treating Nutrition-Related Complications

See Box 15.6 for a list of conditions and behaviors that may cause nutrition-related complications.

Malnutrition

Protein malnutrition or protein–energy malnutrition after WLS is not common but may occur if dietary intake is suboptimal because of confounding circumstances or medical conditions.

BOX 15.5   Recommended Laboratory Assessment After Bariatric Surgery

- Albumin
- CBC with platelets
- Electrolytes
- Glucose
- Iron
- Ferritin
- Lipid profile

- Liver function
- 25-hydroxyvitamin D
- Vitamin B-12
- Optional studies:
  - Folate
  - Intact parathyroid hormone (PTH)
  - Thiamin

Source: Data are from reference 2.

BOX 15.6   Conditions and Behaviors That Can Negatively Affect Nutritional Status After Bariatric Surgery

- Alcohol/drug abuse
- Anorexia
- Depression
- Diarrhea
- Fear of regaining weight
- Food intolerance
- Limited resources for food and/or supplements
- Prolonged vomiting

Micronutrient Deficiencies

Micronutrient deficiencies may occur in all bariatric patients because of a reduction in total food volume, because of intolerances to certain foods or food groups (such as dairy and/or meat), and as a result of altered digestion and/or absorption. Patient must be made aware of the importance of committing to life-long supplementation and monitoring.

THIAMIN DEFICIENCY (16)

Thiamin deficiency may develop in patients with severe, intractable vomiting and decreased intake due to stomal stenosis after RYGB. Deficiency can develop rapidly within a period of weeks or a few months and has been observed as early as 1 to 3 months after surgery.

Decreased serum thiamin is the basis for diagnosis. Symptoms of mild/early deficiency include the following:

- Anorexia
- Weakness
- Parasthesia
- Edema
- Low blood pressure
- Low body temperature

Symptoms of chronic/advanced deficiency include the following:

- Beri beri
- Cardiac failure
- Peripheral neuropathy and myelopathy, moreso in the legs than arms
- Wernicke's encephalopathy
- Wernicke-Korsakoff syndrome

Treatment for patients with neurological symptoms is parenteral thiamin, 100 mg/day for 7 to 14 days, followed by 10 mg oral thiamin per day until symptoms resolve (2).

Note: Do not give IV dextrose solutions to bariatric patients without providing multivitamins that contain thiamin. Thiamin is needed for carbohydrate metabolism, and use of glucose without thiamin can deplete body stores and cause an acute deficiency.

VITAMIN B-12 DEFICIENCY

After surgeries that bypass the lower stomach, vitamin B-12 deficiency may develop because the release of protein-bound vitamin B-12 from food is impaired by reduced gastric acid and enzyme secretion and lack of binding of intrinsic factor with vitamin B-12. Due to enterohepatic recycling and release of vitamin B-12 from hepatic stores, deficiencies are usually not observed in patients earlier than 1 year after surgery.

Diagnosis is determined by the following:

- Low serum vitamin B-12
- Elevated mean corpuscular volume (MCV)
- Increased methylmalonic acid
- Increased homocysteine

Symptoms may include pernicious anemia and numbness or paresthesia in the extremities. Deficiency is treated with intramuscular injection of 1,000 mcg vitamin B-12 per week for 8 weeks followed by 1,000 mcg/month for life (15).

IRON DEFICIENCY

Iron deficiency may develop for the following reasons:

- The site of iron absorption (duodenum and proximal jejunum) is bypassed in the RYGB.
- Stomach acid secretion, which is required for the conversion of iron to its soluble form, is limited by gastric restrictive/intestinal bypass procedures.
- Patients frequently experience intolerances to meat, a primary dietary source of heme iron.

Diagnostic indicators of deficiency include the following:

- Low hemoglobin
- Decreased serum iron
- Decreased serum ferritin

Symptoms may include anemia, fatigue, and pica with compulsive ice-eating. Deficiency is usually treated with oral iron replacement therapy: 3 to 4 iron tablets (50 to 65 mg/tablet) distributed over the day. Iron infusions may be required if oral supplementation is ineffective.

Nutrition Support

The implementation of enteral or parenteral nutrition should be considered when high-risk, critically ill bariatric patients cannot tolerate oral nutrition for more than 5 to 7 days, and when bariatric patients who are not critically ill cannot tolerate oral nutrition for more than 7 to 10 days (2). Standard nutrition support protocols should be followed. See Chapters 19 and 20 for more information on enteral and parenteral nutrition, respectively.

Pregnancy After Weight Loss Surgery

Female patients should be advised to avoid pregnancy for 18 months after surgery or until weight loss has plateaued and nutritional intake is stable. Fertility increases with weight loss, and patients should be counseled regarding appropriate contraception methods. Patients planning to become pregnant should be assessed before pregnancy for micronutrient deficiencies and treated as needed. Prenatal multivitamins may be added to the regimen, and additional iron supplementation may be required.

Conclusion

Bariatric surgery can help morbidly obese individuals lose substantial amounts of weight and resolve comorbidities of obesity. After a bariatric procedure, patients must commit to lifelong changes to their eating practices and food choices, and be prepared to address nutrient deficiencies and adverse effects, which can vary depending on the type of surgical procedure. Regular follow-up with the registered dietitian and other members of the health care team is essential for the patient's long-term success.

References

1. *The Clinical Guidelines on the Identification, Evaluation, and Treatment of Overweight and Obesity in Adults: The Evidence Report*. Rockland, MD: US Department of Health & Human Services; 1998. NIH publication No. 98–4083.
2. AACE/TOS/ASMBS. Clinical practice guidelines for the perioperative nutritional, metabolic, and nonsurgical support of the bariatric surgery patient. *Obesity*. 2013;21(suppl):S1–S25.
3. Buchwald H, Avidor Y, Braunwald E, Jensen MD, Pories W, Fahrbach K, Schoelles K. Bariatric surgery: a systematic review and meta-analysis. *JAMA*. 2004;292:1724–1737.
4. Snyder-Marlow G, Taylor D, Lenhard J. Nutrition care for patients undergoing laparoscopic sleeve gastrectomy for weight loss. *J Am Diet Assoc*. 2010;110:600–607.
5. Sjostrom L, Narbro K, Sjostrom CD, et al. Effects of bariatric surgery on mortality in Swedish obese subjects. *N Engl J Med*. 2007;357(8):741–752.
6. Biesemeier CK, Garland J, eds. *ADA Pocket Guide to Bariatric Surgery*. Chicago, IL: American Dietetic Association; 2009.
7. Kulick D, Hark L, Deen D. The bariatric surgery patient: a growing role for registered dietitians. *J Am Diet Assoc*. 2010;110:593–599.
8. Academy of Nutrition and Dietetics. Nutrition Care Process and Model. www.eatright.org (members-only section). Accessed June 1, 2010.
9. American Dietetic Association. Position of the American Dietetic Association: Weight Management. *J Am Diet Assoc*. 2009;109:330–346.
10. Colles SL, Dixon JB, Marks P, Strauss BJ, O'Brien PE. Preoperative weight loss with a very-low-energy diet: quantitation of change in liver and abdominal fat by serial imaging. *Am J Clin Nutr*. 2006;84:304–311.
11. Guidelines for laparoscopic and open surgical treatment of morbid obesity. (Document adopted by the American Society for Bariatric Surgery and the Society of American Gastrointestinal Endoscopic Surgeons, June 2000.) *Obes Surg*. 2000;10:378–379.
12. DeMaria EJ. Bariatric surgery for morbid obesity. *N Engl J Med*. 2007;356:2176–2183.
13. Beckman L, Beckman T, Earthman C. Changes in gastrointestinal hormones and leptin after Roux-en Y gastric bypass procedure: a review. *J Am Diet Assoc*. 2010;110:571–584.
14. Clinical Issues Committee of the American Society for Metabolic and Bariatric Surgery. Updated position statement on sleeve gastrectomy as a bariatric procedure. *Surg Obes Relat Dis*. 2010;6:1–5.
15. Nocca D, Krawczykowsky D, Bomans B, et al. A prospective multicenter study of 163 sleeve gastrectomies: results at 1 and 2 years. *Obes Surg*. 2008;18:560–565.
16. Allied Health Sciences Section Ad Hoc Nutrition Committee, Aills L, Blankenship J, Buffington C, Furtado M, Parrott J. Bariatric nutrition: suggestions for the surgical weight loss patient. *Surg Obes Relat Dis*. 2008;4(5 suppl):S73–S108.

17. Shen R, Dugay G, Rajaram K, Cabrera I, Siegel N, Ren CJ. Impact of patient follow-up on weight loss after bariatric surgery. *Obes Surg.* 2004;14:514–519.

18. Kellogg T, Bantle J, Leslie D, et al. Postgastric bypass hyperinsulinemic hypoglycemia syndrome: characterization and response to a modified diet. *Surg Obes Relat Dis.* 2008;4:492–499.

19. Institute of Medicine. *Dietary Reference Intakes for Energy, Carbohydrate, Fiber, Fat, Fatty Acids, Cholesterol, Protein, and Amino Acids.* Washington, DC: National Academies Press; 2005. www.nap.edu/catalog .php?record_id=10490. Accessed September 27, 2013.

20. AACE/TOS/ASMBS. Medical guidelines for clinical practice for the perioperative nutritional, metabolic, and nonsurgical support of the bariatric surgery patient. *Obesity.* 2009;17(suppl 1):S1–S70.

PART V

Systemic Disorders and Specific Populations

CHAPTER 16

Obesity

Mary Margaret Huizinga, MD, MPH

The overall aim of the nutrition management of obesity is to promote health. Often a nutrition plan that is aimed at disease management will include help in achieving a healthy weight. This chapter will review some very specialized diets that have been studied with regard to weight loss success. In some cases, it may be appropriate to use these specialized diets to promote weight loss when working with a patient with concomitant gastrointestinal (GI) disease.

Assessment

Nutrition management begins with an assessment of the patient's nutritional status and nutrition needs (see Chapter 3). In the initial assessment, the degree of overweight should be documented, usually by calculating the patient's body mass index (BMI). In addition, the patient's weight history, prior attempts at weight loss (successful and not), and typical eating and drinking habits should be documented. Questions to ask include the following:

- Do you typically snack throughout the day?
- Do you consume large portions at meals?
- How many times each week do you typically eat out?
- Do you consume high-calorie beverages? If so, how often?

Protein requirements and disease-specific medical nutrition therapy (eg, sodium restriction in congestive heart failure) should be addressed.

Assessment can also include exploration of the patient's readiness for change and weight loss objectives. Many patients have unrealistic weight loss goals. The National Institutes of Health recommends an initial goal of 10% of initial body weight (1). Five to ten percent weight loss has been shown to reduce the risk of diabetes, stroke, and cardiovascular disease (2,3).

Types of Dietary Plans

Once the initial assessment is complete, a dietary plan can be chosen. Some patients may prefer a highly specific diet, whereas others may prefer to make gradual changes to their current eating style. Gradual changes may include reducing caloric beverages, replacing processed snack items with healthier options, or reducing the frequency of dining out.

Dietary plans are often defined by either the degree of energy reduction or the macronutrient composition. While some diets may be more beneficial for particular patients, in general, the patient's ability to adhere to the proposed nutrition plan is the most important factor in long-term success (4–6). For this reason, assessment of the patient's history of weight loss attempts may be beneficial. By asking the patient about prior successes and failures, the provider can help the patient select a diet that best meets his or her preferences. In addition, recommending a diet that reflects usual dietary habits may increase adherence to and persistence with the prescribed nutrition plan.

Energy Reduction

There are three primary types of energy-reduction diet plans, defined by the degree of energy reduction (4,7–10):

- Energy-deficit diets reduce calorie intake by 300 to 500 kcal/d from estimated maintenance requirements.
- Low-calorie diets (LCDs) provide energy within the range of 800 to 1,600 kcal/d.
- Very-low-calorie diets (VLCDs) provide energy in the 400 to 800 kcal/d range.

Each diet type will be discussed in this chapter. Energy reduction may be achieved by the use of meal replacements or whole foods, although most VLCDs are comprised solely of meal replacements. The use of meal replacements will be discussed later in this chapter.

ENERGY-DEFICIT DIETS

Energy-deficit diets aim to reduce energy intake by 300 to 500 kcal/d and may be combined with exercise to achieve the energy deficit. Fat is commonly reduced in these dietary plans to less than 30% of the day's total energy intake. The goal is to lose 0.5 to 1.0 pound per week (11). A systematic review of randomized trials found that this type of diet resulted in a 5% weight reduction at 6 months (7). The 1- and 2-year weight reductions were 4.4% and 3%, respectively (7).

Energy deficit can be achieved by alteration of diet, reduction of portion sizes, or the use of meal replacements. Part of energy reduction may be offset by increasing physical activity. This type of weight loss plan can be used with diets designed to treat other diseases, such as the Dietary Approaches to Stop Hypertension (DASH) diet (12).

Often, the reduction of sweetened beverages and high-fat food items are the first steps in this type of diet plan. A "typical day" food history is important to identify potential areas of excess energy intake and to help create a dietary plan that can be adhered to by the patient. Substitution of lower calorie food items may also be used, such as having low-calorie popcorn or vegetables in place of fried potato chips for an afternoon snack.

Reduction of portion sizes can also help reduce the total energy intake. Many people find it challenging to accurately assess portion size even after being taught portion size–estimation skills (13). To monitor portion size, some patients may choose to measure their food. The plate method has been proposed as a way to improve portion size control without measuring and has been shown to be effective in promoting weight loss (14). The use of meal replacements also controls portion size and promotes weight loss if patients are provided information about the interpretation of food labels and guidance about what to look for in a meal replacement (15).

LOW-CALORIE DIETS

The definition of *low-calorie diets* varies. Many people set the calorie range as 800 to 1,200 kcal/d, but some authors allow the range to extend to 1,600 kcal/d (10,16). A meta-analysis shows that LCDs result in 9.7% weight loss in 6 months and an average weight reduction of 5% at 1 and 2 years (16). Low-calorie diets can be low in fat or carbohydrate and can be comprised of conventional foods, meal replacements (discussed later in the chapter), or a mixture of the two.

Patients on LCDs do not require weekly monitoring or intensive screening before participation. Many commercial programs are low-calorie diets and do not require the patient to see a medical professional before starting the diet program (4,10). It is important that patients maintain adequate protein intake, and protein requirements should be calculated for each patient. Requirements are typically 0.8 to 1.5 g protein per kg ideal body weight, depending on the degree of energy restriction. As the total daily energy intake decreases, the percentage of energy from protein will necessarily increase. Some patients, such as those with end-stage renal disease or advanced liver disease, may need to alter their protein intake.

VERY-LOW-CALORIE DIETS

Very-low-calorie diets are defined as diets consisting of less than 800 kcal per day (9,16). They are intensive diet programs that require medical supervision and are reserved for patients with a BMI of 30 or more who have not successfully lost weight with other methods (9,17). At 6 months, weight loss with VLCDs averages 16% (16). However, after 2 years, weight loss from baseline is similar to that seen with LCDs (16). VLCDs are recommended for no longer than 16 weeks (10).

The safety of VLCDs has been questioned. In the 1970s, several people died while on VLCDs because of poor-quality protein; inadequate electrolytes, vitamins, and minerals; and lack of medical supervision (8,10). Currently, an expert panel finds VLCDs to be safe and effective when used under careful medical supervision (8). Despite improvements in the nutritional adequacy of the diets and in their regulation, VLCDs remain potentially harmful, and patients who use them require close monitoring by a physician, usually every other week when undergoing rapid weight loss (10,16,17). The physician should monitor the patient's electrolytes and cardiovascular function, and any potential signs of starvation (10,17). The patient is also at an increased risk of cholelithiasis, dizziness, hair loss, cold intolerance, fatigue, volume depletion, and muscle cramps (8,16,17).

The physician may refer a patient to a registered dietitian (RD) to create a VLCD plan from protein-rich foods such as meat, fish, and poultry, or to assist a patient in adherence to a commercially available program. In addition, RDs help guide patients through a transition phase where they are returning to a more sustainable diet (10,16,17).

Patients should consume 0.8 to 1.5 g protein per kg of ideal body weight per day, with the amount being specified by the supervising physician (8,17). The protein may be from protein-rich foods or from soy-based or milk powder–based liquid protein beverages. In addition to the increased protein requirements to avoid a negative nitrogen balance, patients also require 2 to 3 g potassium daily, multivitamin supplementation, and adequate hydration (usually 2 liters of noncaloric beverages per day) (8,16,18).

MEAL REPLACEMENTS

Meal replacements are prepackaged food items, such as liquids, entrées, or bars. Meal replacements may be produced as dietary aides or for convenience eating; therefore, not all meal replacements are appropriate for weight loss. Nutrition plans may be comprised solely from meal replacements or from a combination of meal replacements and whole foods. Meal replacements are thought to promote weight loss by aiding in the reduction of energy intake through meal planning and portion control (11). Two meta-analyses have found that low-calorie diets with meal replacements are more effective than low-calorie diets without meal replacements for maintaining weight loss at 1 year (net difference 2.6 kg) (7,15).

Macronutrient-Focused Diets

Much attention has been given to the macronutrient composition of the various diets, with most groups advocating low-fat or low-carbohydrate diets. All diets result in a reduction of energy intake, which is the likely source of weight loss; however, some patients may find one type of diet more appealing (4).

LOW-CARBOHYDRATE DIETS

Low-carbohydrate diets have been popular for the last 2 decades, first with the Atkins diet and South Beach diets and more recently with the Paleo diet. The theory behind the weight loss associated with the Atkins diet is that very-low-carbohydrate intake (less than 10% of total daily energy intake) promotes cytogenesis, which leads to increased satiety, lipid peroxidation, and increased energy expenditure (19). Proponents of the Paleo diet attribute weight loss to altered insulin levels.

One concern regarding high-protein diets has been their effect on cardiac risk factors. However, a meta-analysis of research involving 1,141 obese patients showed that a low-carbohydrate diet was associated with significant decreases in body weight (–7.04 kg), BMI, abdominal circumference, blood pressure, plasma triglycerides, fasting plasma glucose, plasma insulin, and plasma C-reactive protein (20). A review of 94 studies found that the weight loss associated with low carbohydrate intake was due to the reduction in energy and not the reduction in carbohydrate (21). A randomized controlled trial of overweight, premenopausal women found that participants on the Atkins diet lost more weight than participants on other diet plans (Ornish, Zone, and LEARN) at 12 months; however, adherence remains a critical variable with any of these diets (6,22).

LOW-FAT DIETS

The Ornish and Pritikin diets are the prototypical very-low-fat diets, with less than 10% to 15% of total daily energy coming from fat. The Ornish diet (23) is vegetarian, and the Pritikin diet (24) allows limited use of very lean animal protein. The Ornish diet was shown to reverse coronary artery disease (23); however, the American Heart Association offered a caution about the use of such diets because of the elevation seen in triglycerides due to the high carbohydrate load in the diet (25). As stated previously, meta-analyses show similar weight loss at 12 months for low-fat and low-carbohydrate diets (20).

BALANCED (40-30-30) DIETS

The Zone diet is an example of a balanced macronutrient diet (26). The premise behind the Zone diet and others like it is that balanced macronutrient intake (moderate carbohydrate, low glycemic load) can result in lower inflammation. The diet's macronutrient composition is 40% carbohydrate, 30% protein, and 30% fat, which purportedly promotes a reduced insulin-to-glucagon ratio leading to lower inflammation; however, there is little scientific evidence to support these claims (27). A randomized controlled trial found similar weight loss for the Zone diet as the Atkins, Ornish, and Weight Watchers diets at 1 year (5). A second randomized controlled trial of overweight, premenopausal women found less weight loss with the Zone diet than the Atkins diet at 1 year (–1.6 kg vs –4.7 kg; $P < .05$); there were no differences between the Zone diet and the Ornish and LEARN diets (22). Patients who were adherent to the diet were more likely to be successful in weight loss (6).

Additional Topics in Obesity Management

The topic of bariatric surgery is covered in Chapter 15. This section briefly reviews several other topics of current interest. These issues are subject to ongoing research, and new information will be forthcoming in the medical literature as studies reach their conclusion.

Glycemic Index

The glycemic index is a way to compare the effect of different foods on blood glucose levels (28). High-glycemic index foods (such as white bread) lead to a sharp, rapid increase in blood glucose, whereas low-glycemic index foods (such as lentils) provide a slower, more consistent source of glucose, resulting in less release of insulin (28,29).

A meta-analysis of six studies (29) found that participants receiving a low–glycemic index diet had more weight loss than those receiving other diets (weighted mean difference –1.1 kg, 95%CI –2.0 to –0.2; P <.05). In addition, low–glycemic index diets resulted in lower total cholesterol and low-density lipoproteins (29). Another meta-analysis of 11 studies comparing low–glycemic index diets to conventional diets in patients with diabetes found that low–glycemic index diets resulted in a significant decrease in glycated hemoglobin (weight mean difference –0.5%, 95%CI –1.0 to –0.1; P = .03) and a reduction in hypoglycemia events (30). Other studies looking at the longer term effects of low–glycemic index diets and their effects on cardiovascular outcomes are underway.

Omega-3 Fatty Acids

Omega-3 fatty acids have been shown to decrease cardiovascular risk (31). Recently, there has been interest in the satiety-inducing effects of omega-3 fatty acids. A study of participants in a weight loss trial found that those with greater intake of long-chain omega-3 fatty acids had increased satiety and decreased hunger immediately after eating and 120 minutes after an energy-restricted meal (32). Another study found that consumption of long-chain omega-3 fatty acids reduced insulin resistance independently of weight loss (33). However, not all data have shown this association, and more research is needed to understand the role of long-chain omega-3 fatty acids in weight loss and metabolic control (34).

Weight Loss Medications

Studies have shown that patients who take prescription weight loss medications in combination with a lifestyle modification program lose more weight than individuals who use either method alone (35–38). The largest randomized controlled trial showed that subjects who received combined lifestyle modification and pharmacological therapy lost more than twice as much as participants who received either therapy alone (38). In addition, participants who regularly recorded their food intake lost much more than those who did not (18.1 ± 9.8 kg vs 7.7 ± 7.5 kg; P = .04). Patients receiving weight loss medications should also receive dietary and other lifestyle modification education to maximize their weight loss.

Weight Loss Maintenance

Long-term weight loss maintenance is the ultimate goal of any weight loss program; however, it is an elusive goal for many. Weight regain commonly occurs after weight loss regardless of the method used to achieve the initial loss (11,39). Much of what we know about the factors associated with successful weight loss maintenance come from the National Weight Control Registry, a volunteer registry of more than 4,000 people who have lost at least 13 kg and maintained the loss for more than 5 years (39,40). Most individuals in the registry eat breakfast daily, exercise, consume diets low in fat (less than 24% of energy intake) and calories (typically 1,300 to 1,500 kcal/d), self-monitor weight and food intake, and control portion size (39,41). Other studies have had similar findings (42,43).

Conclusion

Assisting patients in the nutrition management of obesity can help decrease the severity and/or risk of many chronic illnesses. Obesity is thought to be a cause of metabolic inflammation and may therefore worsen the symptoms of GI disease (44). It is important to set reasonable goals based on the patient's health status and to find a diet that works with the patient's lifestyle to boost adherence. Ability to adhere to the diet is often the most important predictor of successful weight loss. Finally, factors that facilitate long-term weight loss should be discussed early and often during the course of the treatment.

References

1. Executive summary of the Clinical Guidelines on the Identification, Evaluation, and Treatment of Overweight and Obesity in Adults. *Arch Intern Med.* 1998;158(17):1855–1867.

2. Krauss RM, Eckel RH, Howard B, Appel LJ, Daniels SR, Deckelbaum RJ, et al. AHA Dietary Guidelines: revision 2000: a statement for healthcare professionals from the Nutrition Committee of the American Heart Association. *Stroke.* 2000;31(11):2751–2766.

3. Knowler WC, Barrett-Connor E, Fowler SE, Hamman RF, Lachin JM, Walker EA, et al. Reduction in the incidence of type 2 diabetes with lifestyle intervention or metformin. *N Engl J Med.* 2002;346(6):393–403.

4. Tangney CC, Gustashaw KA, Stefan TM, Sullivan C, Ventrelle J, Filipowski CA, et al. A review: which dietary plan is best for your patients seeking weight loss and sustained weight management? *Dis Mon.* 2005;51(5):284–316.

5. Dansinger ML, Gleason JA, Griffith JL, Selker HP, Schaefer EJ. Comparison of the Atkins, Ornish, Weight Watchers, and Zone diets for weight loss and heart disease risk reduction: a randomized trial. *JAMA.* 2005;293(1):43–53.

6. Alhassan S, Kim S, Bersamin A, King AC, Gardner CD. Dietary adherence and weight loss success among overweight women: results from the A TO Z weight loss study. *Int J Obes (Lond).* 2008;32(6):985–991.

7. Franz MJ, VanWormer JJ, Crain AL, Boucher JL, Histon T, Caplan W, et al. Weight-loss outcomes: a systematic review and meta-analysis of weight-loss clinical trials with a minimum 1-year follow-up. *J Am Diet Assoc.* 2007;107(10):1755–1767.

8. Very low-calorie diets. National Task Force on the Prevention and Treatment of Obesity, National Institutes of Health. *JAMA.* 1993;270(8):967–974.

9. Clinical Guidelines on the Identification, Evaluation, and Treatment of Overweight and Obesity in Adults—The Evidence Report. National Institutes of Health. *Obes Res.* 1998;6(Suppl 2):51S–209S.

10. Strychar I. Diet in the management of weight loss. *CMAJ.* 2006;174(1):56–63.

11. Ulen C, Huizinga M, Beech B, Elasy T. Weight regain prevention. *Clin Diabetes.* 2008;26(3):100–113.

12. National Heart, Lung and Blood Institute; National Institutes of Health. Your Guide to Lowering Your Blood Pressure with DASH. Revised 2006. www.nhlbi.nih.gov/health/public/heart/hbp/dash/new_dash.pdf. Accessed June 28, 2010.

13. Huizinga MM, Carlisle AJ, Cavanaugh KL, Davis DL, Gregory RP, Schlundt DG, et al. Literacy, numeracy, and portion-size estimation skills. *Am J Prev Med.* 2009;36(4):324–328.

14. Pedersen SD, Kang J, Kline GA. Portion control plate for weight loss in obese patients with type 2 diabetes mellitus: a controlled clinical trial. *Arch Intern Med.* 2007;167(12):1277–1283.

15. Heymsfield SB, van Mierlo CA, van der Knaap HC, Heo M, Frier HI. Weight management using a meal replacement strategy: meta- and pooling analysis from six studies. *Int J Obes Relat Metab Disord.* 2003;27(5):537–549.

16. Tsai AG, Wadden TA. The evolution of very-low-calorie diets: an update and meta-analysis. *Obesity (Silver Spring).* 2006;14(8):1283–1293.

17. Cummings S, Parham ES, Strain GW. Position of the American Dietetic Association: weight management. *J Am Diet Assoc.* 2002;102(8):1145–1155.

18. Wadden TA, Stunkard AJ, Brownell KD, Day SC. A comparison of two very-low-calorie diets: protein-sparing-modified fast versus protein-formula-liquid diet. *Am J Clin Nutr.* 1985;41(3):533–539.

19. Atkins R. *Dr. Atkins' New Diet Revolution.* New York, NY: Avon Books; 1998.

20. Santos FL, Esteves SS, daCosta Pereira A, et al. Systematic review and meta-analysis of clinical trials of the effects of low carbohydrate diets on cardiovascular risk factors. *Obes Rev.* 2012;13(11):1048–1066.

21. Bravata DM, Sanders L, Huang J, Krumholz HM, Olkin I, Gardner CD, et al. Efficacy and safety of low-carbohydrate diets: a systematic review. *JAMA.* 2003;289(14):1837–1850.

22. Gardner CD, Kiazand A, Alhassan S, Kim S, Stafford RS, Balise RR, et al. Comparison of the Atkins, Zone, Ornish, and LEARN diets for change in weight and related risk factors among overweight premenopausal women: the A to Z Weight Loss Study: a randomized trial. *JAMA.* 2007;297(9):969–977.

23. Ornish D, Scherwitz LW, Billings JH, Brown SE, Gould KL, Merritt TA, et al. Intensive lifestyle changes for reversal of coronary heart disease. *JAMA.* 1998;280(23):2001–2007.

24. Freedman MR, King J, Kennedy E. Popular diets: a scientific review. *Obes Res.* 2001;9(Suppl 1):1S–40S.

25. Lichtenstein AH, Van Horn L. Very low fat diets. *Circulation.* 1998;98(9):935–939.

26. Sears B, Bell S. The Zone diet: an anti-inflammatory, low glycemic-load diet. *Metab Syndr Relat Disord.* 2004;2(1):24–38.

27. Cheuvront SN. The Zone diet phenomenon: a closer look at the science behind the claims. *J Am Coll Nutr.* 2003;22(1):9–17.

28. Jenkins DJ, Wolever TM, Taylor RH, Barker H, Fielden H, Baldwin JM, et al. Glycemic index of foods: a physiological basis for carbohydrate exchange. *Am J Clin Nutr.* 1981;34(3):362–366.

29. Thomas DE, Elliott EJ, Baur L. Low glycaemic index or low glycaemic load diets for overweight and obesity. *Cochrane Database Syst Rev.* 2007(3):CD005105.

30. Thomas D, Elliott EJ. Low glycaemic index, or low glycaemic load, diets for diabetes mellitus. *Cochrane Database Syst Rev.* 2009(1):CD006296.

31. Kris-Etherton PM, Harris WS, Appel LJ. Fish consumption, fish oil, omega-3 fatty acids, and cardiovascular disease. *Circulation.* 2002;106(21):2747–2757.

32. Parra D, Ramel A, Bandarra N, Kiely M, Martinez JA, Thorsdottir I. A diet rich in long chain omega-3 fatty acids modulates satiety in overweight and obese volunteers during weight loss. *Appetite.* 2008;51(3):676–680.

33. Ramel A, Martinez A, Kiely M, Morais G, Bandarra NM, Thorsdottir I. Beneficial effects of long-chain n-3 fatty acids included in an energy-restricted diet on insulin resistance in overweight and obese European young adults. *Diabetologia.* 2008;51(7):1261–1268.

34. Roche HM. Fatty acids and the metabolic syndrome. *Proc Nutr Soc.* 2005;64(1):23–29.

35. Phelan S, Wadden TA. Combining behavioral and pharmacological treatments for obesity. *Obes Res.* 2002;10(6):560–574.

36. Wadden TA, Berkowitz RI, Sarwer DB, Prus-Wisniewski R, Steinberg C. Benefits of lifestyle modification in the pharmacologic treatment of obesity: a randomized trial. *Arch Intern Med.* 2001;161(2):218–227.

37. Wadden TA, Berkowitz RI, Vogt RA, Steen SN, Stunkard AJ, Foster GD. Lifestyle modification in the pharmacologic treatment of obesity: a pilot investigation of a potential primary care approach. *Obes Res.* 1997;5(3):218–226.

38. Wadden TA, Berkowitz RI, Womble LG, Sarwer DB, Phelan S, Cato RK, et al. Randomized trial of lifestyle modification and pharmacotherapy for obesity. *N Engl J Med.* 2005;353(20):2111–2120.

39. Wyatt H, Phelan S, Wing R, Hill J. Lessons from patients who have successfully maintained weight loss. *Obes Manage.* 2005;1(2):56–61.

40. Hill J, Wing R. The National Weight Control Registry. *Permanente J.* 2003;7(3):34–37.

41. Wing RR, Hill JO. Successful weight loss maintenance. *Annu Rev Nutr.* 2001;21:323–341.

42. Byrne S, Cooper Z, Fairburn C. Weight maintenance and relapse in obesity: a qualitative study. *Int J Obes Relat Metab Disord.* 2003;27(8):955–962.

43. Sherwood NE, Jeffery RW, French SA, Hannan PJ, Murray DM. Predictors of weight gain in the Pound of Prevention study. *Int J Obes Relat Metab Disord.* 2000;24(4):395–403.

44. Gregor MF, Hotamisligil GS. Inflammatory mechanisms of obesity. *Annu Rev Immunol.* 2011;29:415–445.

CHAPTER 17

Eating Disorders

Carolyn Coker Ross, MD, MPH, and
Gerard E. Mullin, MD, CNSP, FACN, AGAF

Treatment of individuals with eating disorders is a challenge that requires an integration of psychiatric and nutrition regimens. Psychiatric care is needed to treat the underlying condition that results in distorted self-image and compels patients to engage in disordered behaviors, such as self-imposed limitations on energy intake (dieting or fasting), binge eating, self-induced vomiting, excessive exercise, and the use of cathartics or purgatives. In addition, psychological comorbidities (eg, depression, anxiety, obsessive-compulsive disorders, and substance use disorders), which are common across the spectrum of eating disorders, must be identified and treated. Medical treatment is important in preventing and treating the medical consequences of eating disorder behaviors. In conjunction with medical and psychological treatment, nutrition interventions may be used to address malnutrition and its effects on brain function. Malnutrition has been noted as a contributing factor to the behaviors associated with eating disorders, the concurrent mood and anxiety disorders, and the health consequences of eating disorders.

Ultimately, most individuals with eating disorders develop functional bowel disorders (1) and are at risk for other gastrointestinal (GI) disorders, such as gastroparesis, which may hinder energy intake or cause malabsorption from small intestinal bacterial overgrowth. Coordination of care among the members of the health care team, including mental health professionals, gastroenterologists and other physicians, nurses, pharmacists, registered dietitians (RDs), and others, is essential to improve patient outcomes.

Definitions and Diagnostic Criteria

Eating disorders listed in the *Diagnostic and Statistical Manual of Mental Disorders,* 5th edition (DSM-V; published in 2013) include anorexia nervosa (AN), bulimia nervosa (BN), binge eating disorder (BED), other specified eating disorders, and unspecified eating disorders (ie, eating disorders not otherwise specified [EDNOS]). A patient cannot be diagnosed with more than one of these disorders at one time (2).

Anorexia Nervosa

Anorexia nervosa is a disorder characterized in part by significantly low body weight (defined as a "weight that is less than minimally normal or, for children and adolescents, less than minimally expected") (2).

Before diagnosing a patient with AN, the physician should consider whether weight loss/low body weight has another etiology, such as a GI disease, mental illness, substance abuse, or another type of eating disorder (2).

DSM-V lists three diagnostic criteria for AN (2):

- Restriction of energy intake relative to requirements, leading to significantly low body weight in the context of age, sex, developmental trajectory, and physical health
- Intense fear of gaining weight or of becoming fat, or persistent behavior that interferes with weight gain, even though at a significantly low weight
- Disturbance in the way in which one's body weight or shape is experienced, undue influence of body weight or shape on self-evaluation, or persistent lack of recognition of the acute health risks associated with the current low body weight

Typically, body mass index (BMI) is used to assess weight (eg, BMI ≤17 indicates significantly low weight). However, assessment should be individualized to include a patient's clinical history and psychological profile.

Prior to the publication of DSM-V, presence of amenorrhea for 3 consecutive months was included as a required diagnostic criterion for AN, but this criterion was removed with publication of the DSM-V. This decision was made partially on the basis that amenorrhea is an unreliable measurement of weight status and not of use in assessment of psychiatric comorbidities, outcomes, or clinical factors. A compounding factor was that it meant entire populations—men, prepubescent girls, postmenopausal women, and women prescribed oral contraceptives—could not receive a diagnosis of AN even if it were otherwise appropriate (2–6).

There are two subtypes of AN (2):

- Restricting—ie, "presentations in which the weight loss is accomplished primarily through dieting, fasting, and/or excessive exercise" (2)
- Binge-eating/purging type, which involves recurrent episodes of binge eating or purging behavior (see Boxes 17.1 and 17.2)

When assigning an ICD-10-CM code, the subtype must be specified.

Bulimia Nervosa

DSM-V uses the following five diagnostic criteria for BN (2):

- Recurrent episodes of binge eating occur (see Box 17.1).
- Recurrent inappropriate compensatory behaviors are used to prevent weight gain (see Box 17.2).
- The binge eating and inappropriate compensatory behaviors both occur, on average, at least once a week for 3 months. (**Note:** Prior to the publication of DSM-V, the criterion was set at "at least twice a week for 3 months.)
- Self-evaluation is unduly influenced by body shape and weight.
- The disturbance does not occur exclusively during episodes of AN.

Body weight or BMI is *not* a diagnostic criterion for BN. This eating disorder may affect normal weight, overweight, or obese individuals (2).

BOX 17.1   What Is Binge Eating?

DSM-V defines an episode of binge eating as having two characteristics: (a) "eating, in a discrete period of time (eg, 2 hours), an amount of food that is definitely larger than what most individuals would eat in a similar period of time under similar circumstances"; and (b) a perceived lack of control over eating during the episode.

When assessing whether a patient's intake during an episode qualifies as binge eating, the clinician should consider not just the amount eaten but also the context (eg, an ordinary meal vs a holiday feast), as well as whether the patient felt in control of eating—was he or she capable of not eating or could he or she stop eating once the episode began?

Source: Data are from reference 2.

BOX 17.2   What Are Purging Behaviors?

Examples of purging behaviors (which DSM-V calls "inappropriate compensatory behaviors to prevent weight gain") include self-induced vomiting; misuse of laxatives, diuretics, or other medications; fasting; and excessive exercise.

Source: Data are from reference 2.

Binge Eating Disorder

BED first appeared in the DSM-IV, where it was categorized as an EDNOS. However, a wealth of new studies in recent years has demonstrated consistent diagnostic criteria and treatment outcomes, and BED was classified as an officially recognized disorder in the DSM-V (2–4,6). The DSM-V diagnostic criteria are as follows (2):

- Recurrent episodes of binge eating (see Box 17.1).
- The binge eating episodes are associated with three or more of the following:
  - Eating much more rapidly than usual.
  - Eating until feeling uncomfortably full.
  - Eating large amounts of food when not feeling physically hungry.
  - Eating alone because of feeling embarrassed by how much one is eating.
  - Feeling disgusted with oneself, depressed, or very guilty afterward.
- Presence of marked distress regarding binge eating.
- The binge eating occurs, on average, at least once a week for 3 months.
- The binge eating is not associated with the recurrent use of inappropriate compensatory behavior as in BN and does not occur exclusively during the course of BN or AN.

Patients with BED may be normal weight, overweight, or obese (2).

Other Eating Disorders

DSM-V categories "other specified feeding and eating disorder" and "unspecified feeding or eating disorder" may be used for patients who do not meet all the criteria for AN, BN, or BED but have eating disorder symptoms "that cause clinically significant distress or impairment in social, occupational, or other important areas of functioning" (2). Examples from DSM-V include the following:

- Atypical anorexia nervosa—significant weight loss is present but weight remains within or above the normal range
- Bulimia nervosa (of low frequency and/or limited duration)
- Binge eating disorder (of low frequency and/or limited duration)
- Purging disorder to lose weight (in the absence of bingeing)
- Night eating syndrome

The "unspecified" diagnosis is used in situations where the clinician will not specify the reasons why criteria are unmet or cannot make a specific diagnosis because of lack of information.

Severity of Eating Disorders

Table 17.1 summarizes DSM-V specifications for the severity of AN, BN, and BED. The severity level can be increased to reflect a given patient's symptoms, functional disability, or, in the case of AN, need for supervision (2).

Prevalence

The prevalence of eating disorders varies by type of disorder and by sex (see Table 17.2 on page 216) (7). AN, BN, and BED are most commonly diagnosed in adolescents and young adults, although these disorders may occur earlier or later in life (2).

TABLE 17.1 Severity of Anorexia Nervosa, Bulimia Nervosa, and Binge Eating Disorder

Severity[a]	Anorexia Nervosa[b]	Bulimia Nervosa	Binge Eating Disorder
Mild	BMI ≥17.00	1–3 episodes/wk of inappropriate compensatory behavior[c]	1–3 binge eating episodes/wk
Moderate	BMI 16.00–16.99	4–7 episodes/wk of inappropriate compensatory behavior[c]	4–7 binge eating episodes/wk
Severe	BMI 15.00–15.99	8–13 episodes/wk of inappropriate compensatory behavior[c]	8–13 binge eating episodes/wk
Extreme	BMI <15.00	≥14 episodes/wk of inappropriate compensatory behavior[c]	≥14 binge eating episodes/wk

[a]Severity of diagnosis may be increased based on clinical judgment of other factors, including symptoms or functional disability.
[b]Body mass index (BMI) ranges are based on World Health Organization categories for thinness in adults. Use corresponding BMI percentiles for children and adolescents.
[c]Average incidence.
Source: Data are from reference 2.

TABLE 17.2   Lifetime Prevalence of Eating Disorders in Men and Women

	Women	*Men*
Anorexia nervosa	0.9%	0.3%
Bulimia nervosa	1.5%	0.5%
Binge eating disorder	3.5%	2.0%

Source: Data are from reference 7.

Medical and Nutritional Complications

Table 17.3 lists selected medical complications associated with AN, BN, and BED (8–10). Patients with any of these symptoms or signs should be evaluated for an eating disorder. Box 17.3 presents the GI effects seen in patients with eating disorders. Because the GI tract is a channel for enteral nutrition delivery, compromised digestive function may interfere with the recovery of patients with eating disorders who require nutrition support. See Chapter 19 for more information on indications and contraindications for enteral nutrition.

TABLE 17.3   Medical Risks and Complications of Eating Disorders

	Anorexia Nervosa[a]	*Bulimia Nervosa*	*Binge Eating Disorder*
Cardiac	Nonspecific ST-T wave changes Prolongation of QT interval Severe bradycardia, orthostatic blood pressure changes Peripheral edema Hypoprotenemia Cardiomyopathy Mitral valve prolapse	Low voltage, prolonged QT interval Bradycardia Cardiomegaly (from ipecac toxicity)	Stroke, high blood pressure, and heart disease (secondary to obesity)
Pulmonary	If purging type, same as for bulimia nervosa	Aspiration pneumonia Pneumothorax Subcutaneous emphysema Rib fractures	Sleep apnea
Skin	Lanugo	None	None
Metabolic and orthopedic	Hypoglycemia Hyperlipidemia Loss of bone mineral density Sick euthyroid syndrome (normal TSH, decreased T3 and increased reverse T3)	Hyperlipidemia Hypoglycemia (if restricting) Elevated amylase	Hyperlipidemia Metabolic syndrome Increased risk for diabetes (if obese) Hyperglycemia Insulin resistance
Hematologic	Leukopenia	Hypochloremia, hypokalemia or metabolic acidosis (from vomiting, laxatives, diuretics) Elevated amylase from vomiting	None

[a]Complications of anorexia nervosa can be related to starvation.
Source: Data are from references 8, 9, and 10.

BOX 17.3 Gastrointestinal Manifestations of Eating Disorders

- Abdominal distention or pain
- Barrett's esophagus
- Boerhaave's syndrome
- Cathartic bowel
- Constipation
- Dental caries and loss of dental enamel
- Diarrhea
- Duodenal ulcer
- Dysphagia
- Early satiety
- Esophageal stricture
- Esophagitis
- Functional bowel disorders[a]
- Gastric rupture
- Gastric ulcer (perforated)
- Gastroparesis[b]
- Heartburn/gastroesophageal reflux disease
- Liver disease
- Malabsorptive disorders
- Nausea
- Pancreatitis
- Salivary gland enlargement

---

[a]Patients with functional bowel disorders seem to be at a higher risk for developing eating disorders, and patients with eating disorders seem to be at a higher risk for developing functional bowel disorders.
[b]Gastroparesis is a common problem in this population and may cause long-term consequences for some patients.

Protein-Energy Malnutrition and Micronutrient Deficiencies

Patients diagnosed with eating disorders should be assessed for protein-energy malnutrition (see Boxes 17.4 and 17.5 on page 218) and for micronutrient deficiencies. In studies of diet history and recall, women with AN were found to be at high risk for the following nutrient deficiencies: zinc, calcium, vitamin D, folate, vitamin B-12, magnesium, and copper (11). Correcting abnormal zinc status is often critical for optimal functioning of the GI and neuroendocrine systems, whereas addressing thiamin deficiency is crucial for neuropsychiatric system function.

It is important to note that "normal" laboratory data may not be a reliable indicator of nutritional status or the severity of an eating disorder. Setnick has pointed out that "normal" laboratory results in patients with eating disorders may be due to the following (12):

> The patient's nutritional intake has declined over time, allowing for metabolic changes that maintain homeostasis. Although nutrient *stores* are depleted, blood tests that evaluate *serum* nutrient levels remain within normal limits. [Also,] dehydration increases volume-dependent laboratory values, allowing them to seem normal until the patient achieves normal hydration status. Vitamin and mineral supplements or consumption of fortified foods [can] mask nutritional deficiencies.

For this reason, Setnick encourages RDs to assess laboratory values in the context of a thorough dietary history, which may be more likely to identify potential nutrient deficiencies, as well as nutrition-related physical signs and symptoms (12).

ZINC DEFICIENCY

Patients with AN commonly present with numerous manifestations of zinc deficiency—such as weight loss, appetite loss, specific forms of dermatitis, amenorrhea, and depression (13)—that may be the result of malabsorption of zinc. In protein-energy malnutrition, a disruption of the small intestinal mucosal

---

BOX 17.4   Laboratory Evidence of Malnutrition in Patients with Eating Disorders

- Hematology: Neutropenia; normochromic, normocytic anemia; iron-deficiency anemia; thrombocytopenia
- Chemistry: Elevated liver function tests; hypoalbuminemia; hypoglycemia; prerenal azotemia; renal insufficiency
- Electrolytes/metabolic panel: Hypokalemia, hypomagnesemia, hypocalcemia, hypophosphatemia

---

BOX 17.5   Physical Findings of Malnutrition in Patients with Eating Disorders

- Bradycardia
- Cold extremities
- Dependent edema (may increase during refeeding)
- Dry skin
- Emaciation
- Growth of lanugo hair on the back, arms, and face
- Hair thinning
- Hypotension
- Hypothermia
- Muscle weakness
- Signs of dehydration

---

absorptive capacity results in decreased capability to absorb zinc (14). The acquired zinc deficiency that results consequently induces an altered or "dysfunctional" epithelial barrier and represents a risk for diarrhea, which perpetuates malabsorption (14). In a randomized, double-blinded placebo-controlled trial with 35 female participants with AN, measured increases in BMI demonstrated that zinc supplementation improved the recovery rate (15).

VITAMIN B DEFICIENCIES

Thiamin deficiency should be routinely screened in patients with eating disorders. Factors that can increase thiamin deficiency—namely, abuse of diuretics and alcohol and simple-carbohydrate loading—are commonly seen in individuals with eating disorders. In a study of 37 patients in an eating disorder unit, thiamin deficiency was documented in 14 (38%) of the subjects (16).

Riboflavin deficiency in AN and BN has been documented (17,18). Capo-chichi et al (18) hypothesized that riboflavin deficiency in AN may be due to low triiodothyronine (T3) levels associated with AN, because riboflavin mononucleotide production requires T3. Patients with AN have remained deficient in riboflavin and T3 after refeeding, so consideration should be given to malabsorption and thyroid replacement even in "sick euthyroid syndrome" (18).

Patients with AN may also be deficient in vitamin B-12 or folate (8).

MAGNESIUM DEFICIENCY

In a study of 175 patients with eating disorders (of various types) in an inpatient treatment setting, 25% had documented magnesium deficiency (19). It is noteworthy that among this study population, the heart rhythms of eight patients with low magnesium levels who had cardiac arrhythmias were normalized with magnesium replacement.

ESSENTIAL FATTY ACID DEFICIENCIES

Essential fatty acid deficiencies have been found in patients with AN. They can be caused by the exclusion of sources of dietary fat (20,21).

Treatment Guidelines

The most recent evidence-based practice guideline on the treatment of eating disorders (22) from the American Psychiatry Association (APA) is more than 5 years old (2006) and no longer considered current. However, in 2012, Yager et al reviewed research published on treatment since the APA guideline was issued and concluded that the guideline remained "substantially correct and current in its recommendations" (23). Readers are referred to these publications for additional information about topics such as the choice of treatment setting, medication use, and types of therapy. In addition, the position and practice papers of Academy of Nutrition and Dietetics offer guidance for RDs regarding nutrition interventions for eating disorders (24,25).

Nutrition Management

Within the multidisciplinary approach to treatment, nutrition management is critical. Periodic nutrition assessment by an RD with advanced training and clinical judgment in the area of eating disorders can help the health care team identify appropriate therapies and evaluate the outcomes of interventions (24,25). Qualified RDs may also be involved in nutrition support (enteral or parenteral), meal planning, offering nutrition education and counseling within the parameters of the treatment plan, and coordinating care. For additional information on this topic, see references 12, 24, and 25.

Patients with Anorexia Nervosa

Although care is individualized for each patient, treatment for AN generally involves the gradual increase of energy intake to restore weight. The typical meal plan and dietary guidelines prescribed for patients with AN promote normalization of food intake and eating habits (12,22,25–27). Imposing restrictions on exercise for patients with AN in the interest of accelerating weight gain may be necessary (12).

Patients with Bulimia Nervosa or Binge Eating Disorder

Dietary recommendations for patients with BN and BED vary depending on factors such as the individual's psychological, medical, and nutritional status and the treatment setting. Because restrictive diet regimens can foster disordered eating behaviors, they should not be prescribed to patients with BN or BED (12). Goals of nutritional rehabilitation are the normalization of dietary intake and eating habits (25,26).

Refeeding Syndrome

Management of malnourished patients should include efforts to prevent refeeding syndrome, which represents the clinical complications resulting from refeeding severely malnourished patients too quickly (27). In such circumstances, significant abnormalities in baseline cellular function result from depletion of phosphate. Potential effects include reduced adenosine triphosphate levels (28), which may result in arrhythmias, reduced cardiac stroke volume, and congestive heart failure (29), and complications in the neuromuscular, hematological, metabolic, hepatic, and respiratory functions resulting from abnormal glucose metabolism, hypophosphatemia, hypomagnesemia, hypokalemia, and fluid-balance abnormalities. Ankle edema can be a first sign of refeeding syndrome.

Gradual implementation of a nutritional intake regimen with energy repletion at approximately 20 kcal/kg per day or 1,000 kcal/d during the first 1 to 2 weeks of treatment helps prevent refeeding syndrome (30). Electrolyte abnormalities should be corrected during refeeding, and vitamin and mineral deficiencies should be addressed before and during the first 10 days of refeeding. Thiamin (200 mg to 300 mg/d orally) along with high-potency vitamin B and multivitamin supplements should be given daily. Plasma phosphate, calcium, magnesium, and potassium should be monitored closely along with urine output (31). Carbohydrates introduced into the diet can cause rapid renal excretion of sodium and water. If fluid restoration is then initiated to maintain urine output, patients will develop fluid overload, leading to congestive heart failure, pulmonary edema, and cardiac arrhythmia (32). Therefore, refeeding of severely emaciated patients in a hospital setting is the recommended protocol so that electrolytes and electrocardiograms can be monitored (29).

Conclusion

The primary eating disorders and their associated GI outcomes may be direct causes of nutritional problems among individuals diagnosed with eating disorders. In turn, nutritional deficits can cause or exacerbate behaviors of an eating disorder, the medical consequences, and the concurrent mood and anxiety disorders. However, the etiology of digestive disorders in some individuals with eating disorders may be unrelated to the eating disorder. In fact, these digestive disorders may represent the event that triggers the onset of their eating disorder (12). Correcting nutritional deficiencies associated with eating disorders should involve a well-trained RD as part of an interdisciplinary health care team.

References

1. McClain CJ, Humphries LL, Hill KK, Nickl NJ. Gastrointestinal and nutritional aspects of eating disorders. *J Am Coll Nutr*. 1993;12(4):466–474.
2. American Psychiatric Association. *Diagnostic and Statistical Manual of Mental Disorders*. 5th ed. Arlington, VA: American Psychiatric Publishing; 2013.
3. The DSM-5 Eating Disorders Workgroup [video]. YouTube website. www.youtube.com/watch?v=E4FjiNWmIDM. Accessed August 7, 2013.
4. Walsh BT. DSM-V Video Series: Changes to anorexia nervosa and bulimia nervosa [audio]. American Psychiatric Association website. www.psychiatry.org/practice/dsm/dsm5/dsm-5-video-series-changes-to-anorexia-nervosa-and-bulimia-nervosa. Accessed December 2, 2013.
5. Wilfley DE, Bishop ME, Wilson GT, Agras WS. Classification of eating disorders: Toward DSM-V. *Int J Eat Disord*. 2007;40(Suppl):S123–S129.
6. Moran M. ICD Codes for Some DSM-5 Diagnoses Updated. October 7, 2013. http://psychnews.psychiatry online.org/newsArticle.aspx?articleid=1757346. Accessed November 21, 2013.
7. Hudson JI, Hiripi E, Pope HG, Kessler RC. The prevalence and correlates of eating disorders in the National Comorbidity Survey Replication. *Biol Psychiatry*. 2007;61(3):348–358.
8. de Zwaan M, Mitchell JE. Medical complications of anorexia nervosa and bulimia nervosa. In: Kaplan AS, Garfinkel PE, eds. *Medical Issues and the Eating Disorders: The Interface*. New York, NY: Brunner/Mazel; 1993:60–100.
9. Blomquist KK, Milsom VA, Barnes RD, Boeka AG, White MA, Masheb RM, Grilo CM. Metabolic syndrome in obese men and women with binge eating disorder. *Compr Psychiatry*. 2012;53(7):1021–1027.

10. Binge eating disorder. National Institute of Diabetes and Digestive and Kidney Diseases. http://win.niddk.nih.gov/publications/binge.htm. Accessed December 4, 2013.

11. Hadigan CM, Anderson EJ, Miller KK, et al. Assessment of macronutrient and micronutrient intake in women with anorexia nervosa. *Int J Eat Disord.* 2000;28:284–292.

12. Setnick J. *ADA Pocket Guide to Eating Disorders.* Chicago, IL: American Dietetic Association; 2011.

13. Bakan R. The role of zinc in anorexia nervosa: etiology and treatment. *Med Hypotheses.* 1979;5:731–736.

14. Wapnir RA. Zinc deficiency, malnutrition and the gastrointestinal tract. *J Nutr.* 2000;130(Suppl):1388S–1392S.

15. Birmingham CL, Goldner EM, Bakan R. Controlled trial of zinc supplementation in anorexia nervosa. *Int J Eat Disord.* 1994;15;251–255.

16. Winston AP, Jamieson CP, Madira W, et al. Prevalence of thiamin deficiency in anorexia nervosa. *Int J Eat Disord.* 2000;28:451–454.

17. Rock CL, Vasantharajan S. Vitamin status of eating disorder patients: relationship to clinical indices and effect of treatment. *Int J Eat Disord.* 1995;18:257–262.

18. Capo-chichi CD, Gueant JL, Lefebvre E, et al. Riboflavin and riboflavin-derived cofactors in adolescent girls with anorexia nervosa. *Am J Clin Nutr.* 1999;69:672–678.

19. Hall R, Hoffman CRS, Beresford TP, et al. Hypomagnesemia in patients with eating disorders. *Psychosomatics.* 1988;29:264–272.

20. Langan SM, Farrell PM. Vitamin E, vitamin A and essential fatty acid status of patients hospitalized for anorexia nervosa. *Am J Clin Nutr.* 1985;41:1054–1060.

21. Holman RT, Adams CE, Nelson RA, et al. Patients with anorexia nervosa demonstrate deficiencies of selected essential fatty acids, compensatory changes in nonessential fatty acids, and decreased fluidity of plasma lipids. *J Nutr.* 1995;125:901–907.

22. American Psychiatry Association. Treatment of Patients with Eating Disorders Practice Guideline. 2006. Psychiatry Online website. http://psychiatryonline.org/guidelines.aspx. Accessed December 4, 2013.

23. Yager J, Devlin MJ, Halmi KA, et al. Guideline Watch (August 2012): Practice Guideline for the Treatment of Patients With Eating Disorders, 3rd Edition. Psychiatry Online website. http://psychiatryonline.org/content.aspx?bookid=28&sectionid=39113853. Accessed December 4, 2013.

24. Position of the American Dietetic Association: nutrition intervention in the treatment of eating disorders. *J Am Diet Assoc.* 2011;111:1236–1241.

25. Practice paper of the American Dietetic Association: nutrition intervention in the treatment of eating disorders. www.eatright.org/Members/content.aspx?id=6442464620. Accessed December 5, 2013.

26. Jeejeebhoy KN. Nutritional management of anorexia. *Semin Gastrointest Dis.* 1998;9:183–188.

27. Melchior JC. From malnutrition to refeeding during anorexia nervosa. *Curr Opin Clin Nutr Metab Care.* 1998;1:481–485.

28. Fisher M, Simpser E, Schneider M. Hypophosphatemia secondary to oral refeeding in anorexia nervosa. *Int J Eat Disord.* 2000;28:181–187.

29. Swenne I. Heart risk associated with weight loss in anorexia nervosa and eating disorders: electrocardiographic changes during the early phase of refeeding. *Acta Paediatr.* 2000;89:447–452.

30. Carney CP, Andersen AE. Eating disorders. Guide to medical evaluation and complications. *Psychiatr Clin North Am.* 1996;19:657–679.

31. National Institute for Health and Clinical Excellence. Nutrition Support in Adults. Clinical Guideline CG32. 2006. http://guidance.nice.org.uk/CG32. Accessed April 4, 2014.

32. Veverbrants E, Arky RA. Effects of fasting and refeeding: I. Studies on sodium, potassium and water excretion on a constant electrolyte and fluid intake. *J Clin Endocrinol Metab.* 1969;29:55–62.

CHAPTER 18

Food Allergy and Food Intolerance

John Leung, MD, and

Sheila E. Crowe, MD, FRCPC, FACP, FACG, AGAF

More than 50 million Americans are estimated to have allergies, and up to 15 million of them have food allergies. US health care dollars spent on food allergy approach $25 billion per year (1). Although the vast majority of adverse reactions to food (ARFs) (more than 85%) are not due to true food allergies, one-fifth of the US population self-imposes diet modifications because of perceived ARFs (2). Most ARFs are due to food intolerances that do not involve the immune system (3).

An adverse immune response to proteins in a food—whether a humoral response (immunoglobulin E [IgE] antibody), a cellular response (such as T cells), or both—represents a true food allergy. A clinician's ability to distinguish food allergies from food intolerances is absolutely essential, as prognosis and management of allergy and intolerance require vastly different approaches. This chapter reviews the management of true food allergies and food intolerances.

Prevalence of Food Allergies

Food allergies affect 4% of the adults and 8% of the children in the United States, and the prevalence seems to be on the rise (4–9). In the United States, approximately 200,000 emergency-department visits and 300,000 ambulatory-care visits annually are related to food allergy (10). Eight foods account for 90% of all food allergic reactions in North America: milk, eggs, peanuts, tree nuts, soy, wheat, fish, and shellfish (11).

The most common food allergens affecting adults are shellfish, fish, peanuts, and tree nuts (12). By the time a child reaches school age, allergies to milk, eggs, soy, and wheat have usually (in approximately 80% of cases) abated (13,14).

IgE-Mediated Food Allergies

IgE-mediated responses to food allergy present a variety of clinical manifestations—a spectrum that ranges from self-limited, localized hives to potentially fatal anaphylaxis—and have a rapid onset (15).

Hives and angioedema are the most common symptoms of food allergy. Gastrointestinal (GI), cardiovascular, and/or respiratory systems may also be affected.

The most serious symptom of IgE-mediated food allergy is generalized anaphylaxis. The primary manifestations of a GI allergic reaction are GI anaphylaxis, which typically develops along with allergic symptoms beyond the digestive tract (such as wheezing and urticaria), and oral allergy syndrome (16,17). Moderate to severe nausea, vomiting, diarrhea, and abdominal pain are the most common GI allergy symptoms, which typically present within a span of a few minutes to a couple of hours after ingesting the culprit food (18).

A rare type of anaphylaxis, *food-dependent exercise-induced anaphylaxis* triggers an anaphylactic response when an individual consumes an offending food within 2 to 4 hours of participating in exercise, although no allergic consequences occur if the individual ingests that same food and does not exercise (19).

Symptoms of oral allergy syndrome (also called *pollen-food allergy syndrome*), which is a form of contact hypersensitivity almost entirely confined within the oropharynx, include the rapid onset of pruritus and swelling of the lips, tongue, palate, and throat (20). These symptoms usually resolve within minutes of onset. This syndrome rarely affects other organs. Individuals who have seasonal allergic rhinitis to birch or ragweed pollens commonly show signs of oral allergy syndrome after eating raw fruits and vegetables (21–23).

Other Immune-Mediated Adverse GI Reactions to Food

A heterogeneous group of diseases with seemingly different underlying mechanisms, celiac disease, food protein–induced enterocolitis syndromes (FPIES), and eosinophilic GI disorders (EGID) are examples of conditions with immune-mediated GI ARFs that are not predominantly IgE-mediated. These disorders seem to be affected by multiple components of the immune system, and each of these conditions poses unique nutrition-related challenges. As has been noted with IgE-mediated food allergies, the prevalence of these conditions with immune-mediated ARFs has increased in the first 10 to 15 years of the 21st century. Celiac disease is covered in Chapter 10 of this book. FPIES and EGID are discussed in the following sections of this chapter.

Food Protein–Induced Enterocolitis Syndromes

Typically induced by ingestion of cow's milk-based or soy protein-based infant formula, FPIES are diagnosed most frequently in formula-fed young infants (ages 1 month to 1 year) (24). Symptoms of FPIES in infants typically include protracted vomiting, bleeding, diarrhea, anemia, and failure to thrive. FPIES diagnosis can be challenging, because the symptoms often resemble those of inflammatory bowel disease and a range of other GI infections.

Among infants with non-IgE–mediated cow's milk allergy, 60% will also have an allergic response to soy protein (25). For that reason, an extensively hydrolyzed casein formula should be fed to infants with cow's milk–induced FPIES; these infants should *not* be given soy–protein derived formula as a replacement for cow's milk–based formula.

Eosinophilic Gastrointestinal Disorders

EGID may result from IgE-mediated and/or other immune-mediated food reactions. Eosinophilic infiltration of the esophagus, stomach, and/or intestines with peripheral eosinophilia is detected in as many as 50% of patients with EGID (26–29).

When eosinophilic infiltration is only found in the esophagus, this condition is categorized as eosinophilic esophagitis (EoE). Prevalence of EoE seems to have increased during the past 20 years, with EoE now affecting 0.03% of the US population (30,31). Among patients with EoE, approximately 50% present with atopic symptoms (32–34). Food allergies are responsible for most cases (35). Diagnosis of EoE is made when esophageal eosinophilia (>15 eosinophils per high power field) persists despite a 2-month course of proton pump inhibitor treatment in patients with esophageal dysfunction. Both dietary elimination of foods that cause reactions and topical swallowed steroids (fluticasone or budesonide) can be considered as a first-line therapy (36). Choice of dietary elimination versus topical steroids depends on patient's preference and local expertise (37). Adopting an elimination diet of six foods—cow's milk protein, soy, wheat, egg, peanut, and seafood—can improve symptoms, reduce esophageal eosinophils, and assist in identifying causative foods (38).

Manifestations of eosinophilic gastroenteritis (EGE), which may occur at any age, depend on the layer(s) and extent of bowel involved with eosinophilic infiltration—mucosa, muscle, and/or subserosa (26). When mucosa is involved, nausea, vomiting, diarrhea, and abdominal pain usually occur. Because functional GI disorders such as irritable bowel syndrome (IBS) have symptoms similar to those of EGE, there is a risk of misdiagnosing EGE. When EGE is severe, nutritional deficiency and weight loss caused by malabsorption may occur (36,39). Eosinophilic infiltration of the muscle layer of the GI tract may result in dysmotility and pseudo-obstruction (40,41). Noninfectious eosinophilic ascites typically present in subserosal EGE (39). In the treatment of EGE, systemic corticosteroids are needed (42).

Food Intolerances

More than 85% of perceived ARFs are nonimmunological in origin (13). Given that the prognosis, management, and nutritional implications of food allergies are much different from those related to food intolerances, it is essential that a clinician effectively distinguishes allergy from intolerance. Examples of food intolerances include food toxicity or food poisoning, anaphylactoid or pseudoallergic response to food, and pharmacological reactions, as well as lactose and other carbohydrate intolerances.

Anaphylactoid or Pseudoallergic Food Reactions

Foods that simulate the effects of mast cell degranulation without antibody involvement lead to anaphylactoid or pseudoallergic reactions; for some individuals, this ARF may occur with strawberries or shellfish (43). This type of response also occurs from certain food additives, such as salicylates, benzoates, and tartrazine.

Pharmacological Reactions

Pharmacological reactions are relatively common and may result from consuming certain foods or food additives. For susceptible individuals who have a genetic defect in exogenous histamine metabolism, well-ripened cheese, pickled cabbage, red wine, tuna, or other foods with increased histamine content can induce a spectrum of allergy-like symptoms (44). It has been suggested that deficiencies in diaminoxidase or histamine-N-methyltransferase cause this response (45). In addition, certain individuals who consume amine-rich foods are at risk for developing migraine headaches.

Some ARFs are induced by drug-food interactions. For example, a hypertensive crisis with risk of resulting stroke or cardiac arrhythmia can occur when an individual takes a monoamine oxidase inhibitor (MAOI) antidepressant after consuming a sufficient amount of tyramine-rich foods. By impairing monoamine oxidase function, MAOIs inhibit tyramine breakdown and may cause these life-threatening conditions (46).

Lactose Intolerance

The most common ARF is lactose intolerance. A genetically regulated reduction of intestinal lactase activity occurring in late childhood or early adulthood is the cause of most cases of lactose intolerance (47). Although cases of congenital lactase deficiency have been identified, it is a rare condition, with diagnoses more common in Finnish infants (48).

Bacterial overgrowth and any mucosal injury to the GI tract resulting in villous flattening or intestinal epithelium damage—including celiac disease, inflammatory bowel disease, and viral gastroenteritis—may lead to secondary lactase deficiency (49). Diagnosis may be obtained accurately and noninvasively with a simple lactose breath hydrogen test (50).

Most patients with lactose intolerance can ingest and tolerate small amounts of milk as well as dairy products that are naturally low in lactose, such as hard cheese and yogurt. To reduce symptoms of lactose intolerance, it is acceptable to ingest commercially available lactase enzymes by adding them to foods that contain lactose or to consume them with lactose-containing meals. Most grocery stores stock lactose-free milk products on their shelves. Because low calcium intake is typical among patients with lactose intolerance, additional calcium supplementation in these individuals may be indicated to reduce the risk of osteoporosis and bone fracture (51).

Other Carbohydrate Intolerances

Concerns about fructose malabsorption have grown as high-fructose corn syrups have become a common ingredient in food processing. Patients with IBS and other functional bowel disorders commonly present with fructose malabsorption–related GI symptoms (52). Carbohydrate intolerances resulting from congenital enzyme deficiencies are diagnosed in a minority of patient cases, however. See Chapter 9 for more information on IBS.

Diagnosis and Management of Patients with Adverse Reactions to Food

Because of perceived ARFs, up to 20% of individuals in the United States needlessly self-impose dietary restrictions, which may lead to nutritional deficiencies (53). Individuals who have no need to alter their diet, and thus would not benefit from eliminating foodstuffs, must be differentiated from patients who have a medical necessity to follow any type of elimination diet (ie, those with true food allergy, EoE, celiac disease, or carbohydrate intolerances as well as those following a diet low in fermentable oligosaccharides, disaccharides, monosaccharides, and polyols [FODMAPs] for IBS) (54). (See Chapter 9 for more information about the FODMAPs diet.)

It is also paramount that the clinician considers the differential diagnosis when evaluating patients who present with an ARF (see Box 18.1 on page 226). Obtaining a thorough diet history—an invaluable source of patient information that can determine the need for additional diagnostic tests—is a crucial component of this evaluation.

If clinical history suggests that the patient has a true food allergy, it is reasonable to refer that patient for further evaluation by an allergist and perhaps a gastroenterologist. The diagnostic approach should be individualized on a case-by-case basis. Because patients with functional GI disorders frequently self-report multiple food intolerances, it is important to determine a diagnosis for these particular individuals.

BOX 18.1 Differential Diagnosis of Adverse Reactions to Food

IgE-mediated food allergy
- Generalized anaphylaxis
- Oral allergy syndrome
- GI anaphylaxis
- Food-dependent exercise-induced anaphylaxis
- Latex-food allergy syndrome

Other immune-mediated adverse GI reactions to food
- Celiac disease
- Food protein–induced enterocolitis syndromes
- Eosinophilic esophagitis and eosinophilic gastroenteritis

Food intolerances
- Food toxicity or food poisoning
- Anaphylactoid or pseudoallergic food reactions
- Pharmacological reactions
- Lactose intolerance
- Other carbohydrate intolerances
- Adverse psychological reactions to food
- Physiologic reactions to food
- Other causes of food intolerance

Diagnosis of Food Allergy

Skin prick-puncture and in vitro testing (which have similar sensitivity and specificity) are common approaches to identify food-specific IgE antibodies when evaluating patients for IgE-mediated food allergy (3). The in vitro assays detect serum food-specific IgE antibodies using immunoassays of various forms (eg, Phadia ImmunoCAP system) (55–57). In general, testing for IgE-mediated food allergy demonstrates high negative-predictive values (when results are negative, the test accurately rules out IgE-mediated diseases) and low positive-predictive values (food allergy diagnosis cannot be confirmed if test results are abnormal).

An allergy specialist should perform skin testing because there is a small risk that patients will experience potentially life-threatening allergic reactions (58). Results of this allergy testing must be interpreted in the context of the patient's specific clinical history. A positive test only confirms presence of allergen-specific IgE but not clinical allergy.

As part of the patient evaluation for food allergies, allergists frequently prescribe trial elimination diets or a supervised open-label oral challenge (59,60). The gold standard for food allergy diagnosis is a double-blind, placebo-controlled food challenge, but it is not widely used (61).

Many local and federal health agencies and organizations have issued food allergy evaluation and management guidelines (3,62–66). There are many commercial laboratories that promote expensive in vitro tests for "food allergies" that have not been validated and should not be used in diagnosing true food allergies (67,68).

Management of IgE-Mediated Food Allergy

Managing IgE-mediated and other immune-mediated food allergies involves strictly avoiding an offending food allergen (13). The four Es—elimination, early recognition, epinephrine, and education—form the basis of IgE-mediated food allergy management.

ELIMINATION

Upon confirmation of food allergy, a physician and a registered dietitian experienced in working with this patient population must supervise any elimination diet prescribed to the individual. The prescribed elimination diet should take into account the patient's diet preferences while recognizing that a patient's culture, religion, or other factors might cause reluctance or unwillingness to accept and adhere to diet changes.

The concept of eliminating food proteins from the diet seems simple; however, in practice, it is quite challenging (69–71). Patients must learn how to scan the ingredients listed on food package labels for keywords that identify which products contain offending food proteins (eg, "caramel color" or "nougat" suggests the presence of cow's milk protein whereas "miso" indicates that a product contains soy).

In the United States, consumers have been better able to discern whether a food product contains an allergen since passage of the Food Allergen Labeling and Consumer Protection Act (FALCPA) in 2004. FALCPA dictates that if ingredients in a packaged food contain any of eight ingredients considered major allergens (wheat, milk, eggs, fish, crustacean shellfish, tree nuts, peanuts, and soybeans), then the food label must clearly name the ingredient, either in the ingredients list or in a separate "Contains" statement (72).

EARLY RECOGNITION

Fatal and near-fatal allergic responses are more likely when identification of allergic reactions or administration of epinephrine is delayed (73).

EPINEPHRINE

Prevention of unintended exposure to the offending allergen is a challenge, so patients at risk for severe reactions must get into the habit of always having a means for treatment on hand in case administration is needed in an emergency situation (11). For example, patients may need to carry rapid-acting antihistamines, a self-injection epinephrine device (eg, EpiPen or Auvi-Q), and/or bronchodilators (for patients who have comorbid asthma).

EDUCATION

The signs of early food allergy symptoms and how to administer treatment must be taught to parents, caregivers, and other family members (74,75). All patients with a diagnosed food allergy should consider wearing a medical alert bracelet to identify their food allergy.

Nutrition Issues Related to Specific Food Allergies

As noted earlier, shellfish, peanut, tree nuts, and fish are the most common food allergies in adults (12). These foods are easily replaced in the Western diet, because they typically do not comprise a substantial percentage of dietary intake for most Westerners. Thus, the valuable nutrients in these foods can be obtained from many other foods. Calcium supplements should always be considered in patients with

TABLE 18.1 Alternate Dietary Sources of Nutrients Found in Wheat

Nutrient	Dietary Sources
Carbohydrate	Rice, oat, corn, buckwheat, other grains, potato and other starchy vegetables, legumes
Fiber	Fruits, vegetables, seeds, beans, whole grains
Thiamin (vitamin B-1)	Meat, liver, legumes, nuts, peas, sunflower seeds, brown rice
Riboflavin (vitamin B-2)	Milk, dark green leafy vegetables, cheese, almonds
Niacin (vitamin B-3)	Meat, fish, chicken, legumes, sunflower seeds
Iron	Meat, fish, poultry, broccoli, dried dates, legumes
Folic acid	Beef liver, vegetables, legumes, seeds, orange juice; enriched flours, cereals, pastas, and other grain foods made from grains other than wheat

cow's milk allergy to reduce the risk of osteoporosis and bone fracture (76). Wheat flour—the major product of wheat—is a source of several nutrients, including carbohydrates, fiber, iron, thiamin, riboflavin, niacin, folic acid, vitamin B-6, and magnesium. Alternate dietary sources of these nutrients are shown in Table 18.1.

Conclusion

Most types of food reactions are not immune mediated or life threatening. Patients should be reassured once appropriate testing is done and counseled to not unnecessarily restrict foods that are nutritious. Extreme dietary limitation of foods can have adverse nutritional effects. A registered dietitian and physician should monitor individuals who require restricted diets (eg, those with food allergy, EoE, or celiac disease) to help manage the patient's nutritional intake.

References

1. Gupta R, et al. The high economic burden of childhood food allergy in the United States. *Ann Allergy Asthma Immunol.* 2012;109:A1–A162.
2. Bischoff S, Crowe SE. Gastrointestinal food allergy: new insights into pathophysiology and clinical perspectives. *Gastroenterology.* 2005;128(4):1089–1113.
3. NIAID Expert Panel; Boyce JA, Asa'ad AA, et al. Guidelines for the diagnosis and management of food allergy in the United States: report of the NIAID-sponsored expert panel. *J Allergy Clin Immunol.* 2010;26(6 Suppl):S1–S58.
4. National Institute of Allergy and Infectious Diseases, National Institutes of Health. Report of the NIH Expert Panel on Food Allergy Research. 2006. www3.niaid.nih.gov/topics/foodAllergy/research/ReportFoodAllergy .htm. Accessed April 21, 2014.
5. US Census Bureau. State and County QuickFacts. 2010. quickfacts.census.gov/qfd/states/00000.html. Accessed April 21, 2014.
6. Gupta RS, Springston, MR, Warrier BS, et al. The prevalence, severity, and distribution of childhood food allergy in the United States. *J Pediatr.* 2011;128:e9–e17.
7. Liu AH, Jaramillo R, Sicherer SH, et al. National prevalence and risk factors for food allergy and relationships to asthma: results from the National Health and Nutrition Examination Survey 2005–2006. *J Allergy Clin Immunol.* 2010;126:798–806.

8. Centers for Disease Control and Prevention. QuickStats: percentage of children aged <18 years with food, skin, or hay fever/respiratory allergies—National Health Interview Survey, United States, 1998—2009. 2011. www.cdc.gov/mmwr/preview/mmwrhtml/mm6011a7.htm?s_cid+mm6011a7_w. Accessed April 7, 2014.

9. Centers for Disease Control and Prevention. Trends in allergic conditions among children: United States, 1997–2011. *NCHS Data Brief.* May 2013. www.cdc.gov/nchs/data/databriefs/db121.htm#summary. Accessed October 4, 2013.

10. Clark S, Espinola J, Rudders SA, et al. Frequency of US emergency department visits for food-related acute allergic reactions. *J Allergy Clin Immunol.* 2011;127:682–683.

11. Sicherer SH. Epidemiology of food allergy. *J Allergy Clin Immunol.* 2011;127:594–602.

12. Sicherer SH, Muñoz-Furlong A, Sampson HA. Prevalence of seafood allergy in the United States determined by a random telephone survey. *J Allergy Clin Immunol.* 2004;114:159–165.

13. Sampson HA. Update on food allergy. *J Allergy Clin Immunol.* 2004;113(5):805–820.

14. Wood RA. The natural history of food allergy. *Pediatrics.* 2003;111(6):1631–1637.

15. Sicherer SH, Sampson HA. Food allergy. *J Allergy Clin Immunol.* 2010;125(2 Suppl 2):S116–S125.

16. James JM, Burks AW. Food-associated gastrointestinal disease. *Curr Opin Pediatr.* 1996;8(5):471–475.

17. Crowe SE, Perdue MH. Gastrointestinal food hypersensitivity: basic mechanisms of pathophysiology. *Gastroenterology.* 1992;103(3):1075–1095.

18. Sicherer SH. Clinical aspects of gastrointestinal food allergy in childhood. *Pediatrics.* 2003;111(6 Pt 3): 1609–1616.

19. Du Toit G. Food-dependent exercise-induced anaphylaxis in childhood. *Pediatr Allergy Immunol.* 2007;18(5): 455–46321.

20. Hofmann A, Burks AW. Pollen food syndrome: update on the allergens. *Curr Allergy Asthma Rep.* 2008;8:413–417.

21. Ortolani C, Ispano M, Pastorello EA, Ansaloni R, Magri GC. Comparison of results of skin prick tests (with fresh foods and commercial food extracts) and RAST in 100 patients with oral allergy syndrome. *J Allergy Clin Immunol.* 1989;83(3):683–690.

22. de Groot H, de Jong NW, Vuijk MH, Gerth van Wijk R. Birch pollinosis and atopy caused by apple, peach, and hazelnut; comparison of three extraction procedures with two apple strains. *Allergy.* 1996;51(10):712–718.

23. Pastorello EA, Incorvaia C, Pravettoni V, et al. New allergens in fruits and vegetables. *Allergy.* 1998;53(46 Suppl):S48–S51.

24. Mehr S, Kakakios A, Frith K, Kemp AS. Food protein-induced enterocolitis syndrome: 16-year experience. *Pediatrics.* 2009;123(3):e459–e464.

25. American Academy of Pediatrics. Committee on Nutrition. Hypoallergenic infant formulas. *Pediatrics.* 2000;106(2):346–349.

26. Rothenberg ME. Eosinophilic gastrointestinal disorders (EGID). *J Allergy Clin Immunol.* 2004;113(1):11–28; quiz 29.

27. Rothenberg ME, Mishra A, Collins MH, Putnam PE. Pathogenesis and clinical features of eosinophilic esophagitis. *J Allergy Clin Immunol.* 2001;108(6):891–894.

28. Liacouras CA. Eosinophilic esophagitis in children and adults. *J Pediatr Gastroenterol Nutr.* 2003;37(Suppl 1):S23–S28.

29. Potter JW, Saeian K, Staff D, et al. Eosinophilic esophagitis in adults: an emerging problem with unique esophageal features. *Gastrointest Endosc.* 2004;59(3):355–361.

30. Sealock RJ, Rendon G, El-Serag HB. Systematic review: the epidemiology of eosinophilic oesophagitis in adults. *Aliment Pharmacol Ther.* 2010;32(6):712–719.

31. Noel RJ, Putnam PE, Rothenberg ME. Eosinophilic esophagitis. *N Engl J Med.* 2004;351(9):940–941.

32. Eroglu Y, Lu H, Terry A, et al. Pediatric eosinophilic esophagitis: single-center experience in northwestern USA. *Pediatr Int.* 2009;51(5):612–616.

33. Velázquez V, Camacho C, Mercado-Quiñones AE, Irizarry-Padilla J. Eosinophilic esophagitis and allergies in the pediatric population of Puerto Rico. *Biol Asoc Med P R*. 2009;101(2):21–22.

34. Roy-Ghanta S, Larosa DF, Katzka DA. Atopic characteristics of adult patients with eosinophilic esophagitis. *Clin Gastroenterol Hepatol*. 2008;6(5):531–535.

35. Spergel JM. Eosinophilic esophagitis in adults and children: evidence for a food allergy component in many patients. *Curr Opin Allergy Clin Immunol*. 2007;7(3):274–278.

36. Dellon ES, Gonsalves N, Hirano I, Furuta GT, Liacouras CA, Katzka DA; American College of Gastroenterology. ACG clinical guideline: evidence based approach to the diagnosis and management of esophageal eosinophilia and eosinophilic esophagitis (EoE). *Am J Gastroenterol*. 2013;108(5):679–692.

37. Merves J, Muir A, Modayur Chandramouleeswaran P, et al. Eosinophilic esophagitis. *Ann Allergy Asthma Immunol*. 2014 Feb 21. epub ahead of print.

38. Gonsalves N, Yang G-Y, Doerfler B, et al. Elimination diet effectively treats eosinophilic esophagitis in adults; food reintroduction identifies causative factors. *Gastroenterology*. 2012;142:1451–1459.

39. Talley NJ, Shorter RG, Phillips SF, Zinsmeister AR. Eosinophilic gastroenteritis: a clinicopathological study of patients with disease of the mucosa, muscle layer, and subserosal tissues. *Gut*. 1990;31(1):54–58.

40. Yun MY, Cho YU, Park IS, et al. Eosinophilic gastroenteritis presenting as small bowel obstruction: a case report and review of the literature. *World J Gastroenterol*. 2007;13(11):1758–1760.

41. Landres RT, Kuster GG, Strum WB. Eosinophilic esophagitis in a patient with vigorous achalasia. *Gastroenterology*. 1978;74(6):1298–1301.

42. Lee CM, Changchien CS, Chen PC, et al. Eosinophilic gastroenteritis: 10 years experience. *Am J Gastroenterol*. 1993;88(1):70–74.

43. Reese I, Zuberbier T, Bunselmeyer B, et al. Diagnostic approach for suspected pseudoallergic reaction to food ingredients. *J Dtsch Dermatol Ges*. 2009;7(1):70–77.

44. Maintz L, Novak N. Histamine and histamine intolerance. *Am J Clin Nutr*. 2007;85(5):1185–1196.

45. Götz M. [Pseudo-allergies are due to histamine intolerance]. *Wien Med Wochenschr*. 1996;146(15):426–430.

46. Shulman KI, Fischer HD, Herrmann N, et al. Current prescription patterns and safety profile of irreversible monoamine oxidase inhibitors: a population-based cohort study of older adults. *J Clin Psychiatry*. 2009;70(12):1681–1686.

47. Schirru E, Corona V, Usai-Satta P, et al. Decline of lactase activity and c/t-13910 variant in Sardinian childhood. *J Pediatr Gastroenterol Nutr*. 2007;45(4):503–506.

48. Järvelä I, Torniainen S, Kolho K. Molecular genetics of human lactase deficiencies. *Ann Med*. 2009;41(8):568–575.

49. Montalto M, Curigliano V, Santoro L, et al. Management and treatment of lactose malabsorption. *World J Gastroenterol*. 2006;12(2):187–191.

50. Heyman MB. Lactose intolerance in infants, children, and adolescents. *Pediatrics*. 2006;118(3):1279–1286.

51. Di Stefano M, Veneto G, Malservisi S, et al. Lactose malabsorption and intolerance and peak bone mass. *Gastroenterology*. 2002;122(7):1793–1799.

52. Fedewa A, Rao SS. Dietary fructose intolerance, fructan intolerance, and FODMAPs. *Curr Gastroenterol Rep*. 2014;16(1):370.

53. Sicherer SH, Sampson HA. Food allergy. *J Allergy Clin Immunol*. 2006;117(2 Suppl 2):S470–S475.

54. Halmos EP, Power VA, Shepherd SJ, Gibson PR, Muir JG. A diet low in FODMAPs reduces symptoms of irritable bowel syndrome. *Gastroenterology*. 2014;146(1):67–75.

55. Sampson HA. Utility of food-specific IgE concentrations in predicting symptomatic food allergy. *J Allergy Clin Immunol*. 2001;107(5):891–896.

56. Celik-Bilgili S, Mehl A, Verstege A, et al. The predictive value of specific immunoglobulin E levels in serum for the outcome of oral food challenges. *Clin Exp Allergy*. 2005;35(3):268–273.

57. García-Ara C, Boyano-Martínez T, Díaz-Pena JM, et al. Specific IgE levels in the diagnosis of immediate hypersensitivity to cows' milk protein in the infant. *J Allergy Clin Immunol*. 2001;107(1):185–190.

58. Lockey RF. Adverse reactions associated with skin testing and immunotherapy. *Allergy Proc.* 1995;16(6):293–296.

59. Sicherer SH. Food allergy: when and how to perform oral food challenges. *Pediatr Allergy Immunol.* 1999;10(4):226–234.

60. Agata H, Kondo N, Fukutomi O, Shinoda S, Orii T. Effect of elimination diets on food-specific IgE antibodies and lymphocyte proliferative responses to food antigens in atopic dermatitis patients exhibiting sensitivity to food allergens. *J Allergy Clin Immunol.* 993;91(2):668–679.

61. Sampson HA. Immediate hypersensitivity reactions to foods: blinded food challenges in children with atopic dermatitis. *Ann Allergy.* 1986;57(3):209–212.

62. American Gastroenterological Association medical position statement: guidelines for the evaluation of food allergies. *Gastroenterology.* 2001;120(4):1023–1025.

63. Island Wood School. Food Allergy Guidelines—IslandWood. http://islandwood.org/school_programs/parents/foodallergy. Accessed October 4, 2013.

64. Liberty Public School District. Food Allergies Policy and Guidelines. www.schoolnutrition.org/uploadedFiles/School_Nutrition/104_CareerEducation/ContinuingEducation/Webinars/FoodAllergyWebinar-Allergy_policy_guidelines.pdf?n=9295. Accessed October 4, 2013.

65. Illinois State Board of Education. Food Allergy Guidelines Committee. Food Allergies Guidelines. June 2010. www.isbe.state.il.us/food_allergy/default.htm. Accessed October 4, 2013.

66. FARE Food Allergy Research and Education. Resources for Schools. www.foodallergy.org/resources/schools. Accessed October 4, 2013.

67. Stapel SO, Asero R, Ballmer-Weber BK, et al. Testing for IgG4 against foods is not recommended as a diagnostic tool: EAACI Task Force Report. *Allergy.* 2008;63(7):793–796.

68. Measurement of specific and nonspecific IgG4 levels as diagnostic and prognostic tests for clinical allergy. AAAI Board of Directors. *J Allergy Clin Immunol.* 1995;95(3):652–654.

69. Taylor SL, Hefle SL. Food allergen labeling in the USA and Europe. *Curr Opin Allergy Clin Immunol.* 2006;6(3):186–190.

70. Mills EN, Valovirta E, Madsen C, et al. Information provision for allergic consumers—where are we going with food allergen labelling? *Allergy.* 2004;59(12):1262–1268.

71. Cornelisse-Vermaat JR, Voordouw J, Yiakoumaki V, Theodoridis G, Frewer LJ. Food-allergic consumers' labelling preferences: a cross-cultural comparison. *Eur J Public Health.* 2008;18(2):115–120.

72. US Food and Drug Administration. Food Allergen Labeling and Consumer Protection Act of 2004 Questions and Answers December 12, 2005; Updated July 18, 2006. www.fda.gov/food/guidanceregulation/guidancedocumentsregulatoryinformation/allergens/ucm106890.htm. Accessed April 21, 2014.

73. Sampson HA, Mendelson L, Rosen JP. Fatal and near-fatal anaphylactic reactions to food in children and adolescents. *N Engl J Med.* 1992;327(6):380–384.

74. Gupta RS, Kim JS, Springston EE, et al. Development of the Chicago Food Allergy Research Surveys: assessing knowledge, attitudes, and beliefs of parents, physicians, and the general public. *BMC Health Serv Res.* 2009;9:142.

75. Gupta RS, Springston EE, Kim JS, et al. Food allergy knowledge, attitudes, and beliefs of primary care physicians. *Pediatrics.* 2010;125(1):126–132.

76. Jensen VB, Jørgensen IM, Rasmussen KB, Mølgaard C, Prahl P. Bone mineral status in children with cow milk allergy. *Pediatr Allergy Immunol.* 2004;15(6):562–565.

PART VI

Therapeutic Interventions for Gastrointestinal Disorders

CHAPTER 19

Enteral Nutrition

Angela A. MacDonald, DCN, RD, CNSC

Nutrition support has progressed from adjunctive care provided solely to prevent malnutrition to a proactive therapy designed to prevent oxidative cellular injury and favorably modulate the immune response (1). Enteral nutrition (EN) should usually be attempted before parenteral nutrition (PN) because EN is generally considered safer and more efficacious. See Chapter 20 for additional information on PN. Chapter 21 considers issues related to the use of nutrition support in pediatric patients, and Chapter 22 addresses the use of EN and PN in home care.

Indications for Use

Proposed benefits of EN include the following (2–4):

- Prevention of adverse structural and functional alterations of the gut barrier
- Increased epithelial proliferation
- Maintenance of mucosal integrity
- Decreased gut permeability
- Improved mesenteric blood flow
- Improved local and systemic immune responsiveness

When compared to PN, EN has been shown to reduce cost, septic morbidity, and the rate of infectious complications (5–9). Enteral nutrition is appropriate for patients who cannot eat or cannot eat enough. Other considerations for starting EN are as follows:

- Functional gastrointestinal (GI) tract—"If the gut works, use it!"
- Hemodynamic stability (5):
  - Mean arterial pressure >60 mmHg
  - Stable doses of catecholamine agents (pressors)
  - Access to the GI tract

Contraindications

EN is absolutely contradicted if there is a mechanical obstruction that cannot be bypassed. Relative contraindications include the following (4,10):

- Intractable vomiting or diarrhea refractory to medical management
- Short bowel syndrome (≤100 cm small bowel remaining)
- Paralytic ileus
- High-output fistula
- Peritonitis
- Mild GI bleeding
- Inability to access the GI tract
- Hemodynamic instability

EN may also be contraindicated for ethical reasons, as in the case of a patient with imminently terminal disease who does not desire aggressive intervention. See Chapter 26 for more information on ethical issues.

Potential Complications

If EN is not managed appropriately, it can be associated with serious and potentially fatal complications, including the following (4,11–14):

- Enteral misconnection
- Device misplacements or displacements
- Tube complications
- Bronchopulmonary aspiration
- GI intolerance related to formula contamination
- Drug-nutrient interactions
- Electrolyte abnormalities
- GI ischemia

Complications of EN can be minimized when attention is paid to the following:

- Selecting the appropriate site for delivery
- Timing of EN
- Selecting and ordering the appropriate EN product
- Safe preparation of EN
- Safe delivery of EN
- Safe monitoring of EN

Selecting the Appropriate Site for Delivery

Success of EN depends on careful selection of appropriate enteral access device and placement technique along with proper maintenance and care. Considerations for enteral access device include the following (11,13):

- GI anatomy and motility
- Prior GI surgery
- Patency of the upper GI tract
- Intended uses
- Length of time that EN will be required
- Risks for anesthesia
- Effects of pre-existing comorbidities
- Expected patient outcomes
- Condition of external abdominal wall
- Ability to correct coagulopathies

EN administered into the stomach is acceptable for most patients; however, postpyloric placement may be beneficial for patients who have two or more of the following risk factors (15):

- Prior aspiration
- Decreased level of consciousness
- Neuromuscular disease and structural abnormalities of the aerodigestive tract
- Endotracheal intubation
- Vomiting
- Persistently high gastric residual volumes (GRVs)
- Need for supine positioning

Short-Term Feeding Tubes

Short-term feeding tubes should be used for patients who are expected to receive EN for less than 4 weeks or for whom a long-term feeding tube cannot be placed. Decisions about the placement of the tube will be based on desired tip location and the ability to place the tube nasally or orally (see Tables 19.1 and 19.2 for more information) (16–18). For most patients, gastric feeding is acceptable even during critical illness (9).

TABLE 19.1 Types of Short-Term Feeding Tubes

Tip Location	Types of Tubes	Advantages	Disadvantages
Gastric	• Nasogastric • Orogastric	• Easier to place • Less expensive • TF initiated more quickly	• May increase risk of aspiration[a] • Unable to use in patients with obstruction/need for gastric decompression
Postpyloric	• Nasojejunal • Orojejunal	• Safely feed patients with gastric dysmotility • May allow EN feeding in high-risk patients • SB feedings result in improved nutrient delivery	• Requires special training to place • May delay start of EN

Abbreviations: EN, enteral nutrition; SB, small bowel; TF, tube feeding.
[a]One meta-analysis showed increased risk of ventilator-associated pneumonia with gastric feedings, whereas two others showed no associations (16–18).

TABLE 19.2 Methods to Place Short-Term Feeding Tubes

Method	Advantages	Disadvantages
Blind placement	• Inexpensive • Place at bedside • Lower skill level required to place	• Tube placement errors are higher • Requires X-ray for confirmation • Typically difficult to place postpyloric tubes
Electromagnetic	• May not require X-ray for confirmation • Place at bedside • Allows for postpyloric placement	• Requires specialized equipment for placement • Requires trained personnel to place • More expensive tubes required for placement
Fluoroscopic	• Does not require X-ray for confirmation • Allows for postpyloric placement	• Typically requires transport to fluoroscopy • Requires trained personnel to place • More expensive than blind placement
Endoscopic	• Allows for postpyloric tube placement	• Typically requires transport to endoscopy • Trained personnel to place • Requires X-ray as endoscope can displace tube when removed • More expensive than blind placement
Surgical	• Can be placed at time of surgery • Does not require X-ray for confirmation • Can be gastric or postpyloric placement	• Requires anesthesia and risks associated with surgery • Trained personnel to place • More expensive if tube placement is the sole reason for surgery

---

BOX 19.1   Methods to Check Placement For Blindly Placed Feeding Tubes

X-ray method
• Gold standard for blindly placed feeding tubes (19–21)
• Repeated exposure to radiation can be dangerous

pH method
• Aspirates from different locations in the GI tract have different appearances and pH (not valid for those on gastric acid–suppression therapy) (11)
• Insufficiently accurate to distinguish between gastric and bronchopulmonary placement (11):
  ◦ Pleural space: Pale yellow, serous appearance; pH ≥ 7
  ◦ Gastric fluid: Clear, colorless, or grassy green appearance (fasting); pH ≤ 5 (without gastric acid–suppression therapy)
  ◦ Small bowel, bile stained: pH ≥ 6

Auscultation method
• Relies on sound differences between stomach and lung
• Not accurate

Testing for enzymes in fluid aspirated from tube
• CO_2 detectors (4):
  ◦ Detect CO_2 when tube has been placed inadvertently into the lung
  ◦ Cannot distinguish placement in the esophagus and the stomach

Source: Data are from references 4, 11, and 19–21.

BOX 19.2   Factors in Continuous Postplacement Monitoring of Short-Term Feeding Tubes

- External length of tubing
- Negative pressure when attempting to draw fluid
- Unexpected change in residual volumes
- pH (with intermittent feedings)

Source: Data are from reference 11.

TABLE 19.3   Types of Long-Term Feeding Tubes

Tip Location	Types of Tubes	Advantages	Disadvantages
Gastric	• Percutaneous endoscopic gastrostomy (PEG) • Gastrostomy	• Easier to place • Less expensive • Easier to maintain	• Cannot be used in patients with obstruction/need for gastric decompression
Postpyloric	• Percutaneous endoscopic jejunostomy (PEJ) • Jejunostomy	• Safely feed patients with gastric dysmotility • May allow enteral feeding in high-risk patients	• Tubes may clog more easily because they are typically smaller in diameter

Once the tube has been placed, several methods can be used to determine whether the tip has been successfully placed in the desired location (see Box 19.1) (4,11,19–21). There are also several methods to evaluate whether the tip changes position after placement (Box 19.2) (11).

Long-Term Feeding Tubes

Long-term feeding tubes are used for patients who are going to need either full or supplemental feedings for more than 4 weeks. See Table 19.3 for more information on the types of long-term feeding tubes.

Complications Associated with Feeding Tubes

A number of complications can develop during the placement of short-term and long-term feeding tubes as well as after their placement (see Table 19.4 on page 240). Among these complications are aspiration, which potentially can be fatal, and the common problem of tube occlusion. See Boxes 19.3 and 19.4 (pages 241 and 242, respectively) for more information on these complications associated with EN (4,11,14,22–25).

Timing of Enteral Nutrition

Timing in Critical Illness

In the critically ill, EN should be started within 24 to 48 hours of admission to the intensive care unit (ICU). Do not wait for bowel sounds, passing of flatus, or stool to initiate feeds (5). Early EN is associated with the following benefits (5,9):

- Reduced infectious complications
- Potential reductions in length of stay
- Reduced disease severity
- Improved patient outcomes

Timing After PEG Placement

Studies of patients whose EN is started within 3 to 4 hours after the procedure to place the percutaneous endoscopic gastrostomy (PEG) have concluded that the rates and types of complications are comparable to those observed in patients whose EN is delayed until the next day (26–28).

Timing After Surgery

Traditionally, clinicians required the return of bowel function (flatus/stool) before initiating EN postoperatively. However, several studies have indicated that early EN (within 24 hours of surgery) is safe and may result in fewer infectious complications and reduced length of stay (29). Bowel necrosis is the most serious potential complication, and monitoring for abdominal distension and sepsis or worsening condition should prompt immediate evaluation (11).

Formula Selection

There are many categories of enteral formulas on the market targeted for specific patient populations (see Table 19.5 on pages 243–244) (5,9,30–50). Almost all formulas are nutritionally complete when

TABLE 19.4 Potential Complications Associated with Feeding Tubes

Type of Tube	Placement Complications	Postprocedure Complications
Short-term	• Epistaxis • Aspiration[b] • Circulatory and respiratory compromise	• Inadvertent tube dislodgement[a] • Tube malfunction: breaking, cracking, or kinking • Tube occlusion[c] • Aspiration • Intestinal ischemia
Long-term	• Aspiration[b] • Hemorrhage • Perforation of the GI lumen • Peritonitis/necrotizing fasciitis • Prolonged ileus	• Peristomal infection[d] • Inappropriate equipment usage, such as enteral misconnections • Premature/inadvertent removal, with increased risk of peritonitis within first few weeks of insertion • Accidental catheter tip malposition, leading to leakage of intestinal secretions, gastric/intestinal obstruction, or aspiration • Excessive traction of feeding device, leading to "buried bumper syndrome," pain, tube obstruction, peritonitis, or stomal site drainage

[a]Use of nasal bridle decreases dislodgement rates but may increase risk of nasal septal and nasal tissue trauma.
[b]See Box 19.3 for more information on aspiration.
[c]See Box 19.4 for more information on tube occlusion.
[d]Reduced risk and successful treatment of infection may be achieved by prophylactic antibiotics, early recognition of wound infections, treatment with antibiotics, local wound care, and debridement when indicated.

BOX 19.3 Aspiration Risk Factors and Prevention

Risk factors
- Previous aspiration events
- Decreased level of consciousness
- Significant neuromuscular disease
- Contaminated oropharyngeal environment
- Structural abnormalities of the aerodigestive tract
- Supine positioning
- Persistently elevated gastric residual volumes
- Advanced age
- Need for sedation
- Neurological impairment
- Presence and size of nasogastric tube
- Malposition of feeding tube
- Mechanical ventilation
- Bolus feeding delivery
- Presence of high-risk disease or injury
- Nursing staffing level

Prevention
- Infuse enteral feeding into small bowel instead of the stomach
- Elevate the head of the bed to >45°
- Switch from bolus to continuous feeding
- Oral mouth care including use of chlorhexidine mouthwashes
- Use of prokinetic agents to increase gastrointestinal motility

---

Source: Data are from references 11, 14, and 22.

administered in sufficient quantities. Refer to Table 19.6 (page 245) for information on the ingredients in specialty formulas (3,5,30–32,36,51–57).

Nutrient Composition of Formulas

CARBOHYDRATE

Carbohydrate is the primary macronutrient and energy source, comprising 40% to 90% of calories, in formulas. Carbohydrate contributes to osmolality, digestibility, and sweetness. Most formulas are lactose-free and gluten-free (36).

FAT

Fats are a concentrated energy source. Types of fats found in enteral formulas include the following (36):

- Long-chain triglycerides (LCT) are a source of the essential fatty acids (EFA) linoleic and linolenic acid.
- Medium-chain triglycerides (MCT) are absorbed in portal circulation (do not need bile salts and lipase) and provide no EFA.

- Structured lipids—a mixture of LCT and MCT on the same glycerol molecule. MCT and LCT combined may reduce infection and produce fewer inflammatory eicosanoids compared to LCT alone.
- Omega-3 fatty acids (n-3 FA) have greater anti-inflammatory properties compared to omega-6 fatty acids.

PROTEIN

Protein is a source of nitrogen. Types of protein in enteral formulas are as follows (36):

- Intact proteins, which require normal levels of pancreatic enzymes for digestion and absorption
- Hydrolyzed proteins (di- and tripeptides), which may improve nitrogen absorption compared to free amino acids
- Free amino acids

BOX 19.4   Tube Occlusion Risk Factors, Prevention, and Treatment

Risk Factors
- Diameter of the feeding tube: Risk is greater with small bore than large bore.
- Concentration of the enteral formula: Risk is greater with concentrated formula than with standard.
- Rate of infusion: Slow infusion is riskier than fast.
- Fiber content of the enteral formula: High-fiber formulas are riskier than nonfiber formulas.
- Material of the feeding tube: Risk is greater with silicone than polyurethane.
- Improper administration of medications:
  - Do not mix medications with tube-feeding formulas.
  - Use liquid medications when available and tolerated.
- Tip location: Risk is greater with gastric location vs small bowel (low pH of stomach may cause formula to coagulate; check gastric residuals).
- Tube length: Longer tubes are riskier than shorter tubes.
- Inadequate water flushing.

Prevention
- Flush tube with at least 30 mL water every 4 hours during continuous feeding or before and after infusion during intermittent feedings.
- Flush tube with at least 30 mL water after checking residuals.
- Flush tube with at least 30 mL water before and after each medication.
- Carbonated beverages or cranberry juice are not recommended (23,24).

Treatment methods
- A solution of Viokase (Axcan Pharma, Quebec, Canada) and sodium bicarbonate was found to be the best at dissolving clotted formula in feeding tubes (25).
- Use of a cytology brush.
- Use of an endoscopic retrograde cholangiopancreatography (ERCP) catheter.
- Use of a commercial corkscrew device.

Source: Data are from references 4, 11, and 23–25.

TABLE 19.5 Enteral Product Categories

Product Type and Composition	Specialty Ingredients	Uses, Contraindications, and Other Notes
Standard • 1.0–1.2 kcal/mL • Protein: 14%–19% • CHO: 51%–57% • Fat: 29%–33% • Free H_2O: 82%–85% • Fiber: 0 g/L	Formula containing intact nutrients without the addition of fiber	• Standard formulas without fiber are used for patients who do not tolerate a formula with fiber and those at risk for bowel ischemia (30,31).
Standard with fiber • 1.0–1.2 kcal/mL • Protein: 16%–19% • CHO: 51%–53% • Fat: 29%–33% • Free H_2O: 81%–84% • Fiber: 10–18 g/L	Formula containing intact nutrients with the addition of fiber	• Standard formulas with fiber are used for patients who do not require a specialty formula or one without fiber.
Concentrated • 1.5–2.0 kcal/mL • Protein: 16%–18% • CHO: 39%–54% • Fat: 29%–45% • Free H_2O: 70%–78% • Fiber: 0–22 g/L	Based on a typical healthy diet without additional free H_2O	• Concentrated formulas are used for patients who need a reduced volume due to EN intolerance, cycled feeds, fluid overload, congestive heart failure, renal failure, ascites, or syndrome of inappropriate antidiuretic hormone (32).
Diabetic • 1.0–1.2 kcal/mL • Protein: 17%–20% • CHO: 31%–40% • Fat: 42%–49% • Free H_2O: 81%–85% • Fiber: 14–21 g/L	Lower in CHO and higher in fat; some have added arginine or alpha-linoleic acid	• Research does not support improved outcomes with the use of diabetic formulas over standard with-fiber products in hospitalized or long-term care patients (33–35). • The high fat and high fiber content of diabetic formulas may delay gastric emptying, which may be problematic for patients with gastroparesis (32). • If initial use of standard formulas plus insulin does not adequately manage a patient's glucose levels, use of a diabetic formula may be warranted (36).
Pulmonary • 1.5 kcal/mL • Protein: 17%–18% • CHO: 27%–28% • Fat: 55% • Free H_2O: 78%–79% • Fiber: 0 g/L	Lower in CHO and higher in fat to minimize CO_2 production	• Research does not support benefit of using pulmonary formulas over standard with-fiber products (37). • Overfeeding, rather than higher CHO intake, is associated with increased CO_2 production (38). • May not be well tolerated due to high fat content.
Renal • 1.8–2.0 kcal/mL • Protein: 7%–18% • CHO: 34%–58% • Fat: 35%–48% • Free H_2O: 70%–73% • Fiber: 0–16 g/L	Lower in protein, concentrated to reduce volume, and lower in potassium, phosphorus, and magnesium; some have added arginine.	• Renal formula may be beneficial for patients who cannot tolerate a standard formula due to electrolyte abnormalities (39). • Very low–protein formulas should only be used when goal of care is to avoid RRT (32). Often, protein content of these products is too low to meet the higher protein needs of the patient on RRT.

Continues

TABLE 19.5 Enteral Product Categories *(Continued)*

Product Type and Composition	*Specialty Ingredients*	*Uses, Contraindications, and Other Notes*
Liver • 1.5 kcal/mL • Protein: 11% • CHO: 77% • Fat: 12% • Free H$_2$O: 76% • Fiber: 0 g/L	Higher in BCAA and lower in AAA	• These formulas may be beneficial in hospitalized patients with hepatic encephalopathy refractory to standard treatments (40). • Research does not support the use of these products in all patients with liver disease (41). The lower total protein content of these products may not benefit patients with liver disease who are malnourished (32).
Immune-enhancing • 1.0–1.5 kcal/mL • Protein: 17%–25% • CHO: 28%–53% • Fat: 25%–55% • Free H$_2$O: 85%–87% • Fiber: 0–10 g/L	May contain arginine, glutamine, EPA/DHA, GLA, nucleotides, and/or antioxidants	• In moderately to less severely ill ICU patients, use of immune-enhancing formula is *not* associated with reduced infectious complications, LOS, cost of medical care, days on mechanical ventilation, or mortality (9,42,43). • Use may be associated with increased mortality in severely ill ICU patients (9), especially those with sepsis. • Immune-enhancing products may be beneficial in hospitalized patients with major elective surgery, burns, trauma, or head and neck cancer (5,44,45). • Critically ill patients on mechanical ventilation with acute respiratory distress syndrome or acute lung injury given formulas enriched with EPA, GLA, and antioxidants had fewer days on the ventilator, shorter LOS in ICU, less risk of new organ failure, and lower mortality (5,46–48).
Elemental • 1 kcal/mL • Protein: 8%–20% • CHO: 70%–90% • Fat: 1%–10% • Free H$_2$O: 85%–86% • Fiber: 0 g/L	Completely hydrolyzed nutrients; may contain increased amounts of MCT; may contain arginine and/or glutamine	• Elemental products may be beneficial for patients with malabsorptive syndromes or pancreatic insufficiency who are unable to tolerate a standard formula (32).
Semi-elemental • 1.0–1.5 kcal/mL • Protein: 16%–25% • CHO: 36%–74% • Fat: 9%–39% • Free H$_2$O: 77%–85% • Fiber: 0–10 g/L	Contains small peptides; may contain increased amounts of MCT	• No significant difference found in outcome parameters in critically ill patients receiving semi-elemental compared to polymeric formulas (49). • LOS was found to be reduced in patients with acute pancreatitis receiving a semi-elemental formula as compared to polymeric formulas (50).

Abbreviations: AAA, aromatic amino acids; BCAA, branched-chain amino acids; CHO, carbohydrate; DHA, docosahexaenoic acid; EN, enteral nutrition; EPA, eicosapentaenoic acid; GLA, gamma-linolenic acid; ICU, intensive care unit; LOS, length of stay; MCT, medium-chain triglycerides; RRT, renal replacement therapy.

TABLE 19.6 Specialized Nutrients

Nutrient	Potential Benefits, Uses, and Concerns
Glutamine	• Conditionally essential amino acid. • Has trophic effect on intestinal epithelium (3). • Maintains gut integrity. • Stimulates health and proliferation of epithelial cells. • Stimulates release of heat-shock proteins (stabilizes organ function at distant sites). • Enteral glutamine in an EN regimen reduces hospital and ICU LOS in burn and mixed ICU patients (5,49) and mortality in burn patients (5,51). • Provides 0.3–0.5g/kg/d in 2–3 divided doses per day (5).
Arginine	• Conditionally essential amino acid. • Important for cell growth and proliferation; wound healing; collagen synthesis; immunity via its role as a precursor to nitric oxide (32). • May be associated with increased mortality in severely ill ICU patients.
Fish oils	• Promotes anti-inflammatory cascade under stress conditions by competing with arachidonic acid for the conversion to lipid mediators (32). • May be beneficial in patients with ARDS or severe acute lung injury.
Nucleotides	• Essential in DNA and RNA production during high turnover induced by illness (32).
Selenium	• There are decreased selenium plasma concentrations in critically ill patients especially those with septic shock (52). • Parenteral selenium has shown a trend toward reducing mortality in patients with sepsis or shock (53); no conclusive evidence of benefits of enteral selenium.
Probiotics	• Postulated that immunomodulation results from the interaction of GI probiotic elements, the gut mucosa, and underlying mucosal lymphoid elements (52). • May reduce infection for patients with transplantation, major abdominal surgery, or severe trauma (5). • Differences in species may have different effects with variable impact on patient outcomes. Lack of homogeneity in type of probiotic and populations studied make broad recommendations difficult.
Fiber	• Increases SCFA and fecal microbiota (54). SCFA are a fuel for the colonocytes and help increase intestinal mucosal growth and promote water and sodium absorption (36). • Soluble fiber may be beneficial in the fully resuscitated, hemodynamically stable critically ill patient receiving EN who develops diarrhea. • Insoluble fiber has not been shown to decrease diarrhea but may help decrease transit time by increasing fecal weight (55). • FOS are poorly absorbed carbohydrates that may help maintain large bowel integrity and promote growth of beneficial bacteria (36). • Fiber-containing formulas have been associated with lower glucose values (56). • These formulas may be associated with bowel obstructions in high-risk populations (30,57). • Avoid in hypotensive patients at high risk for developing ischemic bowel (5,31). • Adequate fluid must be delivered to prevent constipation/impaction (32).

Abbreviations: ARDS, acute respiratory distress syndrome; EN, enteral nutrition; FOS, fructo-oligosaccharides; GI, gastrointestinal; ICU, intensive care unit; LOS, length of stay; NPO, nil per os (nothing by mouth); SCFA, short-chain fatty acids.

VITAMINS AND MINERALS

Enteral products provide adequate amounts of vitamins and minerals in 1,000 to 1,500 mL of formula to meet Recommended Daily Intakes (RDI). Disease-specific formulations may have more or less of specific nutrients depending on the disease state (36).

WATER

Water comprises 70% to 85% of an enteral product. The amount of water in EN typically does not provide enough fluid to completely meet hydration needs (36).

Osmolality of Enteral Formulas

Osmolality refers to the concentration of free particles, molecules, or ions in a solution. Enteral formulas range from 270 to 700 mOsm. The osmolality of formula is not related to formula tolerance. Some clear-liquid food items and medications have significantly greater osmolalities than EN (36).

Modular Products

Modular products are available to provide additional energy and/or protein. Typically, modulars are added to meet nutritional needs in patients who have disproportionate requirements for nutrients such as protein (36).

Considerations for Formula Selection

PRODUCT-RELATED CONSIDERATIONS

When selecting a formula for a patient, relevant product-related considerations include the following:

- Digestibility/availability of nutrients
- Nutritional adequacy
- Viscosity
- Osmolality
- Ease of use
- Cost

PATIENT-RELATED CONSIDERATIONS

The following aspects of the patient's medical status will influence the appropriate choice of formula (4):

- Nutritional status and requirements
- Electrolyte balance
- Digestive and absorptive capacity
- Disease state
- Renal function
- Medical or drug therapy
- Routes for administration

Placing the Formula Order

The EN order should contain the following elements (11):

- Patient demographics: including name, location, date of birth, and medical record number
- Formula (either specific name or generic type) and/or modulars/additives
- Route/site of delivery: tube type and location
- Administration method, rate, and time for infusion
- Any additional orders for advancement, transitions, water flushes, head elevations, and monitoring parameters

The Enteral Nutrition Practice Recommendations Task Force recommends that standardized order forms be used to help prescribers meet a patient's individual nutritional needs and to improve order clarity (11).

Delivery of Enteral Nutrition

EN can be delivered by various methods depending on the medical condition, tolerance to feedings, and needs of the patient (see Table 19.7) (4). Most products are available as ready-to-serve with no reconstitution necessary. Formulas should not be diluted because they are at higher risk of microbial contamination due to their lower osmolality and higher pH (11). A few products come in powder form and need to be mixed with water before administration. These powders are not sterile and have a high risk of contamination.

Closed EN systems are available for most formulations. These products are prepackaged in 1- to 1.5-liter containers that can be hung at room temperature for 24 to 48 hours after spiking (11). If the

TABLE 19.7 Types of Enteral Nutrition Delivery

Type of Infusion	Initiation/Advancement	Advantages	Disadvantages
Continuous: Infused for 24 hours with minimal interruptions	• 25–50 mL/h • Increase by 25–50 mL/h every 4–8 hours	• May be better tolerated especially in critically ill patients	• Usually requires a pump for accurate infusion
Cycled: Infused at higher rates during 10- to 12-hour period (usually at night)	• Start with continuous infusion and slowly increase rate and decrease hours infused	• Allows patients time away from pump • Allows oral intakes during the day	• Higher rates may not be well tolerated
Intermittent: Larger volumes (240–480 mL) administered 3–6 times per day, infused over longer periods (30–60 min)	• ½–1 can per feeding • Increase by ½ can per feeding per day to goal	• May result in more adequate volumes being administered • Allows some time off feedings • Gravity feeding system is less expensive than pump	• Higher rates may not be well tolerated
Bolus: Larger volumes (240–480 mL) administered 3–6 times per day over short periods of time (10–15 min)	• ½–1 can per feeding • Increase by ½ can per feeding per day to goal	• Mimics meal delivery • Allows time off feedings • Lower cost	• Larger volume may not be well tolerated • Gastrointestinal symptoms may occur

Source: Data are from reference 4.

containers are opened, the formula can be infused for a maximum of 8 hours, or unused formula from the opened container must be refrigerated, with any remaining formula discarded after 24 hours.

Open systems require a feeding container to be filled with formula (either ready-to-serve or reconstituted) and can be hung at room temperature for a maximum of 4 to 8 hours in the hospital setting or 12 hours at home (11). The recommended maximum hang time for formulas that are reconstituted from powder or contain powder modular additives is 4 hours (11).

Contamination can occur at several points in the preparation process. To decrease the risk of contamination, follow the steps outlined in Box 19.5 (11,58). As Box 19.5 suggests, safe delivery of EN requires that clinicians use aseptic techniques when hanging the containers of EN and avoid touch contamination throughout the infusion process. It is also essential to not confuse EN with intravenous solutions. To prevent potentially fatal errors, an intensive educational campaign should be provided for staff involved in nutrition support (12). Box 19.6 describes the American Society for Parenteral and Enteral Nutrition (A.S.P.E.N.; www.nutritioncare.org) educational campaign that is used to educate professionals on EN safety (59). Note that this campaign suggests elevating the head of the bed by at least 30° whereas other sources recommend 45°.

BOX 19.5   Reducing Risk of Contamination in Enteral Nutrition (EN) Formula Preparation

Open system
1. Wash hands thoroughly before touching any of the cans of enteral formula.
2. Clean the tops of all cans/bottles with isopropyl alcohol and allow to dry prior to opening.
3. Use a sterile EN container.
4. Pour enough formula into the container to last a maximum of 4–8 hours.
5. Label the product (see Labeling guidelines at end of this box).
6. Refrigerate any remaining formula immediately for a maximum of 24 hours or for use within this time frame.
7. Infuse product for 4 hours (reconstituted formula/modulars) to 8 hours (sterile formula) (11). Home EN can hang for 12 hours (11). Discard any remaining formula after this time frame.
8. *Never* add more formula to the container to allow for a longer infusion.
9. Wash container with soap and water and rinse thoroughly.
10. Refill container with enough formula to last a maximum of 4–8 hours.
11. Discard container after 24 hours (11).

Closed system (58)
1. Wash hands thoroughly before touching the container of EN.
2. Unpackage a new spike set.
3. Label the product as described at the end of this box.
4. Turn container upside down and shake vigorously, using a twisting motion, for at least 10 seconds.
5. Lift tab to remove sticker, being careful not to touch spike port.
6. Visually inspect foil for breaks or signs of leakage. If foil is broken, formula should not be used.
7. Close side clamp on feeding set.
8. Remove piercing pin cover.
9. Spike piercing pin completely into port with a sideways (rocking) motion. Once inserted all the way, turn piercing pin one-quarter turn.

Continues

BOX 19.5   Reducing Risk of Contamination in Enteral Nutrition (EN) Formula Preparation *(Continued)*

10. Invert container and suspend using the hanging feature on the bottom of the container.
11. Follow pump priming and operation directions.
12. Discard open, unused formula within 24–48 hours.

Labeling
Labels for both open system and closed system should include:
- Patient demographics
- Formula
- Route/site of delivery
- Administration method, rate, and time for infusion
- Individuals responsible for preparation and hanging
- Time and date that the formula is prepared and/or hung
- "Not for IV Use"

BOX 19.6   The "Be A.L.E.R.T." Plan for Safe Enteral Delivery

Five key practices that nurses and other nutrition support staff should follow to help improve patient safety when administering a tube feeding:
- **A**septic technique
- **L**abel enteral equipment
- **E**levate head of bed ≥30 degrees when clinically possible
- **R**ight patient, right formula, right tube (the three Rs)
- **T**race all lines and tubing back to patient

Source: Data are from reference 59.

Monitoring of Enteral Nutrition

Adequate monitoring is required to ensure the following:

- Tube patency and location (see discussion of tube type and location, earlier in this chapter)
- Prevention of bronchopulmonary aspiration:
  - Elevate head of bed > 45° (5,9).
  - Pause EN if there is overt regurgitation or aspiration.
  - Place feeding tube in distal jejunum if patient is at high risk of aspiration (5).
  - Use continuous infusions rather than bolus or intermittent feeds (5).
  - Use prokinetic medications to promote gastric motility when feasible (5).
  - Use of chlorhexidine mouthwash twice daily may reduce risk of ventilator-associated pneumonia (5).
  - Checking tracheal secretions with glucose oxidase strips is *not* specific or sensitive (60).
  - Blue dye is *not* recommended; presence of blue dye in tracheal aspirations is not a sensitive indicator of aspiration (61), and the harm from blue dye outweighs potential benefits (9).

- Tolerance to EN and management of adverse effects of intolerance (Table 19.8 [5,13,14,62]), such as:
  - Diarrhea (osmotic, secretory, infectious, and noninfectious) (62)
  - Constipation (see Box 19.7 on page 252 for medications that decrease motility) (62)
  - Gastric residuals (GRVs do not correlate well to incidence of pneumonia, measures of gastric emptying, or incidence of regurgitation and aspiration, and should be considered an optional part of EN management) (5)
  - Abdominal distension/pain
  - Nausea and vomiting (occurs in 12% to 20% of patients on EN and may increase risk of pulmonary aspiration, pneumonia and sepsis) (14)
  - Metabolic complications (most metabolic complications from EN are related to malnutrition or an underlying disease process and not due to the EN infusion itself; however, infusion of EN may result in metabolic complications due to pre-existing deficiencies or increased demands to metabolize nutrients; see Table 19.9 on page 253) (49,63–65)
- Adequacy of nutritional intake:
  - Achieve EN goal rates within 24 to 48 hours (4,9); one study showed that starting EN at goal rate in ICU patients improved nutritional delivery, decreased cumulative energy deficit, and did not increase adverse events (66).
  - Monitor actual infused volumes vs prescribed/desired volumes.
  - Holding times and rationales should be monitored for appropriateness.
  - Average intake actually delivered within the first week should be *at least* 60% to 70% of estimated needs, which may be associated with decreased length of stay, fewer days on mechanical ventilation, and lower risk of infectious complications (9).
  - Strategies to improve nutritional intakes include starting at the target rate, a higher threshold for GRVs, use of prokinetics, and small bowel feedings (67).

TABLE 19.8 Management Techniques to Improve Tolerance to Enteral Nutrition

Problem	Potential Causes	Potential Solutions
Diarrhea (14) (>500 mL every 8 hours or >3 stools per day for at least 2 consecutive days)	• Osmotic: Medications (liquid medications containing sorbitol, lactulose, potassium, magnesium, or phosphates); hyperosmolar EN • Secretory: Enterotoxins, IBD, celiac disease, intestinal resection, bile acid malabsorption, fatty acid malabsorption, gastric hypersecretion, intestinal motility disorders, laxative abuse • Infectious: *Clostridium difficile;* contaminated enteral formula • Noninfectious: medications (antibiotics, H$_2$ blockers, antineoplastics, quinidine, prokinetic agents), bolus feeding, hyperosmolar EN, malnutrition, hypoalbuminemia, partial small bowel obstruction	• Avoid medications containing sorbitol. • Check for infectious causes. • Start antidiarrheal medication if no infectious cause is found. • Add/remove fiber. • Use probiotics. • Consider alternate enteral formulas (isotonic, semi-elemental, or elemental). • Ensure proper procedure is followed for preparation and administration of EN.

Continues

TABLE 19.8 Management Techniques to Improve Tolerance to Enteral Nutrition *(Continued)*

Problem	Potential Causes	Potential Solutions
Constipation (14) (excessive waste in the colon)	• Dehydration • Decreased GI motility • Inadequate fiber • Excessive fiber • Inactivity • Medications • Advanced age	• Provide adequate fluid. • Provide adequate fiber. • Medication-related: Add stool softeners, bowel stimulants, laxatives, enemas, and avoid drugs that decrease motility.[a] • Disimpaction.
Gastric residuals[b]	• Ileus/decreased motility • Stress of illness • Gastroparesis • Medications • High-fat formula • Glucose and electrolyte abnormalities (especially potassium and magnesium)	• Medication-related: Add prokinetic agents and avoid drugs that decrease motility.[a] • Concentrate EN to reduce volume. • Place feeding tube postpylorically. • Use low-fat EN. • Correct electrolyte levels.
Abdominal pain/distension	• Constipation/impaction • Obstruction • Ileus • Obstipation • Ascites • Diarrhea • Rapid feeding	• Manage constipation and diarrhea. • Start a prokinetic agent. • Decrease or hold EN.
Nausea and vomiting	• Constipation/impaction • Partial obstruction • Hypotension • Sepsis • Anesthesia • Opiate analgesic medications • Anticholinergics • Excessive rapid infusion of formula • Infusion of a very cold solution or one containing a large amount of fat	• Manage constipation. • Reduce, change, or discontinue all narcotic medications. • Start a prokinetic agent. • Switch to a low-fat formula. • Infuse feeding at room temperature. • Reduce rate of infusion.
Maldigestion/ malabsorption	• Lactose intolerance • Steatorrhea • Short bowel syndrome • Crohn's disease • Diverticular disease • Radiation enteritis • HIV • Pancreatic insufficiency • Celiac disease • Enteric fistulas	• Use of peptide-based formula with greater percentage of fat from MCT. • May need PN or combination of EN and PN if severe. • Test stool for fecal fat.

Abbreviations: EN, enteral nutrition; GI, gastrointestinal; IBD, inflammatory bowel disease; MCT, medium-chain triglycerides; PN, parenteral nutrition.

[a]See Box 19.7.

[b]It is unknown what volume of gastric residuals indicates intolerance. The volume typically ranges from 250 to 500 mL and often requires repeated values to be considered significant (5,13,14).

Source: Data are from references 5, 13, 14, and 62.

BOX 19.7   Medications That May Slow Gastrointestinal Motility

- Sedatives
- Opioid analgesics (morphine, fentanyl, hydromorphone, methadone)
- Catecholamine vasopressors (dopamine, epinephrine, norepinephrine, phenylephrine)
- α-Adrenergic receptor agonists (clonidine, dexmedetomidine)
- Anticholinergics (antihistamines, tricyclic antidepressants, antiparkinsonian agents, phenothiazines)
- Calcium-channel blockers
- Oral or enteral calcium supplements
- Oral or enteral iron supplements
- Calcium- or aluminum-containing antacids

Source: Data are from reference 6.

Feeding Protocols

Enteral feeding protocols may assist in the appropriate ordering, delivery, and monitoring of EN. Feeding protocols should include the following (67):

- Prokinetics at initiation, which may increase GI transit, improve feeding tolerance and EN delivery, and potentially reduce risk of aspiration
- Higher gastric residual volumes (≥250 mL)
- Use of postpyloric feeding tubes

Unfortunately, the implementation of feeding protocols has been met with limited success (68–71). Often, multifaceted practice change strategies must be implemented to achieve compliance with evidence-based nutrition support guidelines. Improvements in compliance with protocols can be achieved by using the following (52):

- Simple algorithms
- Personalized protocols based on staffing, patient population, and resources

Conclusion

Enteral nutrition is clearly regarded as the safest and most beneficial method to support nutritional status in patients who are unable to eat orally. It is associated with improved clinical outcomes and reduced infectious complications and therefore is the preferred method of artificial nutrition support unless its use is contraindicated. Complications associated with EN can be prevented or managed with thoughtful initiation, delivery, and monitoring of EN. Skilled clinicians play an integral role to ensure early and adequate EN is achieved in the critically ill population to minimize complications and improve outcomes.

TABLE 19.9 Common Metabolic Complications Associated with Enteral Nutrition

Metabolic Complication	Causes	Goal	Prevention/Correction
Hyperglycemia	• Diabetes mellitus • Insulin resistance • Stress • Infection • Trauma • Steroids	• Tight (80–110 mg/dL) BG control in critically ill patients may *not* lead to reduced number of days on mechanical ventilation, shorter time in hospital, infectious complications, mortality or cost of medical care (63). • Tight BG control reduces the risk of some types of infectious complication in surgical (primarily cardiac) patients (49). • Hyperglycemia (BG >180 mg/dL) should be avoided in all critically ill patients as it is associated with increased mortality (63). • Aim for BG target of ~125–160 mg/dL (49).	• Treat underlying disease. • Use insulin to maintain optimal BG levels between 140 and 180 mg/dL (63). • Provide OHA as needed.
Hypoglycemia	• Holding EN in patient receiving insulin or OHA	• Do not allow BG to fall below 70 mg/dL.	• Taper EN gradually. • Add dextrose to IV fluids.
Hypernatremia	• Inadequate fluid intakes • Increased fluid loss • Increased sodium intakes	• Maintain serum sodium WNR.	• Increase free H_2O administration. • Decrease exogenous sodium administration from IV solutions.
Refeeding syndrome (64,65)	• Malnutrition	• Maintain serum phosphorus, magnesium, potassium, and thiamin WNR.	• Assess lab values and correct abnormal electrolyte levels prior to starting EN. • Initiate and advance feedings slowly. • Provide exogenous phosphorus, magnesium, potassium, or thiamin to correct/maintain serum levels.
Hyperphosphatemia	• Renal insufficiency	• Maintain serum phosphorus WNR.	• Use low-phosphorus formula. • Start phosphate binder.
Essential fatty acid deficiency	• Inadequate linoleic acid intake	• Adequate fat supply to meet requirements for essential fatty acids.	• Provide at least 4% of energy needs as linoleic acid.

Abbreviations: BG, blood glucose; EN, enteral nutrition; ICU, intensive care unit; IV, intravenous; OHA, oral hypoglycemic agents; WNR, within normal range for institution.
Source: Data are from references 49, 63, 64, and 65.

References

1. Martindale R, McClave SA, Vanek VW, McCarthy M, Roberts P, Taylor B, Ochoa JB, Napolitano L, Cresci G, American College of Critical Care Medicine, A.S.P.E.N. Board of Directors. Guidelines for the provision and assessment of nutrition support therapy in the adult critically ill patient: Society of Critical Care Medicine and American Society for Parenteral and Enteral Nutrition: executive summary. *Crit Care Med.* 2009;37(5):1757–1761.

2. Brantley S. Implementation of the Enteral Nutrition Practice Recommendations. *Nutr Clin Pract.* 2009;24(3):335–343.

3. McClave A, Heyland DK. The physiologic response and associated clinical benefits from provision of early enteral nutrition. *Nutr Clin Pract.* 2009;24(3):305–315.

4. Marian M, McGinnis C. Overview of enteral nutrition. In: Gottschlich M, ed. *The A.S.P.E.N. Nutrition Support Core Curriculum: A Case Based Approach—The Adult Patient.* Silver Spring, MD: American Society for Parenteral and Enteral Nutrition; 2007:187–208.

5. McClave SA, Martindale RG, Vanek VW, McCarthy M, Roberts P, Taylor B, Ochoa JB, Napolitano L, Cresci G, A.S.P.E.N. Board of Directors, American College of Critical Care Medicine. Guidelines for the provision and assessment of nutrition support therapy in the adult critically ill patient: Society of Critical Care Medicine (SCCM) and American Society for Parenteral and Enteral Nutrition (A.S.P.E.N.). *JPEN J Parenter Enteral Nutr.* 2009;33(3):277–316.

6. Trujillo E, Young LS, Chertow GM, et al. Metabolic and monetary costs of avoidable parenteral nutrition. *JPEN J Parenter Enteral Nutr.* 1999;23:109–113.

7. Farber M, Moses J, Korn M. Reducing costs and patient morbidity in the enterally fed intensive care unit patient. *JPEN J Parenter Enteral Nutr.* 2005;29:S562–S569.

8. Koretz R, Avenell A, Lipman TO, Braunschweig CL, Milne AC. Does enteral nutrition affect outcome: a systematic review of the randomized trials. *Am J Gastroenterol.* 2007;102:412–429.

9. Academy of Nutrition and Dietetics Evidence Analysis Library; Malone A, Charney P, Compher C, Halasa-Esper D, Frankenfield D, Hise Brown ME, Kattelmann KK, Marian MJ, Roberts SR, Russell MK. Executive Summary of Recommendations. Critical Illness Nutrition Practice Recommendations. www.andevidence library.com/topic.cfm?cat=3016. Accessed February 2, 2010.

10. McClave A, Change WK. When to feed the patient with gastrointestinal bleeding. *Nutr Clin Pract.* 2005;20:544–550.

11. A.S.P.E.N. Enteral Nutrition Practice Recommendations Task Force: Bankhead R, Boullata J, Brantley S, Corkins M, Guenter P, Krenitsky J, Lyman B, Methany NA, Mueller C, Robbins S, Wessel J, A.S.P.E.N. Board of Directors. Enteral Nutrition Practice Recommendations. *JPEN J Parenter Enteral Nutr.* 2009;33(2):122–167.

12. Guenter P, Hicks RW, Simmons D. Enteral feeding misconnections: an update. *Nutr Clin Pract.* 2009;24(3):325–334.

13. Bankhead R, Fang JC. Enteral access devices. In: Gottschlich M, ed. *The A.S.P.E.N. Nutrition Support Core Curriculum: A Case Based Approach— The Adult Patient.* Silver Spring, MD: American Society for Parenteral and Enteral Nutrition; 2007:233–245.

14. Malone A, Seres DS, Lord L. Complications of enteral nutrition. In: Gottschlich M, ed. *The A.S.P.E.N. Nutrition Support Core Curriculum: A Case Based Approach— The Adult Patient.* Silver Spring, MD: American Society for Parenteral and Enteral Nutrition; 2007:246–263.

15. McClave A, Demeo MT, DeLegge MH, et al. North American Summit on Aspiration in the Critically Ill consensus statement. *JPEN J Parenter Enteral Nutr.* 2002;26(6 Suppl):S80–S85.

16. Heyland D, Drover JW, Dhaliwal R, Greenwood J. Optimizing the benefits and minimizing the risks of enteral nutrition in the critically ill: role of small bowel feeding. *JPEN J Parenter Enteral Nutr.* 2003;26(6 Suppl):S51–S57.

17. Marik P, Zaloga GP. Gastric versus post-pyloric feeding: a systematic review. *Crit Care.* 2003;7:R46–R51.

18. Ho K, Dobb GJ, Webb SAR. A comparison of early gastric and post-pyloric feeding in critically ill patients: a meta-analysis. *Intensive Care Med.* 2006;32:639–649.

19. Methany N, Meert KL. Monitoring feeding tube placement. *Nutr Clin Pract.* 2004;19:487–495.

20. Methany N, Meert KL, Clouse RE. Complications related to feeding tube placement. *Curr Opin Gastroenterol.* 2007;23:178–182.

21. Baskin W. Acute complications associated with bedside placement of feeding tubes. *Nutr Clin Pract.* 2006;21:40–55.

22. Methany N. Risk factors for aspiration. *JPEN J Parenter Enteral Nutr.* 2002;26(6 Suppl):S26–S31.

23. Nicolau D, Davis SK. Carbonated beverages as irrigants for feeding tubes. *DICP.* 1990;24(9):840.

24. Wilson M, Haynes-Johnson V. Cranberry juice or water? A comparison of feeding-tube irrigants. *Nutr Support Serv.* 1987;7:23–24.

25. Marcuard S, Stegall KL, Trogdon, S. Clearing obstructed feeding tubes. *JPEN J Parenter Enteral Nutr.* 1989;13:81–83.

26. Brown D, Miedema BW, King PD, Marshall JB. Safety of early feeding after percutaneous endoscopic gastrostomy. *J Clin Gastroenterol.* 1995;21:330–331.

27. Choudhry U, Barde CJ, Markert R, Gopalswamy N. Percutaneous endoscopic gastrostomy: a randomized prospective comparison of early and delayed feeding. *Gastrointest Endosc.* 1996;44:164–167.

28. McCarter T, Condon SC, Aguilar RC, et al. Randomized prospective gastrostomy placement. *Am J Gastroenterol.* 1998;93:419–421.

29. Lewis S, Egger M, Sylvester PA, Thomas S. Early enteral feeding versus "nil by mouth" after gastrointestinal surgery: systematic review and meta-analysis of controlled trials. *BMJ.* 2001;323:1–5.

30. McIvor A, Meguid MM, Curtas S, Kaplan DS. Intestinal obstruction from cecal bezoar: a complication of fiber containing tube feedings. *Nutrition.* 1990;6:115–117.

31. McClave A, Change WK. Feeding the hypotensive patient: does enteral feeding precipitate or protect against ischemic bowel? *Nutr Clin Pract.* 2003;18:279–284.

32. Chen Y, Peterson SJ. Enteral nutrition formulas: Which formula is right for your adult patient? *Nutr Clin Pract.* 2009;24(3):344–355.

33. Leon-Sans M, Garcia-Luna PP, Planas M, et al. Glycemic and lipid control in hospitalized type 2 diabetic patients: evaluation of 2 enteral nutrition formulas (low carbohydrate-high monounsaturated fat vs high carbohydrate. *JPEN J Parenter Enteral Nutr.* 2005;29:21–29.

34. Mesejo A, Acosta JA, Ortega C, et al. Comparison of a high-protein disease-specific enteral formula with a high-protein enteral formula in hyperglycemic critically ill patients. *Clin Nutr.* 2003;22:295–305.

35. Craig L, Nicholson S, Silverstone FA, Kennedy RD. Use of a reduced carbohydrate, modified fat enteral formula for improving metabolic control and clinical outcomes in long-term care residents with type 2 diabetes. *Nutrition.* 1998;14:529–534.

36. Lefton J, Esper DH, Kochevar M. Enteral formulations. In: Gottschlich M, ed. *The A.S.P.E.N. Nutrition Support Core Curriculum: A Case Based Approach— The Adult Patient.* Silver Springs, MD: American Society for Parenteral and Enteral Nutrition; 2007:209–232.

37. Vermeeren M, Wouters EF, Nelissen LH, van Lier A, Hofman Z, Schols AM. Acute effects of different nutritional supplements on symptoms and functional capacity in patients with chronic obstructive pulmonary disease. *Am J Clin Nutr.* 2001;73:295–301.

38. Talpers S, Romberger DJ, Bunce SB, Pingleton SK. Nutritionally associated increased carbon dioxide production: excess total carbohydrate vs high proportion of carbohydrate calories. *Chest.* 1992;102:551–555.

39. Russell M, Charney P. Is there a role for specialized enteral nutrition in the intensive care unit? *Nutr Clin Pract.* 2002;17:156–168.

40. A.S.P.E.N. Guidelines for the use of parenteral and enteral nutrition in adult and pediatric patients. *JPEN J Parenter Enteral Nutr.* 2002;26(1 Suppl):1SA–128SA.

41. Als-Nielsen B, Koretz RL, Kjaergard LL, Gluud C. Branched-chain amino acids for hepatic encephalopathy. *Cochrane Database Syst Rev.* 2003;2:CD001939.

42. Kieft H, Roos AN, van Drunen JDE, et al. Clinical outcome on immunonutrition in a heterogeneous intensive care population. *Intensive Care Med*. 2005;31:524–532.

43. Heyland D, Dhaliwal R. Immunonutrition in the critically ill: from old approaches to new paradigms. *Intensive Care Med*. 2005;31:501–503.

44. Consensus recommendations from the US Summit on Immune-Enhancing Enteral Therapy. *JPEN J Parenter Enteral Nutr*. 2001;25(2 Suppl):S61–S62.

45. Waitzberg D, Saito H, Plank LD, et al. Postsurgical infections are reduced with specialized nutrition support. *World J Surg*. 2006;30:1592–1604.

46. Gadek J, DeMichele SJ, Karlstad MD, et al. Effect of enteral feeding with eicosapentaenoic acid, gamma-linolenic acid and antioxidants in patients with acute respiratory distress syndrome. *Crit Care Med*. 1999;27:1409–1420.

47. Singer P, Theilla M, Fisher H, et al. Benefit of an enteral diet enriched with eicosapentaenoic acid and gamma-linolenic acid in ventilated patients with acute lung injury. *Crit Care Med*. 2006;34:1033–1038.

48. Pontes-Arruda A, Aragao AM, Albuquerque JD. Effects of enteral feeding with eicosapentaenoic acid, y-linolenic acid, and antioxidants in mechanically ventilated patients with severe sepsis and septic shock. *Crit Care Med*. 2006;34:2325–2333.

49. Heyland D, Dhaliwal R, Drover JW, Gramlich L, Dodek P, Canadian Critical Care Clinical Practice Guidelines Committee. Canadian clinical practice guidelines for nutrition support in mechanically ventilated, critically ill adult patients. *JPEN J Parenter Enteral Nutr*. 2003;27:355–373.

50. Tiengou L, Gloro R, Pouzoulet J, et al. Semi-elemental formula or polymeric formula: is there a better choice for enteral nutrition in acute pancreatitis? Randomized comparative study. *JPEN J Parenter Enteral Nutr*. 2006;30:1–5.

51. Garrel D, Patenaude J, Nedelec B, et al. Decreased mortality and infectious morbidity in adult burn patients given enteral glutamine supplements: a prospective, controlled, randomized clinical trial. *Crit Care Med*. 2003;31:2444–2449.

52. Taylor B, Krenitsky J. Nutrition in the intensive care unit: year in review 2008–2009. *JPEN J Parenter Enteral Nutr*. 2010;34(1):21–31.

53. Crimi E, Liguori A, Condorelli M, et al. The beneficial effects of antioxidant supplementation in enteral feeding in the critically ill patients: a prospective, randomized, double-blind, placebo-controlled trial. *Anesth Analg*. 2004;99:857–863.

54. Schneider S, Girard-Pipau F, Frame F, et al. Effects of total enteral nutrition supplemented with a multi-fibre mix on faecal short-chain fatty acids and microbiota. *Clin Nutr*. 2006;25:82–90.

55. Malone A. Enteral formula selection: a review of selected product categories. *Pract Gastroenterol*. 2005;24:44–74.

56. Kagansky M, Rimon E. Is there a difference in metabolic outcome between different enteral formulas? *JPEN J Parent Enteral Nutr*. 2007;31:320–323.

57. Scaife C, Saffle JR, Morris SE. Intestinal obstruction secondary to enteral feedings in burn and trauma patients. *J Trauma*. 1999;47:859–863.

58. Ready-to-Hang. Suggested Setup Procedure. Columbus, OH: Abbott Laboratories; 2010. http://static.abbott nutrition.com/PHB/09-27-2010-01-29-43_READY-TO-%20HANG-SETUP-PROCEDURE.pdf. Accessed on February 3, 2014.

59. Nestlé HealthCare Nutrition and Medical Professionals Unite to Improve Patient Safety "Be A.L.E.R.T." Initiative Complements New Tube-Feeding Best-Practice Recommendations (press release). February 3, 2009. American Society for Parenteral and Enteral Nutrition website. www.nutritioncare.org/Press_Room /Press_Releases/Be_A_L_E_R_T__Initiative_Complements_New_Tube-Feeding_Best-Practice _Recommendations. Accessed February 3, 2014.

60. Methany N, Dahms TE, Stewart BJ, Stone KS, Frank PA, Clouse RE. Verification of inefficacy of the glucose method in detecting aspiration associated with tube feedings. *Med Surg Nurs*. 2005;14:112–121.

61. Methany N, Dahms TE, Stewart BJ, et al. Efficacy of dye-stained enteral formula in detecting pulmonary aspiration. *Chest*. 2002;122:276–281.

62. Btaiche I, Chan LN, Pleva M, Kraft MD. Critical illness, gastrointestinal complications, and medication therapy during enteral feeding in critically ill adult patients. *Nutr Clin Pract*. 2010;25(1):32–49.

63. Academy of Nutrition and Dietetics Evidence Analysis Library. Critical Illness (CI) 2012 Evidence-Based Nutrition Practice Guideline. www.andevidencelibrary.com. Accessed February 3, 2014.

64. Kraft M, Btaiche IF, Sacks GS. Review of the refeeding syndrome. *Nutr Clin Pract*. 2005;20:625–633.

65. Stanga Z, Brunner A, Leuenberger M, et al. Nutrition in clinical practice— the refeeding syndrome: illustrative cases and guidelines for prevention and treatment. *Eur J Clin Nutr*. 2008;62:687–694.

66. Desachy A, Clavel M, Vuagnat A, Normand S, Gissot B, Francois B. Initial efficacy and tolerability of early enteral nutrition with immediate or gradual introduction in intubated patients. *Intensive Care Med*. 2008;34:1054–1059.

67. Heyland D, Dhaliwal R, Drover JW, Gramlich L, Dodek P, Canadian Critical Care Clinical Practice Guidelines Committee. Canadian Clinical Practice Guidelines: Summary of Topics and Recommendations. www.criticalcarenutrition.com/docs/cpg/srrev.pdf. Accessed January 30, 2010.

68. McClave S, Sexton LK, Spain DA, Adams JL, Owens NA, Sullins MB, Blandford BS, Snider HL. Enteral tube feeding in the intensive care unit: factors impeding adequate delivery. *Crit Care Med*. 1999;27(7):1252–1256.

69. Mackenzie S, Zygun DA, Whitmore BL, Doig CJ, Hameed SM. Implementation of a nutrition support protocol increases the proportion of mechanically ventilated patients reaching enteral nutrition targets in the adult intensive care unit. *JPEN J Parent Enteral Nutr*. 2005;29(2):74–80.

70. Pinilla J, Samphire J, Arnold C, Liu L, Thiessen B. Comparison of gastrointestinal tolerance to two enteral feeding protocols in critically ill patient: A prospective, randomized controlled trial. *JPEN J Parenter Enteral Nutr*. 2001;25(2):81–86.

71. Jain M, Heyland D, Dhaliwal R, Day AG, Drover J, Keefe L Gelula M. Dissemination of the Canadian clinical practice guidelines for nutrition support: Results of a cluster randomized controlled trial. *Crit Care Med*. 2006;34(9):2362–2369.

CHAPTER 20

Parenteral Nutrition

Jennifer C. Lefton, MS, RD, CNSC, FAND,
Annette M. Carpenter, RD, CNSC, Jennifer R. Carter, RD, CNSC,
and Suzanne M. Lugerner, MS, RN, LDN, CNSC, CNS

This chapter briefly reviews the topic of parenteral nutrition (PN)—"the infusion of intravenous nutrients via peripheral or central veins" (1). A more detailed discussion of patient selection and the initiation, advancement, and monitoring of PN is beyond the scope of this publication. Readers are encouraged to explore the references and other resources on this topic. For information about the use of PN in pediatric patients, see Chapter 21. Refer to Chapter 22 for coverage of home parenteral nutrition, and Chapter 26 for discussion of legal and ethical matters related to nutrition support.

Indications for Use

Indications for the use of PN include the following:

- Bowel obstruction
- Severe necrotizing pancreatitis
- Short bowel syndrome
- Malabsorption
- High-output GI fistulas
- Hemodynamic instability
- Paralytic ileus
- Intolerance to enteral feedings

PN is reserved as a last resort for patients who are unable to be fed enterally (2,3). (See Chapter 19 for more information on enteral nutrition.) Recent guidelines suggest that if critically ill patients cannot be fed enterally, then no nutrition support should be provided for the first 7 days. However, if patients have pre-existing malnutrition, it is appropriate to initiate PN as soon as possible once the patient has been adequately resuscitated. Additionally, PN should be initiated in postoperative patients only if it is anticipated that the patient will need at least 7 days of nutrition support (4).

Venous Access

Parenteral nutrition may be infused via a peripheral or central line. Peripheral PN (PPN) often delivers less than adequate nutrients in large amounts of fluid because of restraints in the osmolarity of the solution. Patients must have good peripheral venous access and be able to tolerate large volumes of fluid to receive PPN. Therefore, patients with renal, cardiac, or liver failure are not good candidates for PPN.

Most patients have PN administered through a central line. It is ideal to have a dedicated line for delivery of PN. The tip of the catheter should be confirmed to be in the superior vena cava prior to administering a central PN formulation.

Box 20.1 summarizes selected factors involved in decisions regarding venous access routes for PN infusion (1).

Parenteral Nutrition Formulation

Parenteral nutrition is a very complex mixture containing as many as 40 different components. Recommendations for safe practices for ordering, compounding, and administering PN have been published by the American Society for Parenteral and Enteral Nutrition (A.S.P.E.N.) (5,6).

Amino Acids

Crystalline amino acids provide 4 kcal/g and are available in concentrations of 3% to 15%. Specialized amino acid formulations targeted toward liver and renal failure patients are available but are rarely used because of a lack of research demonstrating their efficacy. See Table 20.1 for additional information on PN products. There is no need to start with lesser amounts of amino acids and incrementally increase toward a goal. Amino acids can be prescribed in goal amounts with the initial PN order.

Dextrose

Anhydrous dextrose monohydrate provides 3.4 kcal/g. Dextrose is typically initiated at half of the goal requirement in order to monitor glucose tolerance and avoid the electrolyte disturbances that may occur when initiating nutrition support with excessive amounts of dextrose. Once glucose levels are in a normal range and stable, dextrose amounts in the PN can be adjusted toward goal requirements.

See Box 20.2 for an example of dextrose calculations. Glucose infusion rates (GIR) of more than 4 to 5 mg/kg/min should be avoided in the critically ill population (7,8).

Fat

Intravenous fat emulsion (IVFE) may be provided within the PN as a total nutrient admixture (TNA) or as a separate infusion. IVFE provide 9 kcal/g. Fat intake should be limited to 20% to 35% of total energy or less than 1 g/kg/d.

There are circumstances when IVFE should not be added to the PN formulation. IVFE is contraindicated in patients with egg allergy. Patients receiving propofol for sedation may not require additional IVFE because propofol is delivered in a 10% lipid emulsion providing 1.1 lipid kcal/mL. Additionally, IVFE should be avoided in patients with hypertriglyceridemia-induced pancreatitis or a triglyceride level in excess of 400 mg/dL (9). See Table 20.2 (page 262) for information on IVFE products.

BOX 20.1   Factors to Consider in the Selection of an Access Route for Parenteral Nutrition (PN)

Length of therapy/available access route
- **Peripheral catheters** access the peripheral vessels and are among the simplest catheters to place for short-term access (≤10 to 14 days). To minimize the risk of phlebitis, peripheral catheters are rotated every 72 hours. Peripheral access should only be used for PN solutions with lower osmolarity (<900 mOsm/L). The inclusion of IV fat emulsions in the PN formula may also minimize the risk of phlebitis.
- **Central venous catheters** (CVC) access large veins, and their distal tip lies in the distal vena cava or right atrium. CVCs are most commonly placed in the jugular, subclavian, femoral, cephalic, and basilic veins. They may be single- or multi-lumen. The three categories of CVC are as follows:
  - **Nontunneled**: Percutaneous nontunneled central catheters are used in the acute setting for short-duration therapies. Catheters are most often placed utilizing the subclavian, jugular, and femoral veins. Higher infection risk is present with these catheters, so they are not recommended for home care. Peripherally inserted central catheter (PICC) lines are a form of nontunneled CVC used in acute and home-care settings. These catheters are inserted into the basilic, cephalic, or brachial vein and threaded up so that the tip lies in the superior vena cava. Although peripherally inserted, PICCs are considered central lines.
  - **Tunneled**: Tunneled catheters are surgically tunneled through the skin so that the exit point of a tunneled catheter is remote from the actual vein entry point. A tunneled catheter is used when long-term vascular access is required. Broviac, Hickman, and Groshong are commonly used tunneled catheters. Tunneled catheters have a cuff that has antimicrobial qualities and acts to prevent migration of the catheter. Access to tunneled catheters is external.
  - **Implanted**: Implanted ports are entirely internal and are accessed through piercing the skin. Implanted ports are best utilized for long intermittent therapies such as chemotherapy but can be used for PN.

Osmolarity/concentration of solution
- PN solutions with a final dextrose concentration more than 10% are extremely hypertonic and must be infused into a large vein to avoid damage to the vein.
- Solutions with osmolarity of 900 mOsm/L or more should be infused via CVC.

Anatomical considerations
- Accessing the desired placement site can be difficult.

Clinician expertise
- PICCs may be placed by specially trained nurses.
- Implanted ports are placed by surgical staff or interventional radiology staff.

Considerations for Home PN:[a]
- For home PN patients, when determining the insertion site and the catheter type consider:
  - Activity
  - Lifestyle
  - Quality of life

[a]Refer to Chapter 22 for additional information on home PN.

Source: Adapted with permission from Parenteral nutrition. In: Academy of Nutrition and Dietetics Nutrition Care Manual. 2013. www.nutritioncaremanual.org. Accessed November 15, 2013.

TABLE 20.1 Amino Acid Products for Parenteral Nutrition

Product	Manufacturer	Indication	Concentration, %
Aminosyn[a]	Hospira	Standard	3.5, 5, 7, 8.5, 10
Aminosyn II[a]	Hospira	Standard	7, 8.5, 10, 15
Aminosyn—Hepatic Formula (HF)	Hospira	Hepatic failure	8
Aminosyn—High Branched-Chain (HBC)	Hospira	Metabolic stress	7
Aminosyn—Pediatric Formula (PF)[b]	Hospira	Pediatric	7, 10
Aminosyn—Renal Formula (RF)	Hospira	Renal failure	5.2
BranchAmin	Baxter	Metabolic stress	4
Clinisol[a]	Baxter	Fluid restriction	15
Hepatasol[a]	Baxter	Hepatic failure	8
Premasol[b]	Baxter	Pediatric	6, 10
Prosol	Baxter	Fluid restriction	20
RenAmin	Baxter	Renal failure	6.5
Travasol[a]	Baxter	Standard	10

[a]Preferred for use in adults, available for use in pediatric patients.
[b]Preferred for use in pediatric patients.

BOX 20.2   Sample Dextrose Calculations

Calculating the maximum dextrose tolerance

Patient Weight (kg) × Desired GIR × 1,440 (min/d)/1,000 = Grams of Dextrose per Day

For example:

65 kg × 4 × 1,440 min/1,000 = 374 g dextrose

Calculating the dextrose infusion rate

Dextrose (g)/Patient Weight (kg)/1,440 min/d × 1,000 = Infusion Rate (mg/kg/min)

For example:

400 g dextrose/65 kg/1,440 × 1,000 = 4.3 mg/kg/min

Abbreviation: GIR, glucose infusion rate.

Electrolytes

Sodium, potassium, chloride, acetate, phosphorus, calcium, and magnesium can all be added to PN solutions in various amounts, as determined by the individual patient's requirements. Standard electrolyte requirements are shown in Table 20.3 on page 262 (5). Sodium and potassium may be added as chloride, acetate, or phosphate salts. Bicarbonate is never added to PN solutions because it poses stability concerns. Acetate is provided for base needs and it is converted into bicarbonate once in the body. The amounts of phosphorus and calcium that can be added to PN solutions also are of concern for PN stability and institution-specific guidelines should be followed.

TABLE 20.2 Lipid Products for Use in Parenteral Nutrition

Product	Manufacturer	Concentration, %
Liposyn II[a]	Hospira	10, 20
Liposyn III[a]	Hospira	10, 20, 30
Intralipid[a]	Baxter	20, 30

[a]Approved for use in both adult and pediatric patients.

TABLE 20.3 Standard Electrolyte Requirements for Adult Parenteral Nutrition Formulations

Electrolyte	Standard Requirement
Sodium	1–2 mEq/kg
Potassium	1–2 mEq/kg
Chloride	As needed to maintain acid-base balance
Acetate	As needed to maintain acid-base balance
Calcium	10–15 mEq
Magnesium	8–20 mEq
Phosphorus	20–40 mmol

Source: Adapted from Mirtallo J, Canada T, Johnson D, et al. Safe practices for parenteral nutrition. *JPEN J Parenter Enteral Nutr.* 2004;28(6 Suppl):S39–S70. Copyright ©2004 *Journal of Parenteral and Enteral Nutrition.* Used by permission of SAGE Publications.

Vitamins and Minerals

Vitamins and minerals should be added to PN solutions daily. Tables 20.4 and 20.5 show parenteral requirements for vitamins and trace elements (5). In some instances, changes to the formulation may be necessary. For example, patients with excessive small bowel losses from fistula or ostomies should receive an additional 12 mg zinc per liter of loss (10), and patients with hepatobiliary disease may need to have the copper and manganese removed from the PN solution because of impaired excretion (5).

Calculating the Parenteral Nutrition Prescription

Refer to Box 20.3 (on page 264) for an example of how to calculate the PN prescription for a critically ill woman.

PN Complications

Complications associated with PN fall into several categories: infectious, mechanical, metabolic, and gastrointestinal. Infectious complications are most often related to catheter and aseptic technique. Refer to Box 20.4 (on page 264) for examples of the complications from the other categories. Additional information about acute and long-term complications may be found in reference 11.

TABLE 20.4 Daily Requirements for Adult Parenteral Vitamins[a]

Vitamin	Requirement
Thiamin (B-1)	6 mg
Riboflavin (B-2)	3.6 mg
Niacin (B-3)	40 mg
Folic acid	600 mcg
Pantothenic acid	15 mg
Pyridoxine (B-6)	6 mg
Cyanocobalamin (B-12)	5 mcg
Biotin	60 mcg
Ascorbic acid	200 mg
Vitamin A	3,300 IU
Vitamin D	200 IU
Vitamin E	10 IU
Vitamin K	150 mcg

[a]Food and Drug Administration requirements for marketing an effective adult parenteral vitamin product.
Source: Reprinted from Mirtallo J, Canada T, Johnson D, et al. Safe practices for parenteral nutrition. *JPEN J Parenter Enteral Nutr.* 2004;28(6 Suppl):S39–S70. Copyright ©2004 *Journal of Parenteral and Enteral Nutrition.* Reprinted by permission of SAGE Publications.

TABLE 20.5 Daily Trace Element Supplementation to Adult PN Formulations[a]

Trace Element	Standard Intake
Chromium	10–15 mcg
Copper	0.3–0.5 mg
Iron	Not routinely added
Manganese[b]	60–100 mcg
Selenium	20–60 mcg
Zinc	2.5–5 mg

[a]Standard intake ranges based on generally healthy people with normal losses.
[b]The contamination levels in various components of the PN formulation can significantly contribute to total intake. Serum concentrations should be monitored with long-term use.
Source: Reprinted from Mirtallo J, Canada T, Johnson D, et al. Safe practices for parenteral nutrition. *JPEN J Parenter Enteral Nutr.* 2004;28(6 Suppl):S39–S70. Copyright ©2004 *Journal of Parenteral and Enteral Nutrition.* Reprinted by permission of SAGE Publications.

BOX 20.3 Sample Parenteral Nutrition Calculation for a 3-in-1 Formulation

A critically ill female patient will require parenteral nutrition. She weighs 64 kg and is 67 inches tall. Her energy needs are estimated to be 25 kcal/kg/d (~1,600 kcal/d) and her protein requirements are 1.5 g/kg/d (~100 g/d).[a]

To calculate the PN prescription, the following steps are suggested:
1. *Determine grams of protein (as amino acids) and calculate calories provided as protein:*

$$100 \text{ g protein} \times 4 \text{ kcal/g} = 400 \text{ protein kcal}$$

2. *Determine calories left to be provided as dextrose and IVFE:*

$$1,600 \text{ kcal desired} - 400 \text{ protein kcal} = 1,200 \text{ kcal}$$

3. *Determine amount of calories to be provided as fat (usually about 30% or less of nonprotein calories):*

$$1,200 \text{ kcal} \times 0.30 = 360 \text{ kcal/d}$$

$$360 \text{ kcal/d} \div 9 \text{ kcal/g} = 40 \text{ g lipids}$$

4. *Determine calories left to be provided as dextrose:*

$$1,600 \text{ kcal desired} - (400 \text{ protein kcal} + 360 \text{ fat kcal}) = 840 \text{ dextrose kcal}$$

$$840 \text{ dextrose kcal} \div 3.4 \text{ kcal/g} = 247 \text{ or } {\sim}250 \text{ g dextrose}$$

The final PN prescription would include:
- 100 g amino acids
- 40 g lipids
- 250 g dextrose

Abbreviations: IVFE, intravenous fat emulsion; PN, parenteral nutrition.
[a]Refer to Chapter 4 for information on estimating energy and protein requirements in critically ill patients.

BOX 20.4 Potential Mechanical, Metabolic, and Gastrointestinal Complications of Parenteral Nutrition

Mechanical
- Pneumothorax
- Hemothorax
- Subclavian artery injury or thrombosis
- Catheter occlusion

Continues

BOX 20.4   Potential Mechanical, Metabolic, and Gastrointestinal Complications of Parenteral Nutrition *(Continued)*

Metabolic
- Hyperglycemia[a]
- Hypoglycemia[b]
- Electrolyte and fluid disorders related to shifts in electrolytes and fluid that may occur from movement between intracellular and extracellular spaces
- Hypertriglyceridemia[c]
- Acid-base disorders
- Refeeding syndrome[d]

Gastrointestinal
- Hepatic steatosis
- Cholestasis

---

[a]May be related to severe stress, trauma, corticosteroid therapy, overfeeding, or diabetes.
[b]Related to the administration of insulin.
[c]May be due to overfeeding or intravenous fat emulsion (IVFE) administration.
[d]The metabolic and physiologic consequences of depletion, repletion, compartmental shifts, and interrelationships of phosphorus, potassium, magnesium, glucose metabolism, vitamin deficiency, and fluid resuscitation—a serious complication resulting from overzealous nutritional resuscitation of the severely malnourished patient, which can result in sudden decompensation and death.

Conclusion

Parenteral nutrition can be a useful and life-sustaining therapy when a patient's GI tract is dysfunctional. Nutrition assessment and nutrition monitoring and evaluation of the patient on PN are essential to ensure safe and efficacious use of PN therapy. Registered dietitians are an integral part of the nutrition care for patients on PN therapy.

References

1. Parenteral nutrition. In: Academy of Nutrition and Dietetics Nutrition Care Manual. 2013. www.nutritioncaremanual.org. Accessed November 15, 2013.
2. Academy of Nutrition and Dietetics. Critical Illness 2012 Evidence-Based Nutrition Practice Guideline. www.andevidencelibrary.com. Accessed November 15, 2013.
3. Critical Care Nutrition. Canadian Clinical Practice Guidelines. 2013. www.criticalcarenutrition.com/index.php. Accessed November 15, 2013.
4. McClave SA, Martindale RG, Vanek VW, et al. Guidelines for the provision and assessment of nutrition support therapy in the adult critically ill patient: Society of Critical Care Medicine (SCCM) and American Society for Parenteral and Enteral Nutrition (A.S.P.E.N.). *JPEN J Parenter Enteral Nutr.* 2009;33:277–316.
5. Mirtallo J, Canada T, Johnson D, et al. Safe practices for parenteral nutrition. *JPEN J Parenter Enteral Nutr.* 2004;28(suppl):S39–S70.
6. Boullata JI, Gibert K, Sacks G, et al. A.S.P.E.N. Clinical Guidelines: Parenteral Nutrition Ordering, Order Review, Compounding, Labeling, and Dispensing. *JPEN J Parenter Enteral Nutr.* Feb 14, 2014. epub ahead

of publication. http://pen.sagepub.com/content/early/2014/02/13/0148607114521833. Accessed February 26, 2014.

7. Cresci G, Martindale R. Nutrition support in trauma. In: Gottsclich MM, ed. *The Science and Practice of Nutrition Support: A Case-Based Core Curriculum.* Dubuque, IA: Kendall/Hunt Publishing; 2000:445–460.

8. Rosmarin D, Wardlaw G, Mirtallo J. Hyperglycemia associated with high, continuous infusion rates of total parenteral nutrition. *Nutr Clin Pract.* 1996;11:151–156.

9. American Society for Parenteral and Enteral Nutrition (A.S.P.E.N.) Board of Directors and the Clinical Guidelines Task Force. Guidelines for the use of parenteral and enteral nutrition in adult and pediatric patients. *JPEN J Parenter Enteral Nutr.* 2002;26(1 Suppl):1SA–138SA.

10. Jeejeebhoy K. Zinc: an essential trace element for parenteral nutrition. *Gastroenterology.* 2009;137(suppl):S7–S12.

11. Charney P, Malone AM. *ADA Pocket Guide to Parenteral Nutrition.* Chicago, IL: American Dietetic Association; 2007.

CHAPTER 21

Pediatric Enteral and Parenteral Nutrition

Jenifer L. Thompson, MS, RD, LDN, CSP,
and Tiffani Lynn Hays, MS, RD, LDN

Many pediatric patients with gastrointestinal (GI) disease require nutrition support in the form of enteral or parenteral nutrition. This chapter focuses on the use of such interventions in pediatrics and the unique challenges of nutrition support for children. See Chapter 19 for more information on enteral nutrition (EN) and Chapter 20 for more information on parenteral nutrition (PN).

Pediatric Enteral Nutrition

Enteral nutrition is the delivery, via oral administration or feeding tube, of liquid nutrition to the GI tract. Compared with PN, EN is a more physiologic approach to delivery of nutrition support—one that more effectively preserves GI tract integrity and functioning and incurs lower medical costs. If the gut is functioning, it should be used in the digestive process. For these reasons, when treating pediatric patients, EN is the preferred delivery method of nutrition support.

For patients who cannot meet their nutrient needs via oral intake (eg, where there is a clinical condition that requires increased energy, an anatomic interference with ability to consume orally, or an altered metabolism and/or absorption function that necessitates specialized delivery of nutrients), clinical nutrition delivery via feeding tube is indicated (1,2). EN may also be beneficial in pediatric patients who show signs of malnutrition, including poor weight gain and decreased linear growth. Box 21.1 (page 268) lists indications and contraindications for EN in the pediatric population.

Routes of Enteral Nutrition Delivery

There are several routes of administration for EN via a feeding tube: nasogastric (NG), oral-gastric (OG), gastrostomy (GT), nasoduodenal (ND), nasojejunal (NJ), or jejunostomy tube (JT). Feedings can be continuous, intermittent (bolus), or a combination of the two (2,3). See Chapter 19 for additional information on feeding routes and their advantages and disadvantages.

BOX 21.1   Indications and Contraindications for Enteral Nutrition in Children

Indications
- Unable to meet ≥80% of estimated energy needs by mouth
- Prematurity
- Burns, trauma, sepsis
- Cystic fibrosis
- Bronchopulmonary dysplasia
- Cleft palate
- Congenital heart disease
- Facial trauma
- Esophageal atresia or tracheo-esophageal fistula
- Cerebral palsy
- Short bowel syndrome
- Chronic diarrhea
- Inflammatory bowel disease
- Anorexia nervosa

Potential contraindications
- Compromised gut perfusion (eg, necrotizing enterolcolitis)
- Gastrointestinal obstruction
- Intestinal atresia
- Severe inflammatory bowel disease
- Acute pancreatitis

Initiation and Advancement of Enteral Nutrition in Children

Patient age, clinical condition, and route of feeding delivery affect EN initiation and advancement. Simultaneous increases in feeding rate and formula concentration are not recommended. See Table 21.1 for suggested feeding initiation and advancements (2,4).

Formula Selection

Human Milk vs Infant Formula

The World Health Organization and the American Academy of Pediatrics (AAP) recommend that human milk be the sole nutrition source for the first 6 months of an infant's life and that it continue to be used throughout the following 6 months as solid foods are introduced (5). Advantages to feeding human milk include the following:

- Strengthened infection resistance
- Enhanced mother-infant bonding
- Decreased risks of overfeeding
- Improved GI tract maturation
- Reduced costs related to feeding

Infants solely fed human milk will need a vitamin D supplement. Of note, human milk contains lactose and is therefore not recommended for patients with galactosemia.

Although human milk consumption yields numerous benefits, it is not a viable option for all infants. Appropriate formulas must be available for those cases. Formula manufacturers have put in much effort to develop products that offer the same nutritional and immunological qualities available in human milk.

TABLE 21.1 Advancement of Enteral Nutrition in Children

Age of Patient	Initiation Rates and Volumes	Advancement Rates
Continuous feeding		
Preterm infant	0.5–1 mL/kg/h	10–25 mL/kg/d
Full-term neonate (0–12 mo)	1–2 mL/kg/h	0.5–1 mL/kg/h Increase every 4–24 h
Age 1–6 y	1–2 mL/kg/h	0.5–1 mL/kg/h Increase every 4–12 h
Age 7–13 y	1–2 mL/kg/h	1 mL/kg/h Increase every 4–12 h
Intermittent feeding (bolus)		
Preterm infant	2–4 mL/kg/feed	2–4 mL/feed
Full-term neonate (0–12 mo)	10–15 mL/kg every 2–4 h	10–30 mL/feed
Age 1–6 y	5–10 mL/kg every 3–4 h	30–45 mL/feed
Age 7–13 y	90–120 mL every 3–4 h	60–90 mL/feed

Source: Data are from references 2 and 4.

However, the goal is not merely to manufacture a facsimile of the contents of human milk; rather, formula is intended as a product rich in nutrients that acts in infant development the same way that human milk does. Compared with formula, human milk yields a higher bioavailability of many nutrients; therefore, formulas are manufactured with a higher nutrient concentration to supply comparable nourishment to growing infants.

Regulation of Infant Formula

Optimal growth and development requirements for infants from birth to 1 year of age serve as the basis for quality control and nutrient level standards in infant formula. In the United States, the quality control standards for all infant formulas are dictated by the Infant Formula Act, which was enacted in 1980 and amended in 1986, and the nutrient level standards are set by the US Food and Drug Administration (4).

Preparation of Infant Formulas

Infant formulas are manufactured in ready-to-feed, concentrate, and powder forms. To resemble the approximate energy content provided in human breastmilk, standard dilution and preparation of formula (see Table 21.2 on page 270) will yield 20 kcal/oz (0.67 kcal/mL). If a higher concentration is clinically indicated (eg, in infants with elevated metabolic needs or strict restrictions related to fluid intake), it is acceptable to add less water to formula. However, because increased formula concentration results in increased renal solute load and osmolality, a concentration that exceeds 27 kcal/oz is generally not recommended unless modular fat, modular carbohydrate, or both are added (1).

Types of Formulas

COW'S MILK–BASED FORMULAS
With casein and whey from nonfat cow's milk serving as the protein source, standard cow's milk–based formulas are constituted to meet the nutritional needs of healthy full-term infants from birth to 1 year of

TABLE 21.2 Standard Formula Preparation[a]

	Ready-to-Feed	*Concentrate*	*Powder*
20 kcal/oz	No preparation needed	1:1 dilution (1 oz concentrate + 1 oz water)	1 scoop[b] powder + 2 oz water

[a]Most infant formulas.
[b]Use only the scoop that was included in the formula container.

age. Additionally, because they are fortified with iron, standard cow's milk–based formulas can prevent iron-deficiency anemia from developing in newborns. Carbohydrate and fat in cow's milk–based infant formulas are provided through lactose and vegetable oil, respectively. Because of the added lactose, this type of formula is not used for infants with galactosemia.

Cow's milk–based formulas include organic and lactose-free products. For a formula to be certi-fied and labeled as organic, its ingredients must meet regulations established by the US Department of Agriculture; specifically, production processes must have been free of pesticides, antibiotics, and growth hormones.

It is not possible to guarantee that cow's milk–based formulas—even the lactose-free types—are 100% free of all lactose. For this reason, infants with galactosemia should not be fed lactose-free formula. Infants with lactose intolerance may consume lactose-free formula; however, diagnosis of congenital lac-tase deficiency in infants is extremely rare. Secondary lactose deficiency may occur on a temporary basis, typically a result of an acute gastrointestinal illness.

SOY-BASED FORMULAS

Manufacturers developed formulas from soy protein as an alternative for infants diagnosed with intoler-ance or allergy to cow's milk and as an option for infants whose caregivers preferred a vegetarian formula in the baby's diet. Soy protein is of lower biological value compared with casein, but soybeans nevthe-less yield a high-quality protein. To improve the biological value and enhance the amino acid profile of soy-based formulas, manufacturers supplement these formulas with L-methionine and taurine.

It should be noted that the allergenicity of soy protein is comparable to that of cow's milk protein, and there is a high incidence (10% to 42%) of concomitant allergy to both proteins (6–8).

The phytic acid present in soy protein isolate decreases the bioavailability of phosphate, zinc, and iron. Therefore, these minerals are supplemented in soy formulas (9).

Premature infants fed soy protein formulas demonstrated decreased bone mineralization and poor weight gain when compared with premature infants fed cow's milk–based formula. Thus, soy protein formulas are contraindicated in premature infants, and the AAP issued a policy statement that states, "Soy protein–based formulas are not designed or recommended for premature infants who weigh less than 1,800 grams" (10).

Sucrose, corn syrup solids, and/or maltodextrin provide the carbohydrate in soy-based infant formu-las. Because soy-based formulas contain no lactose, they are recommended for infants with galactosemia.

PROTEIN-MODIFIED FORMULAS

Altered protein formulas, structured as partially and extensively hydrolyzed casein and/or whey, and free amino acid–based (elemental) formulas have been developed (see Table 21.3).

Several extensively hydrolyzed formulas, with slight variations in their nutrient make–up, are avail-able. Some have a mixture of medium-chain triglycerides (MCT) and long-chain triglycerides (LCT) as the fat source, and some have just LCT. Some formulas provide carbohydrate via sucrose and corn syrup

TABLE 21.3 Protein-Modified Formulas

Formula Type	Protein Size	Hypoallergenic?	Indication	Price	Includes MCTs?
Partially hydrolyzed	Peptides	No	Potential allergy prevention	$	No
Extensively hydrolyzed	Di- and tripeptides, amino acids	Yes	Cow's milk protein allergy	$$	Varies
Free amino acid (elemental)	Free amino acids	Yes	Severe allergy, severe malabsorption	$$$	Varies

solids. All extensively hydrolyzed formulas are lactose-free and considered hypoallergenic and appropriate for infants with cow's milk–protein allergy.

Partially hydrolyzed formulas are, by definition, hydrolyzed to a lesser extent than extensively hydrolyzed formulas. They are not hypoallergenic and are not indicated for the treatment of cow's milk–protein allergy. There is some evidence that they may play a role in allergy prevention.

Free amino acid–based formulas are indicated for severe allergies or severe malabsorption. Due to the amino acids, these formulas are quite expensive and have a higher osmolarity than other formulas.

FOLLOW-UP FORMULAS

For infants transitioning to solid foods—typically from age 9 to 10 months through 24 to 36 months—follow-up formulas, also called *toddler formulas* or *next-step formulas*, are recommended. These formulas, which offer slightly higher protein and mineral contents than standard infant formula, are available in both cow's milk and soy formulations.

There is no real advantage to replacing standard infant formula with follow-up formula, even though such compositions are nutritionally complete (9,11). After 1 year of age, it is appropriate to feed cow's milk to an infant.

SPECIALIZED INFANT FORMULAS

Many specialized formulas have been developed for use in patients with certain medical conditions and disease states. For example:

- Increased levels of protein, calcium, and phosphate are added to formulas for premature infants to optimize bone mineralization.
- Infants with rare lipid metabolism disorders, lymphatic transport disorders, and chylothorax may be fed reduced-fat or modified-fat formulas; however, when these formulas are administered, patients require careful monitoring to ensure they are meeting essential fatty acid requirements.
- Patients with specific inborn errors of metabolism may be given formulas that are available in formulations with each offending amino acid(s) appropriately manipulated. Blenderized formulas (homemade formulas using a mixture of formula and foods) can also be used when monitored closely for micro- and macronutrient completeness.

PEDIATRIC FORMULAS

Pediatric patients who require EN support after the first year of life can be given formulas—available in cow's milk, soy protein, partially hydrolyzed protein, and free amino acid formulations—that are specifically designed for older children. Pediatric formulas are typically designed to meet the Dietary Reference

Intakes (DRIs) for children 1 to 10 years of age in volumes of 1,000 mL/d to 1,100 mL/d. The standard energy concentration of pediatric formulas is 30 kcal/oz (1 kcal/mL); the typical protein load is 30 g/L.

It is acceptable to administer adult formulas to meet the nutritional needs of older children (at least 10 years of age) and adolescents who require EN support. Careful monitoring of nutrient levels to ensure all DRIs are met is essential, particularly in cases where the patient's energy needs are decreased and a lower total formula volume is administered.

Recent Innovations in Infant Formulas

Research is ongoing, and new developments continually improve the ability of infant formulas to mimic both the nutrient content and the function of human milk in infant development. All additives in infant formula have been deemed safe; however, studies of the long-term clinical benefits of additives in infant formulas continue and their inclusion in formulas vary by company and product composition (see Table 21.4) (12–15).

Pediatric Parenteral Nutrition

PN is the intravenous administration of nutrients. Central PN (CPN) is PN delivered into a large-diameter vein, usually the superior vena cava, whereas peripheral PN (PPN) is PN delivered into a peripheral vein, usually in the hand or forearm.

PN should not be considered unless EN is not a viable option for nutrition support or EN has failed. As is the case when treating adult patients, deliberation regarding whether to use PN in pediatric patients must take into account the inherent risk of nosocomial infections while giving equal consideration to the gravity of the development and consequences of malnutrition. Because neonates and young children have limited fat and protein stores and additional energy needs for growth, earlier administration of PN (possibly as an adjunct to EN) is worth considering on an individual basis.

Age, disease state, and current nutritional status inform the decision as to when it is appropriate to begin PN administration in pediatric patients (see Table 21.5). Box 21.2 lists indications and contraindications for PN in pediatric patients (16–25).

Cycling PN, or delivering the solution in less than 24 hours, may be considered for long-term PN patients and/or home PN patients to allow for time off the infusion. Cycling PN should be considered only if the patient has stable fluid and electrolyte balance. Blood glucose levels should initially be monitored to ensure tolerance. See Chapter 22 for additional information on PN in the home setting.

TABLE 21.4 Formula Additives

Additive	Amount Added	Potential Benefits
DHA and ARA	Variable; amount similar to human milk	Role in cognitive and visual function; increased benefit seen with preterm infants (12)
Nucleotides	Variable; amount similar to human milk	DNA and RNA synthesis
Prebiotics	Variable	Increased concentration of bifidobacteria (13)
Probiotics	Variable	Adequate growth, Improvement in infectious diarrhea (14,15)

Abbreviations: DHA, docosahexaenoic acid; ARA, arachidonic acid.
Source: Data are from references 12–15.

TABLE 21.5 Timeline for Initiating Parenteral Nutrition in Pediatric Patients

Patient Age and Nutritional Status	Estimated Time Patient Will Be NPO
Neonate	3 days
Neonate, malnourished or very low birth weight	Consider PN immediately
Well-nourished child, age 2–10 y	3–5 days
Well-nourished child, age >10 y	≥7 days
Malnourished child (any age)	3–5 days

Abbreviations: NPO, nil per os (nothing by mouth); PN, parenteral nutrition.

BOX 21.2   Indications and Contraindications for Parenteral Nutrition in Children

Potential indications
- Gastrointestinal obstruction
- Severe gut injury—this may include (but is not limited to) atresias, gastroschisis, ileus, intestinal perforation, mucositis, necrotizing enterocolitis , omphalocele, and short bowel syndrome (16–21)
- Severe prematurity/low birth weight (22,23)
- Potentially compromised gut perfusion, hemodynamic instability/use of vasopressors (24), and extracorporeal membrane oxygenation
- Severe acute pancreatitis
- Severe inflammatory bowel disease

Contraindications
- Anticipated need for nutrition support ≤3 days
- Lack of vascular access
- Fungal line infection
- End-of-life care (because PN is an aggressive therapy, it may not be an ethical course of treatment)
- Potential contraindication: intravenous fat emulsion (IVFE) in patients with egg allergy (requires administration of test dose of IVFE) (25)

Source: Data are from references 16–25.

Risks and Complications of PN in Children

Acute risks and complications of PN in children mimic those seen in adults (see Chapter 20); however, PN–associated cholestasis, a potentially life-threatening complication of long-term PN administration, is more common in children. Because of the risks associated with PN, it is essential that practitioners continually monitor these patients' vital signs, electrolytes, and liver function tests for the duration of PN administration (see Monitoring Pediatric Patients Receiving Parenteral Nutrition section later in this chapter).

Selecting the PN Solution

When selecting the appropriate PN solution, vascular access is the first route that should be considered. In most children, adequate PN delivery requires central access; if the need for PN support is projected to be longer than 7 days, central access should be attempted. To avoid infiltration, the osmolality of peripheral solutions should not exceed 900 mOsm/kg (26). Fluid allowance, other infusions, estimated nutrient needs, electrolyte requirements, and advancement of nutrients according to patient tolerance are other factors that must be taken into account when determining which PN solution to use (see Table 21.6) (27).

FLUID

To determine the volume allotted for PN, subtract the volume of all other necessary infusions from the patient's total fluid allowance. Concentrating other infusions administered to the patient may be needed to maximize PN volume.

ENERGY

The goal energy level is set by using indirect calorimetry or appropriate equations that take into account the patient's age and growth (such as the DRI or World Health Organization equations). Estimated energy requirements for patients on PN are often 5% to 10% lower than estimates for those on EN because patients on PN do not expend energy on digestion and absorption.

PROTEIN

Determination of the protein goal for individual patients receiving PN is based on the DRI for protein, which is determined by age, growth, activity, and injury factors and adjusted for known or suspected protein losses. Prevention of lean body mass loss and promotion of healing and growth in the pediatric patient is the ultimate goal of protein delivery. While monitoring for azotemia, it is recommended to start the patient at 1.5 to 3 g protein per kg of body weight per day and then increase it by 0.5 to 1 g/kg/d as tolerated until the protein goal is reached (see Table 21.6) (27).

For patients younger than 1 year who are receiving PN, the clinician should administer specialized pediatric amino acid solutions, as they provide amino acids that are conditionally essential in infants and have a lower pH, which allows for increased calcium and phosphorus concentrations.

FAT

Essential fatty acid deficiency can develop in children within 1 to 3 weeks. Therefore, supplementing fat during PN support is essential. To provide sufficient essential fatty acids, between 2% and 4% of the total energy should come from LCT delivered as 0.5 to 1 g fat per kg of body weight per day (27). As an additional source of adequate energy, fat generally provides 30% to 40% of total energy.

In children, fat is often delivered as an intravenous fat emulsion (IVFE), separate from delivery of dextrose and protein. Separation of these nutrients enhances PN solution stability and compatibility. While monitoring the patient for hypertriglyceridemia, the clinician should initiate IVFE administration at 1 g/kg/d and advance by 1 g/kg/d as tolerated until the goal for fat intake is reached (see Table 21.6) (27).

CARBOHYDRATE

To maintain euglycemia in neonates and to meet all pediatric patients' energy needs, carbohydrate delivery is required. When initiating carbohydrate delivery, the level should match or be slightly higher than the dextrose concentration of the current intravenous fluids. This concentration is increased in neonates by 1 to 2 mg/kg/min each day and in children by 2% to 5% dextrose per day, as tolerated, until the goal for energy intake is reached. Patients should be monitored for hyperglycemia (see Table 21.6) (27).

A glucose infusion rate (GIR) of 5 to 18 mg/kg/min is typically the maximum that pediatric patients can tolerate (27). Insulin may be needed to maintain blood glucose at or less than 150 mg/dL while meeting the energy goal.

TABLE 21.6 General Recommendations for Advancement of Parenteral Nutrients in Children

Nutrient	Premature Infants	Children
Dextrose	Begin 5% dextrose. Advance 1–2 mg/kg/min/d when glucose is within desired range.	Begin 10% dextrose. Advance 5% per day.
Amino acids	Begin 1.5–3 g/kg/d. Increase by 1 g/kg/d to goal of 3–4 g/kg/d.	Begin 1–2 g/kg/d. Increase by 1 g/kg/d to goal of 1.5–3 g/kg/d.
Fat	Begin 1 g/kg/d. Increase by 0.5–1 g/kg/d to goal of 3 g/kg/d.	Begin 1–2 g/kg/d. Increase by 0.5–1 g/kg/d to goal of 2–3 g/kg/d.

Source: Data are from references 30, 31, 34, 39, 40, and 42–46.

VITAMINS

All patients on PN should receive daily parenteral multivitamins provided in doses based on the patient's weight. Dependent on the patient's age, a pediatric-designated multivitamin solution may be recommended. When severe renal or hepatic dysfunction or excessive losses are present, or if the patient is on long-term PN, modifications to vitamin administration may be considered (28).

TRACE ELEMENTS

Parenteral trace elements should be delivered daily to all pediatric patients receiving PN. The solution should be a pediatric-designated one, because pediatric solutions may differ from adult trace element solutions. Modifications to trace element administration may be considered when a patient has severe renal or hepatic dysfunction or excessive losses or is on long-term PN, (28). Iron infusions should be considered for patients on long-term exclusive PN who are unable to receive enteral iron.

ELECTROLYTES

Daily monitoring of electrolytes and any necessary related PN adjustments should continue as needed until electrolyte levels are stable. Once the electrolyte levels are stable, they should be monitored weekly.

MEDICATIONS

Some medications are incompatible with PN solutions, IVFE solutions, or both, but some common medications (eg, ranitidine and insulin) may be added to the PN solution during compounding. Pharmacy departments should be able to provide information about solution-medication compatibility. Once a medication is added to the PN solution, it is necessary to make sure that all previous orders for that medication are discontinued.

Monitoring Pediatric Patients Receiving Parenteral Nutrition

When managing a patient receiving PN, it is essential to monitor blood chemistries and metabolic panels. Before initiating PN, baseline measurements of magnesium, phosphorus, and triglyceride levels should be documented and a basic metabolic panel obtained. Then these measurements should be obtained daily throughout the process of advancing PN to the patient's goal. The clinician should also perform weekly monitoring of the hepatic panel and bilirubin level. Once the patient is stable at the goal PN, laboratory testing may be performed at a reduced frequency, with comprehensive metabolic panel and triglyceride levels tested weekly. Once PN support has been administered for 3 months, the clinician should evaluate vitamin and trace mineral laboratory values and then re-evaluate those values every 3 to 12 months while PN continues. For patients receiving long-term PN at home, this same timetable for monitoring vitamins and trace elements should be used, although, depending on a patient's clinical status, it is acceptable to schedule routine metabolic monitoring once every 1 to 3 months. Additional laboratory testing of these values is indicated when changes to the solution are made or when clinical symptoms of nutrient-related problems become evident (27).

In hospitalized pediatric patients receiving PN, progress toward goals established during the Nutrition Care Process should be evaluated at least weekly. Growth trends; input/output data; clinical signs or symptoms of PN intolerance, fluid status, or nutrient excess or deficiency; and any changes in GI function are clinical measurements to assess and monitor. Laboratory results and any recommended changes to the nutrition support plan based on those values should be documented (28,29).

Special Considerations for Parenteral Nutrition in Pediatric Patients

PARENTERAL NUTRITION–ASSOCIATED CHOLESTASIS (PNAC)

PNAC is a condition of impaired bile secretion. The first sign of PNAC is an increased level of bilirubin (conjugated bilirubin concentration > 2 mg/dL) after PN has been administered for at least 2 weeks, potentially followed by elevated levels of aminotransferase. Pediatric patients receiving PN are more likely than adult patients to have PNAC. Liver failure often results from continued PN (30). Lack of enteral feedings (31), sepsis (32,33), length of bowel (34,35), and prematurity and low birth weight (36) are other clinical factors that have been associated with PNAC. The following factors specific to PN administration are associated with development of PNAC: total energy (in particular, overfeeding) (37), amino acid dose (38,39), taurine deficiency (40), aluminum toxicity (41), IVFE dose and source (34,42–46), and continuous vs cyclic infusion (47,48). See Box 21.3 for recommendations to help minimize PNAC.

DIALYSIS

PN considerations for pediatric patients on dialysis depend on the route of dialysis (see Table 21.7) (27).

BOX 21.3   Recommendations to Help Minimize Parenteral Nutrition–Associated Cholestasis (PNAC) When Parenteral Nutrition Is Anticipated to Be ≥3 Months

- Initiate trophic enteral feeds as soon as possible and advance enteral feedings as often as patient tolerates (able to maintain fluid and electrolyte balance).
- Advance dextrose as tolerated to goal energy, while avoiding overfeeding.
- Limit intake of protein intake to 2.5–3 g/kg/d in infants, or the minimum needed to maintain protein status.
- Use appropriate amino acid solutions for infants <1 y of age.
- If PN is anticipated to be long term (>3months), limit fat to 1 g/kg/d and consider providing an omega-3 fatty acid source (if available).
- Once patient is clinically stable and growing well, consider cycling parenteral nutrition.

TABLE 21.7 Parenteral Nutrition Modifications for Pediatric Patients on Dialysis

PN Component	Predialysis	Hemodialysis	Peritoneal Dialysis
Fluids	Match urine output	Ultrafiltration+ urine output + insensible losses	Fluid restriction normally not needed
Energy	DRI + catch-up growth	Based on clinical status	Account for energy absorbed from dialysate (~7–10 kcal/kg/d)
Protein	DRI	DRI + 0.2g/kg/d	DRI + 0.4g/kg/d
Electrolytes	Restrict in PN according to blood chemistries	Discuss with renal team before adjusting in PN	Discuss with renal team before adjusting in PN

Abbreviations: DRI, Dietary Reference Intake; PN, parenteral nutrition.
Source: Data are from reference 27.

FLUID RESTRICTION

Fluid restriction often severely limits nutrient delivery in pediatric patients. To concentrate nutrients for PN administration, central venous access is required and nutrient levels must be increased proportionately as tolerated by the patient. Typically, central PN solutions can provide at least 1 kcal/mL. Clinicians can consider concentrating other intravenous fluids and medications to provide energy in all available fluids.

HYPERAMMONEMIA

Hyperammonemia may occur in liver failure and metabolic diseases. To decrease the total aromatic amino acids crossing the blood-brain barrier, specialized amino acid solutions with elevated levels of branched-chain amino acids can be administered. Patients with metabolic diseases may require customized amino acid solutions.

HYPERGLYCEMIA

Risk of hyperglycemia is increased in pediatric patients on PN support who are under stress or receiving steroid treatment. Gradually increasing the GIR minimizes the effects of hyperglycemia. If hyperglycemia persists, it is appropriate to administer insulin as a means to maintain PN while controlling blood glucose levels. However, with tight glucose control, the risk of hypoglycemia increases. Therefore, caution should be used if administering insulin (49). Clinical guidelines issued in 2009 by the American Society for Parenteral and Enteral Nutrition state that "aggressive glycemic control cannot be recommended as yet in the critically ill child" (50), but recent studies have investigated hyperglycemia protocols for the pediatric intensive care unit (51,52).

HYPERTRIGLYCERIDEMIA

Hypertriglyceridemia, which is common in patients under stress, is caused by IVFE intolerance. Monitoring triglyceride levels as IVFE is gradually increased will help prevent hypertriglyceridemia (see Table 21.8 on page 278).

OSTEOPENIA

Neonates who receive long-term PN support commonly have osteopenia. Specialized infant amino acid solutions have been developed to allow for increased calcium and phosphorus delivery. To determine the best approach to maximize the delivery of phosphorus and calcium via the parenteral solution for

TABLE 21.8   Intravenous Fat Emulsion Modifications Based on Triglyceride Levels

TG level, mg/dL	Modification to IVFE
>400	Discontinue IVFE and recheck TG.
	Restart IVFE at 0.5–1 g/kg/d once TG <250 mg/dL.
	Need ~1 g/kg 3 times each week, or 0.5 g/kg/d, to avoid EFAD.
250–400	Decrease by 1 g/kg/d and recheck.
<250	Advance by 1 g/kg/d to goal.

Abbreviations: IVFE, intravenous fat emulsion; TG, triglyceride; EFAD, essential fatty acid deficiency.

an individual patient, consult with the pharmacy department. Vitamin D status should be monitored and vitamin D supplemented as needed.

REFEEDING SYNDROME

There is a risk of refeeding syndrome when specialized nutrition support is initiated in acutely or severely malnourished pediatric patients. Potentially fatal hypophosphatemia, hypokalemia, and hypomagnesemia result from providing substrate and creating adenosine triphosphate (ATP) drive anions in the cells.

Gradual, slow advancement of the level of energy in the PN—with an initial goal of 50% to 60% of estimated energy requirements—helps reduce electrolyte disturbance. As the energy levels in PN are advanced, phosphorus, potassium, and magnesium levels must be monitored (2). If levels are low, discontinue caloric advancement until the electrolytes are promptly repleted and their levels are rechecked and confirmed to be restored. Once electrolytes are stable for several days, it is appropriate to restore advancement of energy levels to the estimated energy requirement.

TRANSITIONING TO ENTERAL FEEDS

To support growth and development in pediatric patients and neonates on long-term PN, it is necessary to maintain adequate provision of parenteral nutrient during the transition to enteral feedings. Decreases in the parenteral provision of energy, protein, or fluid should only occur in conjunction with increases in enteral nutrients. Providing micronutrients during the transition to enteral feedings is also worth considering, since the patient's needs for some or all nutrients may increase due to malabsorption. To maintain electrolyte stability and patient growth, patients with severe malabsorption transitioning to enteral feedings may require 1.5 to 3 times the nutrient levels they were receiving via PN.

Conclusion

When human milk is not available for infant feeding, clinicians should carefully deliberate which formula to choose, taking into account factors such as the infant's age, clinical condition, and possible food allergies or intolerances. For patients older than 12 months, there are pediatric formulas that meet the nutrient needs of older children and younger adolescents. Attempts to make improvements to the quality of formula—especially in mimicking the function of human milk on development—have been ongoing among manufacturers.

For pediatric patients who cannot meet their nutritional needs orally, as evidenced by poor weight gain, decreased linear growth, or other signs of malnutrition, EN is indicated. Inadequate intake may be due to disease state resulting in elevated energy needs, anatomic anomalies that interfere with adequate oral consumption, or the need to be fed a specialized nutrition therapy best delivered via a tube.

The pediatric patient population requires a different approach to EN initiation and advancement compared with adults receiving EN support. The age and weight of the child are major considerations in initiation and advancement decisions. Simultaneous increases in the feeding rate and concentration are not recommended.

When EN is not a viable treatment option or has failed in a pediatric patient, PN should be considered early. Indications for PN in most pediatric patients (with the exception of neonates) are similar to those in adult patients. Delivery of adequate PN in children usually requires central access. Goals for nutrient levels, which are often substantially higher for pediatric patients than the estimated needs of adult patients, are based on the patient's weight. Solutions that specifically meet pediatric protein needs deliver conditionally essential amino acids for infants and increase the solubility of calcium and phosphorus. To improve the PN solution's stability and compatibility, fat is often provided to the patient separately from protein, carbohydrate, and electrolytes. Pediatric patients have an elevated risk of developing PNAC; to minimize this risk, those who are writing the PN prescription must frequently monitor levels of bilirubin in patients receiving long-term PN.

References

1. Green-Corkins K, Sentongo T. Infant formulas and complementary feeding. In: Corkins MR, ed. *The A.S.P.E.N. Pediatric Nutrition Support Core Curriculum*. Silver Spring, MD: American Society for Parenteral and Enteral Nutrition; 2010:129–142.
2. Courtney E, Grunko A, McCarthy T. Enteral nutrition. In: Hendricks KM, Duggan C, eds. *Manual of Pediatric Nutrition*. Hamilton, ON: BC Decker; 2005:252–316.
3. American Dietetic Association. Enteral nutrition: feeding methodology. Pediatric Nutrition Care Manual. 2010. www.nutritioncaremanual.org/content.cfm?ncm_content_id=90957. Accessed September 11, 2010.
4. Nevin-Folino N, Miller M. Enteral nutrition. In: Samour PQ, Helm KK, Lang CE, eds. *Handbook of Pediatric Nutrition*. Sudbury, MA: Jones and Bartlett Publishers, Inc; 2004:513–549.
5. American Academy of Pediatrics. Breastfeeding and the use of human milk. *Pediatrics*. 2005;115:496–506.
6. Zeiger RS, Sampson HA. Soy allergy in infants and children with IgE-associated cow's milk allergy. *J Pediatr*. 1999;134:614–622.
7. Klemola T, Vanto T, Juntunen-Backmanm K. Allergy to soy formula and to extensively hydrolyzed whey formula in infants with cow's milk allergy: a prospective, randomized study with a follow-up to the age of 2 years. *J Pediatr*. 2002;140:219–224.
8. Sicherer SH, Eigenmann PA, Sampson HA. Clinical features of food protein-induced enterocolitis syndrome. *J Pediatr*. 1998;133:175–176.
9. Chang T, Kleinman R. Standard and specialized enteral formulas. In Walker WA, Watkins JB, Duggan C, eds. *Nutrition in Pediatrics*. Hamilton, ON: BC Decker; 2003:935–944.
10. Committee on Nutrition, American Academy of Pediatrics. Soy protein-based formulas: recommendations for use in infant feeding. *Pediatrics*. 1998;101:148–153.
11. American Dietetic Association. Normal nutrition: types of infant formulas. Pediatric Nutrition Care Manual. 2010. www.nutritioncaremanual.org/content.cfm?ncm_content_id=91959. Accessed September 11, 2010.
12. American Dietetic Association. Position of the American Dietetic Association and Dietitians of Canada: Dietary Fatty Acids. *J Am Diet Assoc*. 2007;107:1599–1611.
13. Rao S, Srinivasjois R, Patole S. Prebiotic supplementation in full-term neonates: a systemic review of randomized controlled trials. *Arch Pediatr Adolesc Med*. 2009;163:755–764.
14. Saavedra JM, Abi-Hanna A, Moore N, Yolken RH. Long-term consumption of infant formulas containing live probiotic bacteria: tolerance and safety. *Am J Clin Nutr*. 2004;79:261–267.
15. Guandalini S. Probiotics for children with diarrhea: an update. *J Clin Gastroenterol*. 2008;42(suppl):S53–S57.

16. Axelrod D, Kazmerski K, Iyer K. Pediatric enteral nutrition. *JPEN J Parenter Enteral Nutr.* 2006;30(1 suppl):S21–S26.

17. Samour PQ, King K. *Handbook of Pediatric Nutrition.* 3rd ed. Lake Dallas, TX: Helm Publishing; 2005.

18. Watkins JB, Walker W, Duggan C. *Nutrition in Pediatrics: Basic Science and Clinical Applications.* 3rd ed. Hamilton, ON: BC Decker; 2003.

19. Abad-Sinden A, Sutphen J. Nutrition management of pediatric short bowel syndrome. *Pract Gastroenterol.* 2003;12:28–48.

20. Serrano M, Schmidt-Sommerfeld E. Nutrition support of infants with short bowel syndrome. *Nutrition.* 2002;18:966–970.

21. Okada A. Clinical indications of parenteral and enteral nutrition support in pediatric patients. *Nutrition.* 1998;14(1):116–118.

22. Puntis JW. Nutritional support in the premature newborn. *Postgrad Med J.* 2006;82:192–198.

23. Groh-Wargo S, Thompson M, Cox J, eds. *Nutritional Care for High-Risk Newborns, Revised.* 3rd ed. Chicago, IL: Precept Press; 2000.

24. Pettignano R, Heard M, Hart M, Davis R. Total enteral nutrition versus total parenteral nutrition during pediatric extracorporeal membrane oxygenation. *Crit Care Med.* 1998;26(2):358–363.

25. Intralipid 20%, A 20% I.V. Fat Emulsion [package insert]. Clayton, NC: Kabi Pharmacia; 1991.

26. American Academy of Pediatrics, Committee on Nutrition. Commentary on parenteral nutrition. *Pediatrics.* 1983;71(4):547–552.

27. Corkins M, ed. *The A.S.P.E.N. Pediatric Nutrition Support Core Curriculum.* Silver Spring, MD: American Society for Parenteral and Enteral Nutrition; 2010.

28. American Society for Parenteral and Enteral Nutrition Board of Directors and Task Force on Standards for Specialized Nutrition Support for Hospitalized Pediatric Patients. Standards for specialized nutrition support: hospitalized pediatric patients. *Nutr Clin Pract.* 2005;20:103–116.

29. A.S.P.E.N. Board of Directors and the Clinical Guidelines Task Force. Guidelines for the use of parenteral and enteral nutrition in adult and pediatric patients. *JPEN J Parenter Enteral Nutr.* 2002;26(1 Suppl):1SA–138SA.

30. Kumpf VJ. Parenteral nutrition-associated liver disease in adult and pediatric patients. *Nutr Clin Pract.* 2006;21:279–290.

31. Kelly DA. Liver complications of pediatric parenteral nutrition: epidemiology. *Nutrition.* 1998;14:153–157.

32. Wolf A, Pohlandt F. Bacterial infection: the main cause of acute cholestasis in newborn infants receiving short-term parenteral nutrition. *J Pediatr Gastroenterol Nutr.* 1989;8:297–303.

33. Chung C, Buchman AL. Postoperative jaundice and total parenteral nutrition-associated hepatic dysfunction. *Clin Liver Dis.* 2002;6:1067–1084.

34. Cavicchi M, Beau P, Crenn P, Degott C, Messing B. Prevalence of liver disease and contributing factors in patients receiving home parenteral nutrition for permanent intestinal failure. *Ann Intern Med.* 2000;132:525–532.

35. Teitelbaum DH, Drongowski R, Spivak D. Rapid development of hyperbilirubinemia in infants with the short bowel syndrome as a correlated to mortality: possible indication for early small bowel transplantation. *Transplant Proc.* 1996;28:2699–2700.

36. Beale EF, Nelson RM, Bucciarelli RL, Donnelly WH, Eitzman DV. Intrahepatic cholestasis associated with parenteral nutrition in premature infants. *Pediatrics.* 1979;64:342–347.

37. Quigley EMM, Marsh MN, Shaffer JL, Markin RS. Hepatobiliary complications of total parenteral nutrition. *Gastroenterology.* 1993;104:286–301.

38. Vileisis RA, Inwood RJ, Hunt CE. Prospective controlled study of parenteral nutrition-associated cholestatic jaundice: effect of protein intake. *J Pediatr.* 1980;96:893–897.

39. Sankaran K, Berscheid B, Verma V, Zakhary G, Tan L. An evaluation of total parenteral nutrition using Vamin and Aminosyn as protein base in critically ill preterm infants. *JPEN J Parenter Enteral Nutr.* 1985;9:439–442.

40. Spencer AU, Yu S, Tracy TF, et al. Parenteral nutrition-associated cholestasis in neonates: multivariate analysis of the potential protective effect of taurine. *JPEN J Parenter Enteral Nutr.* 2005;29:337–344.

41. Klein GL, Berquist WE, Ament ME, et al. Hepatic aluminum accumulation in children on total parenteral nutrition. *J Pediatr Gastroenterol Nutr.* 1984;3:740–743.

42. Chung PH, Wong KK, Wong RM, et al. Clinical experience in managing pediatric patients with ultra-short bowel syndrome using omega-3 fatty acids. *Eur J Pediatr Surg.* 2010;20:139–142.

43. de Meijer VE, Gura KM, Le HD, Meisel JA, Puder M. Fish oil-based lipid emulsions prevent and reverse parenteral nutrition-associated liver disease: the Boston experience. *JPEN J Parenter Enteral Nutr.* 2009;33:541–547.

44. Diamond IR, Steresca A, Pencharz PB, Kim JH, Wales PN. Changing the paradigm: Omegaven for the treatment of liver failure in pediatric short bowel syndrome. *J Pediatr Gastroenterol Nutr.* 2009;48:209–215.

45. Gura KM, Lee S, Valim C, et al. Safety and efficacy of a fish-oil based fat emulsion in the treatment of parenteral nutrition-associated liver disease. *Pediatrics.* 2008;121:e678–e686.

46. Lee S, Valim C, Johnston P, Le HD, et al. Impact of fish-oil based lipid emulsion on serum triglyceride, bilirubin, and albumin levels in children with parenteral nutrition-associated liver disease. *Pediatr Res.* 2009;66(6):698–703.

47. Blaiche IF, Khalidi N. Parenteral nutrition-associated liver complications in children. *Pharmacotherapy.* 2002;22:188–211.

48. Hwang TL, Lue MC, Chen LL. Early use of cyclic TPN prevents further deterioration of liver functions for the TPN patients with impaired liver function. *Hepatogastroenterology.* 2000;47:1347–1350.

49. Srinivasan V, Spinella PC, Drott HR, et al. Association of timing, duration, and intensity of hyperglycemia with intensive care unit mortality in critically ill children. *Pediatr Crit Care Med.* 2004;5(4):329–336.

50. Mehta NM, Compher C, A.S.P.E.N. Board of Directors. A.S.P.E.N. clinical guidelines: nutrition support of the critically ill child. *JPEN J Parenter Enteral Nutr.* 2009;33:260–276.

51. Vlasselaers D, Milants I, Desmet L, et al. Intensive insulin therapy for patients in paediatric intensive care: a prospective, randomized controlled study. *Lancet.* 2009;373:547–556.

52. Agus MSD, Hirshberg EL. Pediatrics: intensive insulin therapy in critically ill children. *Nature Rev Endocrinol.* 2009;5(7):360–362.

CHAPTER 22

Home Parenteral and Enteral Nutrition

Therese L. Austin, MS, RD, LD, CNSC, and
Karen M. Sexton-Hamilton, MS, RD, LD, CNSC

Home parenteral and enteral nutrition support (HPEN) is appropriate for patients who no longer require acute care but still require nutrition support due to their underlying gastrointestinal (GI) dysfunction (1). The goals of HPEN are to promote nutritional rehabilitation, avoid therapy-related complications associated with specialized nutrition support, and minimize therapy dependence as tolerated and improve patient quality of life. Refer to Chapters 19, 20, and 21 for additional information about nutrition support.

Hospital Discharge Considerations

Selecting a Home Care Provider

When transitioning a patient from hospital or rehabilitation to home with HPEN therapy, it is important to recognize that both the patient management and therapy goals for home nutrition support are substantially different from those in the acute-care setting (see Table 22.1). To facilitate a smooth discharge, the patient and hospital personnel should evaluate objective qualitative and quantitative data and select a provider that has experience with similar patients, achieves positive outcomes, and otherwise meets the needs of the specific individual (see Table 22.2). Once selected, the home care provider then assists with the evaluation of the patient and his or her particular situation to determine whether the patient is an appropriate candidate for HPEN (see Box 22.1 on page 284) (2).

TABLE 22.1 Care Management Differences in Acute and Home Care

	Acute Care	Home Care
Individual referenced as	Patient	Consumer
Management type	Crisis/stabilize	Long-term/quality-of-life
Therapy goals	Nutrition maintenance by best-tolerated route	Nutrition repletion and transition to most physiologic therapy with GI adaptation or primary disease resolves
Potential complications	• Catheter or tube: infectious and mechanical • Metabolic • GI intolerance	• Catheter or tube: infectious and mechanical • Metabolic • Long-term parenteral nutrition issues: metabolic bone disease, liver dysfunction, and micronutrient abnormalities • Noncompliance • Coping
Therapy provision	Dependent and managed by clinicians	Independent and managed by consumer and caregiver with periodic oversight by clinicians
Reimbursement	Generally covered as part of the bed day rate	Variable coverage depending upon the plan and insurer
Provider	Hospital at which the patient is admitted	Choice of a variety of local, regional, and national home-infusion providers
Environment	Tightly controlled and managed by clinicians	Must meet basic safety and compliance criteria with periodic clinician monitoring

TABLE 22.2 Selection of a Home Parenteral and Enteral Nutrition Provider

Consideration	Types of Data to Evaluate
Patient population	• Patient demographics (eg, patient age, gender, primary and secondary diagnoses, average length of therapy, and concurrent therapies) • History with the ordering physician and insurance provider
Clinical outcomes	• Rehospitalization rate • Rates of catheter complications (catheter sepsis, exit-site infection, thrombus, occlusion, and mechanical issues) • Patient satisfaction with care and services • Reasons for discharge • Complications associated with therapy provision
Provider profile	• Size and geographic coverage • Years in operation • Accreditation status
Provider availability and services	• 24-hour availability • Ability to troubleshoot pump or therapy complications • Proximity to patient • Ability to accommodate patient work or travel schedule • Knowledge to reinforce patient teaching • Patient monitoring and nursing care
Reimbursement/payment issues	• Private insurance contracts • Reimbursement by public payers (eg, Medicare) • Indigent care policy

---

BOX 22.1 Criteria for Selecting Home Nutrition Support Patients

- Hemodynamic and clinical stability
- Long-term intravenous or enteral access established
- Capable and willing care partner
- Consumer consent to home therapy
- Safe and adequate home environment: refrigeration, electricity, clean water supply, access to a telephone, storage space, clean work space for therapy preparation, safety issues identified and resolved
- Adequate insurance coverage for prescribed therapy

Source: Data are from reference 2.

Selecting the HPEN Device

Before discharge, the physician and other members of the nutrition support team must select the appropriate access device for the patient who requires HPEN.

- For patients who require home enteral nutrition (HEN), device selection criteria include the intended length of therapy and the patient's current GI anatomy. Common HEN devices include percutaneous endoscopic gastrostomy (PEG), percutaneous endoscopic jejunostomy (PEJ), and gastrojejunostomy (G-J) tubes. Jejunostomy or Mic key button are often used for pediatric patients.
- For patients who require home parenteral nutrition (HPN), device selection criteria include the intended length of therapy, other intravenous needs, vascular history, caregiver availability, patient preference, and formula osmolarity. Common HPN devices include Hickman, peripherally inserted central catheter (PICC), or ports. Broviac catheters are generally reserved for pediatric patients.

Predischarge and Postdischarge HPEN Education

Education prior to discharge home builds patient independence and promotes the provision of safe and effective therapy. During predischarge education, valuable information about safety, therapy administration, and supply management is imparted to the patient; questions from the patient are answered; any misconceptions are corrected; and, ideally, all of the consumer's fears about HPEN are alleviated. Topics to cover in predischarge education include the following (3):

- Rationale for HPEN prescription
- Anticipated length of therapy
- Pumps, equipment, and procedures
- The catheter and its care
- Aseptic (sterile) techniques necessary for safe therapy administration
- Nutritional formulations and additives and their storage and preparation
- Precautions to prevent and treat complications (self-monitoring)
- Development of an emergency plan

The consumer's and caregivers' learning needs, capabilities, and readiness to learn should be assessed before education begins, and the teaching techniques and materials should then be tailored to the particular consumer or caregiver. A combination of written, verbal, and demonstration techniques can be used in patient education. The patient should be taught with the equipment and supplies that will be used in the home setting (3).

Patient and caregiver education should continue once the patient is discharged, with the goal that the patient or care partner will be able demonstrate how to safely and effectively administer feeding and medications, care for the access device, and, if applicable, use a pump.

Discharge Orders

Prior to discharge, physician orders for the HPEN therapy are received and reviewed by the home care clinicians to ensure the orders are appropriate for the individual patient's needs and make therapy administration as easy as possible (see Box 22.2). At this time, the insurance coverage for the prescribed therapy should be verified.

BOX 22.2   Discharge Order Information for Home Parenteral and Enteral Nutrition (HPEN)

Information for all HPEN patients
- Basic physician information (name, contact information, etc)
- Patient name, age, gender, and other relevant demographic/general health data
- Medication profile
- Allergy history
- HPEN therapy prescription
- Reason for therapy, including ICD-10 code(s)
- Insurance policy information
- Monitoring parameters, including laboratory orders and frequency

Information specific to the home enteral nutrition (HEN) prescription
- Product name
- Number of cans/day or dosage
- Rate and duration
- Days per week
- Method of administration (bolus, intermittent, continuous)
- Tube type, French size, and placement
- Pump choice
- Flushing regimen

Information specific to the home parenteral nutrition (HPN) prescription
- Catheter type, number of lumens, and flushing protocol
- Macronutrient content
- Specialty amino acid product specifications as needed
- Volume and infusion schedule
- Electrolyte content
- Additives (multivitamin, trace element, insulin, H_2-blocker, heparin, etc)

Formula Selection

ENTERAL FORMULAS

Factors to consider when choosing an enteral formula for the patient at home include the following (4):

- Current GI anatomy and digestive capability
- Nutrient requirements
- Fluid requirements
- Any disease-specific considerations such as specific nutrient(s) malabsorbed and GI motility

The nutrition support team should also evaluate the patient's schedule at home (work, family care, and medical treatment schedule) in order to develop a prescription that promotes both patient compliance and quality of life.

PARENTERAL FORMULAS

Most home care providers have the ability to customize an HPN formula to the patient's unique needs, including the following:

- His or her energy and nutrient requirements (eg, is formula intended to replete nutrient stores or promote weight loss?)
- Individual tolerances (monitor closely)
- Compatibility and stability guidelines related to the weekly compounding regimen
- Cycling of HPN (which can allow for activities of daily living and reduce stress)
- Increased losses
- HPN as a supplement to oral or enteral nutrition

Reimbursement

Before the patient is discharged, registered dietitians (RDs) based in hospitals and rehabilitation facilities should work with the discharge case manager and the selected home care provider to ensure reimbursement of HPEN. The home care provider may also be able to assist in guiding the discharge team to the required documentation to obtain insurance authorization.

MEDICARE COVERAGE

Medicare covers HPEN under Part B of the Prosthetic Device Benefit. Only specific medical conditions qualify for Medicare coverage of HPEN. The most common conditions that qualify for Medicare coverage of HEN include oral, esophageal, gastric, or proximal small bowel obstruction; severe dysphagia; Crohn's disease or pancreatitis where intact nutrients are malabsorbed; and failure to thrive (in children). The most common conditions that qualify for Medicare coverage of HPN include malabsorption due to functional, anatomical, or mechanical small bowel issues; postsurgical or disease-related requirement for bowel rest; and small bowel obstruction.

Regardless of the underlying initial diagnosis, most patients who require HPEN have a dysfunction of their GI tract. Medicare acknowledges this and requires specific objective documentation to prove medical necessity (see Box 22.3). Medicare will *not* bear the cost of coverage in the following circumstances (5):

- HPEN as a supplement to another route of nutrition support
- HPEN required because of refusal to take adequate nutrition (psychological or anorexia due to medication)
- HPEN therapy required for <90 days

BOX 22.3   Medicare Part B Criteria for Coverage of Home Parenteral and Enteral Nutrition

Home enteral nutrition (HEN)
- **Permanence**: Determined by the attending physician and substantiated in the medical record that the condition is of long and indefinite duration (at least 3 months).
- **Functional capacity**: The condition is either anatomic or due to a motility disorder. Need objective evidence of GI dysfunction.
- **Pumps**: Must be medically justified (ie, jejunostomy tube or malabsorption diagnosis).
- **Specific nutrients**: Elemental or disease-specific formulas must be medically justified.

Home parenteral nutrition (HPN)
- **Permanence**: Same as for HEN.
- **Malabsorption of nutrients**: A condition involving the small intestine and or its exocrine glands that impairs absorption, or a motility disorder that impairs the ability of nutrients to be transported through the GI tract.
  - Criteria A: Patient has undergone recent massive small bowel resection within the last 3 months and has ≤5 feet of bowel beyond the ligament of Treitz.
  - Criteria B: Short bowel syndrome is severe enough that the patient has net GI fluid and electrolyte malabsorption exceeding 50% of oral/enteral intake (2.5–3 L/d) and urine output <1 L/d.
  - Criteria C: The patient requires bowel rest for at least 3 months and is receiving intravenously 20–35 kcal/kg/d for treatment of symptomatic pancreatitis with/without pancreatic pseudocyst, severe exacerbation of regional enteritis, or a proximal enterocutaneous fistula where tube feeding distal to the fistula is not possible.
  - Criteria D: Patient has complete mechanical small bowel obstruction and surgery is not an option.
  - Criteria E: Patient is significantly malnourished (>10% weight loss in 3 months and albumin ≤3.4 g/dL) and has severe fat malabsorption evidenced by a 72-hour fecal fat test consisting of >50% fecal fat output on a standard 50-g fat diet.
  - Criteria F: The patient is significantly malnourished (>10% weight loss in 3 months and albumin is ≤3.4 g/dL) and has a severe motility disturbance of the small intestine, and/or stomach that is unresponsive to prokinetic medication and is demonstrated by motility studies.
  - Criteria G and H: G = The patient is malnourished (10% weight loss over 3 months and serum albumin <3.4 g/dL), and H = The patient has a disease/clinical condition that has been documented as present and has not responded to altering the manner of delivery of appropriate nutrients.
- Additional documentation may be required to support the care when required to support the medical necessity of (a) energy intake <20 or >35 kcal/kg/d; (b) protein intake <0.8 or >1.5 g/kg/d; (c) dextrose concentration <10%; (d) lipids >1,500 g/mo (>50g/d) 10% or 20%; (e) TPN infusion <7 days per week; (f) a need for special nutrients.

Source: Data are from reference 5.

MEDICAID COVERAGE

Medicaid coverage for HPEN varies from state to state. Refer to the state policy for details.

PRIVATE PAYERS AND HOME PARENTERAL NUTRITION

Most commercial insurers will pay for HPN with documentation of medical necessity and a physician's prescription. Some commercial insurers require a member to use Medicare criteria for coverage to demonstrate the medical necessity of HPN. In some cases, prior authorization of HPN services is required; however, it is not a guarantee of payment.

PRIVATE PAYERS AND HOME ENTERAL NUTRITION

Commercial insurance coverage for HEN is variable. HEN coverage may be covered under the pharmacy benefit, as is HPN, or it may be covered under the Durable Medical Equipment (DME) benefit. Under some plans, only HEN supplies and equipment may be covered, leaving the patient to pay out of pocket for formula.

Home Initiation of HPEN

For a subset of patients, initiation of HPEN can occur in the home, which allows the patients to avoid hospitalization. Although the American Society for Parenteral and Enteral Nutrition (A.S.P.E.N.) Standards for Specialized Nutrition Support: Home Care Patients, Safe Practices for Parenteral Nutrition, and A.S.P.E.N. Guidelines for the Use of Parenteral and Enteral Nutrition in Adult and Pediatric Patients do not contain specific information about the initiation of HPEN, it has been successfully initiated in the home since the early 1990s (1,3,6). Considerations for safe home initiation of HPEN include the following:

- The patient was recently examined by the prescribing physician.
- The patient is clinically stable (eg, no congestive heart failure, renal failure, or substance abuse).
- Access device is established and appropriate for formula.
- Baseline laboratory values (ie, comprehensive metabolic panel, complete blood count, phosphorus, and magnesium) indicate metabolic stability.
- The home environment and care partner are suitable.
- The patient consents to therapy.

Appropriate candidates for HEN initiation are those who have a feeding tube placed in an endoscopy suite or other outpatient setting and are not severely debilitated by malnutrition or disease. Appropriate candidates for initiation of HPN include the following:

- Patients who have failed enteral feedings
- Those who have GI diseases without excessive GI losses
- Those with an oncology diagnosis and inability to tube feed

HPEN initiation in the home is contraindicated for infants and very young children as well as patients of all ages with severe kidney or liver disease, uncontrolled diabetes, or uncorrectable fluid and electrolyte abnormalities

Refeeding Syndrome

Refeeding syndrome is a concern related to the initiation of HPEN, but it can be prevented when patients are properly evaluated and managed before HPEN begins. Management includes rehydration with fluid and electrolytes before the initiation of HPEN as needed to normalize blood chemistry. HPN initiation should start with a moderate-volume, low-carbohydrate solution compounded with optimal potassium, phosphorus, and magnesium content (7,8). Starting HEN at a volume of 50% of estimated needs may be indicated to prevent the negative sequelae of refeeding syndrome. For both HPN and HEN, gradual advancement of the formula over 7 to 10 days to goal is ideal.

Continuation of Care

Ultimately, the goal of HPEN is to promote nutritional rehabilitation and quality of life through the prevention of therapy-related complications (Table 22.3) and reduction of HPEN dependency. To achieve these goals, ongoing nutrition assessment and monitoring are required (see Box 22.4 on page 292 for parameters to monitor), and patient education must be provided periodically.

Ongoing Nutrition Assessment and Monitoring of HPN Patients

The RD can provide initial and periodic follow-up nutrition assessments of HPN consumers via phone, outpatient clinic visit, or home visit. Assessment parameters in home care are similar to assessment in the acute care setting. However, there are a few unique considerations, including the patient's increased physical activity, bowel adaptation, and potential for complications related to long-term therapy (such as liver and metabolic bone disease and micronutrient deficiency and toxicity). The RD's assessment should also evaluate the patient's need to complete essential activities of daily living, such as the following:

- Increased physical activity (indoors and outdoors)
- Care for self and other family members
- Traveling for medical reasons or pleasure
- Managing household chores and home maintenance
- Required medical treatments/procedures for underlying disease
- Self-care activities, including ostomy care, wound care, and administration of multiple oral or IV medications

Follow-up assessments should be scheduled as needed based on patient acuity, plan of care goals, frequency of laboratory testing (Table 22.4), and the patient's response to therapy (see Box 22.4). Formula and supply needs should be reviewed regularly to determine patient compliance to the therapy prescription and need for additional education.

TABLE 22.3 Complications of Home Parenteral and Enteral Nutrition

Complication	Symptoms	Intervention
Mechanical—enteral nutrition (EN)		
Damage	Visible break or crack in feeding tube	Clamp the tube between the damaged area and the stoma.
	Leaking from the feeding tube	Check and reinforce all connections.
	Burning or discomfort at stoma site	Avoid tension on feeding tube. Never use force to irrigate.

Continues

TABLE 22.3   Complications of Home Parenteral and Enteral Nutrition *(Continued)*

Complication	*Symptoms*	*Intervention*
Mechanical—enteral nutrition (EN) *(continued)*		
Occlusion	Inability to infuse formula	Check flow control clamps. Check feeding tube for kinks.
	Inability to irrigate feeding tube	Flush feeding tube with warm water as prescribed and before and after medications.
	Pump alarming occlusions	Check pump for malfunction. Secure the administration set to prevent kinks and accidental disconnection.
Tube dislodgement	Complaints of coughing, gagging, dyspnea, cyanosis	Assess feeding tube placement prior to each feeding.
	Complaints of bloating, pain, or fullness	Elevate head of bed at least 30 degrees to avoid coughing and vomiting, which can dislodge tube.
	Leakage of formula around feeding tube	Secure feeding tube to prevent pulling or tension.
Aspiration	Paroxysmal coughing, fever, chills, dyspnea, wheezing	Seek medical attention at a medical facility.
Mechanical—parenteral nutrition (PN)		
Clotting or blockage of catheter	Resistance or inability to infuse PN Unable to flush the catheter	Check that clamps are open. Assess need to declot catheter with tissue plasminogen activator.
Air embolism	Coughing, shortness of breath, chest pain	Clamp catheter immediately. Lie on left side. Seek medical attention.
Thrombosis	Swelling of arm, shoulder, neck, or face accompanied by eye tearing or runny nose	Hold PN infusion. Seek immediate medical attention.
Catheter dislodgement	Pain or discomfort in neck or chest especially when infusing	Hold PN infusion. Confirm catheter tip placement by X-ray.
Catheter breakage	Blood or fluids leaking from catheter	Clamp catheter between the patient and breakage. Pursue catheter repair or replacement.
Infectious—EN		
Local infection	Redness, swelling, tenderness at stoma site	Increase frequency of feeding tube changes. Obtain order for topical antibiotic treatment. Adhere to good hand-washing skills.
Feeding tube–related systemic sepsis	Fever, chills, malaise, diaphoresis	Seek medical attention at medical facility.
Infectious—PN		
Exit-site infection	Redness, swelling, tenderness, drainage at exit site	Contact managing physician for antibiotic treatment for catheter salvage.
Tunnel infection	Redness, swelling, tenderness along the catheter track	Catheter removal and replacement and IV antibiotics.
Intravenous catheter segment infection	Fever, chills, malaise, diaphoresis	Stop PN infusion. Seek medical attention at medical facility.

Continues

TABLE 22.3 Complications of Home Parenteral and Enteral Nutrition *(Continued)*

Complication	Symptoms	Intervention
Metabolic—EN		
Diarrhea	Frequent, loose, watery stools	Gradually increase feedings to goal rate. Use fiber-containing formula. Use antidiarrheals as appropriate.
Constipation	Infrequent or hard stools, bloating, distension	Adequate water flushes, use fiber-containing formula. Use stool softeners/laxatives as appropriate.
Vomiting and abdominal distension	Increased gastric residual, bloating, abdominal pain	Decrease flow rate or discontinue feeding. Reinitiate gradually. Administer antiemetics as appropriate.
Refeeding syndrome	Hypophosphatemia, hypokalemia, hypomagnesemia, shortness of breath, muscle spasms, pulmonary congestion	Initiate feeding gradually. Monitor serum electrolytes closely and replete as necessary. Gradually increase feedings to goal fluid requirement.
Metabolic—PN		
Hypoglycemia	Symptomatic low blood glucose	Increase to 2-h taper down at end of cycle. Decrease insulin. Closely monitor blood glucose levels.
Hyperglycemia	Blood glucose >140 mg/dL	Reduce dextrose rate or reduce dextrose concentration. Ensure accurate fluid volume delivery. Rule out infection. Administer insulin.
Electrolyte abnormalities	Sodium, potassium, chloride, phosphorus, magnesium elevation above or reduction below laboratory reference range, with or without clinical symptomology	Identify and treat the underlying cause for increase or decrease of the electrolyte(s). Monitor intake and output. Replete or withhold individual electrolyte(s) as indicated.
Dehydration	Intravascular reduction of fluid volume causing clinical symptoms of thirst, weight loss, and dry mucous membranes	Monitor intake and output. Assess and treat underlying cause. Replete fluids as indicated.
Fluid retention	Intravascular or third spacing of fluids as evidenced by weight gain or edema	Monitor intake and output. Assess and treat underlying cause. Withhold or reduce fluids as indicated.
Liver dysfunction	Elevated liver function test (LFT) values or total bilirubin, jaundice, hepatomegaly	Avoid overfeeding total calories. Keep lipid <1 g/kg. Initiate enteral feedings if possible.
Essential fatty acid deficiency	Dermatitis, alopecia	Provide a minimum of 8%–10% of calories as lipid to prevent deficiency.
Micronutrient deficiency/toxicity	Changes in skin, hair, or nails; altered taste; poor wound healing; anemia	Periodic monitoring of micronutrient levels and dose in PN based on results. Assess for physical signs and symptoms.
Refeeding syndrome	Hypophosphatemia, hypokalemia, hypomagnesemia, shortness of breath, muscle spasms, pulmonary congestion	Initiate feeding gradually, monitor serum electrolytes closely and replete as necessary. Gradually increase to goal fluid requirement.

BOX 22.4   Ongoing Monitoring Parameters for Home Parenteral and Enteral Nutrition Patients

- Current weight and progress toward goal weight
- Vital signs/history of fever
- Hydration status
- Gastrointestinal, metabolic, or mechanical complications
- Equipment and supply issues
- Completion of pediatric growth charts
- Patient compliance
- Medication changes
- Tube and stoma site assessment or vascular access device assessment (redness, drainage, or tube patency)
- Insurance changes
- Quality-of-life measure—functional performance status

TABLE 22.4   Laboratory Monitoring of Home Parenteral Nutrition Patients

Tests	Monitoring Frequency
Electrolytes, blood glucose, and renal function: sodium, potassium, chloride, bicarbonate, glucose, BUN, creatinine, calcium, phosphorus, magnesium	Weekly until stable, then monthly for 3 months, then every other month if stable
CBC	Baseline; monthly for 3 months, then every other month
Triglycerides	Baseline; monthly for 3 months, then every other month if stable
Liver function: AST, ALT, ALP, total bilirubin, PT, INR	Every 3–6 months
Albumin	Baseline; then every 3 months
Vitamins, minerals, trace elements	Every 6–12 months based on facility policy or if clinical evidence suggests deficit or toxicity
Iron studies	Baseline, at 3 months, and then every 6 months or if clinical evidence suggests deficit or toxicity

Abbreviations: BUN, blood urea nitrogen; CBC, complete blood count; AST, aspartate aminotransferase; ALT, alanine aminotransferase; ALP, alkaline phosphatase; PT, prothrombin time; INR, international normalized ratio.

Ongoing Nutrition Assessment and Monitoring of HEN Patients

HEN patients generally require less frequent monitoring than HPN patients. However, periodic follow-up should be completed to review the patient's response to therapy and evaluate whether nutrition goals are being met (see Box 22.4). The following are reasons why patients may require more frequent monitoring:

- Use of jejunostomy tube
- Use of a condition-specific formula
- Malabsorptive disease
- Risk for refeeding syndrome
- Significant malnutrition
- Evidence of a micronutrient deficiency
- Glucose intolerance
- A history of complications requiring a hospital admission

Ongoing Education and Patient Quality of Life

Ongoing patient/consumer education on disease process and therapy helps patients maintain a desired quality of life (9,10), particularly if they will require HPEN for years or for the rest of their life. The education and support needs for the chronic intestinal failure patient differ from those of short-term HPEN consumers. In addition to requiring education for the prevention of potential long-term HPEN therapy complications, long-term HPEN consumers face insurance coverage and coping issues that differ from those of the short-term consumer. See Box 22.5 for a variety of resources and support groups for long-term HPEN consumers.

BOX 22.5   Educational Resources for HPEN Consumers

- American Society for Parenteral and Enteral Nutrition (A.S.P.E.N.): www.nutritioncare.org
- Association of Gastrointestinal Motility Disorders (AGMD): www.agmd-gimotility.org
- Celiac Disease Foundation (CDF): www.celiac.org
- Coping Well: www.copingwell.com
- Crohn's & Colitis Foundation of America: www.ccfa.org
- Digestive Disease National Coalition (DDNC): www.ddnc.org
- International Foundation for Functional Gastrointestinal Disorders (IFFGD): www.iffgd.org
- Oley Foundation: www.oley.org
- Patient Advocate Foundation (PAF): www.patientadvocate.org
- Patients on Intravenous and Nasogastric Therapy: www.pinnt.co.uk
- Tef Vater Support Network: www.tefvater.org
- United Ostomy Associations of America (UOAA): www.uoaa.org

Transitioning Off Home Parenteral or Enteral Nutrition

Patients should be transitioned off HPEN when they are able to tolerate 60% of their new form of nutrition (11). The transition may involve switching from enteral or parenteral nutrition to oral nutrition or from PN to EN. Factors to consider when weaning a patient from nutrition support include the following (4,12):

- Current GI anatomy:
  - Remaining bowel length
  - Presence of residual disease in the remnant bowel
  - Ileocecal valve present
  - Colon incontinuity
- Is enteral intake at least 1 L/d greater than enteral output?
- Is urine output greater than 1,000 mL/d?

The potential for bowel adaptation and intestinal rehabilitation efforts should be assessed if the patient's dependence on EN or PN can eventually be minimized or discontinued. The integrity of the remaining bowel is important to consider as well as the part of the small bowel that is retained. Patients have better absorption with an intact ileum vs the jejunum (12). Evaluation of weight, intake, and output records and laboratory data, including electrolytes, blood urea nitrogen (BUN), and creatinine, are also necessary to ensure adequate hydration during the transition process (12,13).

Patients can be weaned from EN by gradually eliminating intermittent or bolus feedings or by decreasing the infusion period of a continuous feeding based on the patient's tolerance to oral intake. PN can be reduced by decreasing the volume or calorie content, or by reducing the number of infusions as appropriate given the patient's oral or enteral intake.

Patients should have continued follow-up for a period of time after discontinuation of HPEN to ensure tolerance to the new form of nutrition. Continued monitoring of intake and output and body weight should be conducted. Patients should also be evaluated for the need for oral vitamin and mineral supplementation.

Conclusion

HPEN provides nutrition support for patients whose GI dysfunction prevents sufficient intake of calories and nutrients from oral intake. For HPEN to succeed, clinicians must provide careful instruction to patients in the discharge/initiation stages; help consumers select an appropriate home care provider and obtain reimbursement; and follow-up periodically to assess patients' nutritional/health status, quality of life, and risk for complications. Patients should be transitioned off HPEN if possible. Those individuals who must remain on HPEN for the long term will require ongoing education and monitoring to ensure that their nutrition care plan remains adequate and appropriate.

References

1. A.S.P.E.N. guidelines for the use of parenteral and enteral nutrition in adult and pediatric patients. *JPEN J Parenter Enteral Nutr.* 2002;26(1 Suppl):1SA–138SA.
2. Fung S, Reyen L. Setting the stage for hospital discharge on parenteral nutrition. *Support Line.* 2007;29:8–12.
3. A.S.P.E.N. Board of Directors and the Clinical Guidelines Task Force. Standards of practice. Standards for specialized nutrition support: home care patients. *Nutr Clin Pract.* 2005;20:579–590.

4. Seidner DL, Ramasamy D. Enteral nutrition in intestinal failure. In: Matarese LE, Steiger E, Seidner DL, eds. *Intestinal Failure and Rehabilitation A Clinical Guide*. Boca Raton, FL: CRC Press; 2005:209–227.

5. Centers for Medicare & Medicaid Services. www.cms.hhs.gov. Accessed October 28, 2013.

6. A.S.P.E.N. Board of Directors and the Clinical Guidelines Task Force. Safe practices for parenteral nutrition. *JPEN J Parenter Enteral Nutr*. 2004;28(suppl):S39–S70.

7. Kraft M, Btaiche I, Sacks G. Review of the refeeding syndrome. *Nutr Clin Pract*. 2005;20:625–633.

8. Miller SJ. Pivotal Paper: Death resulting from overzealous total parenteral nutrition: the refeeding syndrome revisited. *Nutr Clin Pract*. 2008;23:166–171.

9. Smith C. Quality of life in long-term total parenteral nutrition patients and their family caregivers. *JPEN J Parenter Enteral Nutr*. 1993;17:501–506.

10. Winkler M. Quality of life in adult home parenteral nutrition patients. *JPEN J Parenter Enteral Nutr*. 2005;29:162–170.

11. A.S.P.E.N. Board of Directors and the Clinical Guidelines Task Force. Standards of practice. Nutrition support dietitians. *Nutr Clin Pract*. 2000;15:53–59.

12. Parekh N, Seidner D. Advances in enteral feeding of the intestinal failure patient. *Support Line*. 2006;28:18–24.

13. Rhoda K, Chhatriwalla E, Parekh N. Transitional feeding: challenges and approaches. *Support Line*. 2008;30:21–28.

CHAPTER 23

Drug-Nutrient Interactions with Gastrointestinal Drugs

Carol J. Rollins, MS, PharmD, RD, BCNSP, FASPEN

This chapter reviews several types of gastrointestinal (GI) drugs that can interact with nutrients and affect nutritional status. Each section provides a brief overview of the potential for drug-nutrient interactions and identifies examples of the type of drug. Most sections also offer more specific interaction notes and recommendations for particular medications.

Antacids

The rate and/or extent of drug absorption may be altered by antacids because of effects on GI transit time and binding or chelating of the drug. Nutrients, at least theoretically, may be influenced in the same way. Antacids increase gastric pH. This could affect nutrients requiring an acid environment for absorption, such as calcium and iron.

Examples

Drugs in this category include:

- Aluminum-containing antacids (carbonate, hydroxide, phosphate)
- Calcium-containing antacids (carbonate)
- Magnesium-containing antacids (carbonate, hydroxide, oxide, trisilicate)
- Magaldrate
- Sodium bicarbonate

Interaction Notes

ALUMINUM-CONTAINING ANTACIDS (CARBONATE, HYDROXIDE, PHOSPHATE)
Phosphate binding in the GI tract leads to increased bone loss and increased urinary calcium loss (1).

SODIUM BICARBONATE
Urinary potassium losses are increased through physiologic effects on the kidneys.

Recommendation

Administer antacids 1 to 2 hours apart from mineral supplements.

Adsorbents

Adsorbents are not selective for substances that can be removed by adsorption. Vitamins, minerals, amino acids, and other nutrients can be adsorbed from the GI tract.

Example

Drugs in this category include activated charcoal.

Recommendation

Reserve activated charcoal for use in acute poisonings. Activated charcoal, per US Food and Drug Administration (FDA) classification, lacks substantial evidence of efficacy for treatment of GI disorders, including flatulence and diarrhea, or as a digestive aid. The limited duration of use in the setting of acute poisoning is not expected to result in clinically relevant loss of nutrients.

Antidiarrheal Agents

The rate and/or extent of drug absorption may be altered by antidiarrheal agents because of effects on GI transit time. Nutrients, at least theoretically, may be influenced in the same way, although studies are lacking. Decreased GI tract motility and increased contact time of intestinal contents with the absorptive surface within the GI tract is likely to improve absorption of drugs and nutrients compared to the rapid GI transit associated with diarrhea, although it is difficult to predict the exact effect.

Losses of electrolytes, especially sodium, potassium, and magnesium, may be reduced with decreased stool volume. Effects on electrolytes are difficult to predict because electrolyte losses can vary depending on the etiology, volume, and consistency of diarrhea. Specific drug-nutrient interactions may also occur with particular antidiarrheal agents based on the pharmacology and metabolism of the agent.

Examples

Drugs in this category include:

- Diphenoxylate
- Loperamide
- Opium preparations: Paregoric (camphorated opium tincture) and opium tincture deodorized

Interaction Notes

St. John's wort or valerian used concurrently with loperamide may increase the risk of delirium, based on one case report of such an interaction (2).

Antiflatulents

Agents classified as antiflatulents work on gas bubbles within the GI lumen and are not absorbed from the GI tract. There is no evidence that drug or nutrient absorption is altered with concomitant use.

Example

Drugs in this category include simethicone.

Cathartics and Laxatives

All agents classified as cathartics or laxatives increase GI tract motility and reduce the time intestinal contents are in contact with the absorptive surface of the GI tract. Reduced absorption of drugs and nutrients may occur with rapid transit through the GI tract, although it is difficult to predict the exact effect.

Examples

Drugs in this category include:

- Bulk-forming laxatives: Malt soup extract, methylcellulose, and psyllium hydrophilic mucilloid
- Stimulant laxatives: Anthraquinone laxatives (senna preparations), bisacodyl, and castor oil
- Hyperosmotic laxatives: Glycerin and sorbitol
- Mineral oil
- Saline laxatives
- Stool softeners: Docusate salts

Interaction Notes

BULK-FORMING LAXATIVES

- The emollient gel or viscous solution produced by bulk-forming laxatives may trap drugs or nutrients that are in the GI lumen and reduce their absorption. For example, cellulose is known to bind certain drugs in the GI tract, reducing serum concentrations of the drugs.
- Chronic use of bulk-forming laxatives has been associated with reduced serum cholesterol concentrations, likely as the result of cholesterol and bile acids being trapped within the gel matrix produced when bulk-forming laxatives mix with water. Substances trapped within the gel matrix are removed in the feces rather than being absorbed.
- Other drugs or nutrients present in the GI tract could potentially be removed in the feces as well, although data for specific nutrient losses are lacking.

STIMULANT LAXATIVES

- Laxative dependence may occur with long-term use.
- Electrolyte abnormalities, including hyponatremia, hypokalemia and hypocalcemia, and malabsorption with protein-losing enteropathy may occur with chronic long-term use of these drugs.
- In addition, chronic use can result in "cathartic" colon from damage to enteric nerves and colectomy may be required, especially with the anthraquinone laxatives.

HYPEROSMOTIC LAXATIVES

- Laxatives in this category are generally administered rectally and, as such, act low in the GI tract where interference with nutrient absorption should be negligible.
- If administered orally, reduced absorption of drugs and nutrients may occur due to rapid GI transit.
- Infrequent use of hyperosmotic laxatives is unlikely to result in clinically relevant changes in drug or nutrient absorption.

MINERAL OIL

Absorption of fat-soluble nutrients (vitamins A, D, E, K, and beta-carotene) may be impaired with chronic use of mineral oil. Short-term, infrequent use of small doses is unlikely to have a clinically significant effect on fat-soluble vitamin status, although beta-carotene serum concentrations may be more readily decreased than other fat-soluble vitamins (3).

SALINE LAXATIVES

- Electrolytes used in these laxatives can be absorbed and may result in serious, potentially life-threatening electrolyte abnormalities with excessive doses and/or prolonged periods of use.
- Patient with poor renal function may be at increased risk of electrolyte abnormalities.
- Hypermagnesemia can occur with magnesium-containing saline laxatives because approximately 15% to 20% of an orally administered dose is absorbed.
- Hypertonic sodium phosphate laxatives can cause hyperphosphatemia with resultant hypocalcemia. The hypocalcemia results from precipitation of calcium-phosphate into soft tissue. Renal failure is a potential consequence of calcium-phosphate precipitation in the kidneys. Other systemic effects may also occur depending on the tissues where precipitation occurs.
- Absorption of rectally administered sodium phosphate is variable, with 1% to 20% potentially absorbed.

STOOL SOFTENERS

- Theoretically, absorption of many oral medications may be increased with concomitant use of an orally administered stool softener.
- Drugs with a narrow range between therapeutic efficacy and toxicity are of particular concern, and some clinicians suggest that these drugs should not be administered concurrently with a stool softener.
- Absorption of micronutrients provided as supplements may be enhanced, but data are lacking. Trace elements would be of most concern because they have a relatively narrow range between safety and toxicity.

Recommendations

BULK-FORMING LAXATIVES

Some practitioners recommend at least a 3-hour separation period between drugs known to be bound by these agents and the bulk-forming laxative itself. This same separation period would be reasonable for vitamin and mineral supplements to avoid the potential for trapping nutrients within the gel matrix, although there are no studies documenting loss of vitamins and minerals with bulk-forming laxatives.

STIMULANT LAXATIVES

- Use stimulant laxatives infrequently for self-care.
- Long-term use (eg, with chronic opiate use for pain management) should be under the supervision of a physician.
- Laxative use should be stopped or the dose/frequency reduced if loose stools are occurring. Appropriate use and dosage adjustment of stimulant laxatives should limit nutritional adverse consequences.
- With long-standing laxative abuse, evaluation for systemic effects of malabsorption, protein-losing enteropathy, and colonic dysfunction may be appropriate.
- Bisacodyl:
  - Tablets are enteric-coated; do not crush or chew.
  - Separate oral administration of bisacodyl by at least 1 hour from milk or antacid ingestion.

MINERAL OIL

- Administer mineral oil on an empty stomach.
- Use mineral oil without medical supervision for a maximum of 1 week.
- Check fat-soluble vitamin status with chronic use of mineral oil over several months.

SALINE LAXATIVES

- Limit use to a single dose with infrequent intervals when used for self-care.
- Monitor appropriate serum electrolytes when multiple doses or frequent use of a saline laxative are ordered by the health care provider.
- Consider other laxative agents when frequent use or multiple doses are necessary.

STOOL SOFTENERS

- Separating administration of stool softener and drugs with a narrow range between efficacy and toxicity by 2 to 3 hours is suggested by some clinicians. It would be reasonable to apply this same suggestion to trace element supplements (zinc, copper, manganese, chromium, and selenium) to avoid potentially enhanced absorption of the supplement and subsequent risk of toxicity when a stool softener is used routinely.
- Infrequent use of a stool softener would be unlikely to have a clinically significant effect. Clinical relevance of this potential drug-nutrient interaction is unclear because there are no studies that address the interaction.

Cholelitholytic Agents

Secretion of cholesterol by the liver and reabsorption of cholesterol from enterohepatic recycling are reduced by cholelitholytic agents. Over several weeks to months, the cholesterol content of bile and bile stones is reduced, and cholesterol gallstones are dissolved.

Example

Drugs in this category include ursodiol (ursodeoxycholic acid).

Recommendations

- Take ursodiol with food.
- Aluminum antacids should be taken at least 2 hours after ursodiol. Antacids containing calcium and magnesium do not seem to interact with ursodiol, and there are no reported drug-nutrient interactions.

Digestants

Agents classified as digestants provide pancreatic enzymes, primarily lipase with some amylase and protease, for the treatment of malabsorption resulting from pancreatic insufficiency. Enzyme replacement should improve absorption of fat-soluble vitamins when pancreatic insufficiency is the cause of malabsorption and when the dose of enzymes is adequate. See Chapter 12 for more information on pancreatic enzyme replacement therapy.

Examples

Drugs in this category include pancreatic enzymes: Creon, Pancreaze, and Zenpep.

Antiemetics

Significant nutrient depletion occurs when vomiting is frequent and prolonged because food intake and retention is inadequate to meet nutritional requirements. Antiemetic agents, when effective, allow food to be retained for digestion and absorption. In addition, effective antiemetic therapy reduces the fluid and electrolyte losses associated with vomiting.

Examples

Drugs in this category include:

- Antihistamines: Dimenhydrinate, meclizine, prochlorperazine, and trimethobenzamide
- 5-HT3 receptor antagonists: Dolasetron, granisetron, ondansetron, and palonosetron
- Antiemetics, miscellaneous: Aprepitant, diphenidol, phenothiazine, promethazine, and scopolamine

Interaction Notes

ANTIHISTAMINE—PROCHLORPERAZINE

- Coenzyme Q may be depleted by several drugs in the same class as prochlorperazine (phenothiazines), based on in vitro studies using animal hearts. No in vivo data in humans are available to confirm or refute the animal data (4).
- Riboflavin excretion in the urine may be increased by drugs in the same class as prochlorperazine, including chlorpromazine and some tricyclic antidepressant drugs (eg, amitriptyline, imipramine). There are structural similarities between the phenothiazine ring and riboflavin that may be responsible for the interaction (5,6).

5-HT3 RECEPTOR ANTAGONIST—DOLASETRON

- Drugs and dietary supplements inhibiting or inducing cytochrome P-450 (CYP) isoenzymes can change the clearance of dolasetron and potentially alter its efficacy. There are no specific drug-nutrient interactions reported; however, there is the potential for such interactions.
- Other 5-HT3 receptor antagonists are less likely than dolasetron to result in CYP-related interactions.

ANTIEMETICS, MISCELLANEOUS

- Aprepitant: Drugs and dietary supplements inhibiting or inducing isoenzyme CYP3A4 can change the clearance of aprepitant and potentially alter its efficacy. Aprepitant can potentially alter the clearance of other drugs and dietary supplements by inhibiting or inducing CYP3A4 and by increasing metabolism of CYP2C9 substrates. There are no specific drug-nutrient interactions reported based on altered CYP activity, but the potential exists for such interactions.
- Promethazine: Coenzyme Q may be depleted by several drugs in the same class as promethazine (phenothiazines), based on in vitro studies using animal hearts. No in vivo data in humans are available to confirm or refute the animal data (4). Riboflavin excretion in the urine may be increased by drugs in the same class as promethazine, including chlorpromazine and some tricyclic antidepressant drugs (eg, amitriptyline, imipramine). There are structural similarities between the phenothiazine ring and riboflavin that may be responsible for the interaction (5,6).
- Phenothiazine: Coenzyme Q interactions—*see* Promethazine. Riboflavin interactions—*see* Promethazine. Concurrent use of evening primrose oil requires caution because there may be a potential for increased risk of seizures; studies are small and data are conflicting regarding this risk (7,8).

Antiulcer Agents and Acid Suppressants

Drugs used to treat ulcers either suppress gastric acid production or reduce proteolytic enzyme (pepsin) production. Most antiulcer agents decrease gastric acid production.

Gastric acid plays an important role in the solubility of minerals, activation of proteolytic enzymes, and release of nutrients from foods, thereby making the nutrients available for absorption. Drugs causing suppression of gastric acid may result in poor release of nutrients from food (eg, vitamin B-12, iron) and an elevated pH in the upper GI tract.

Minerals such as calcium, magnesium, and iron are usually absorbed in the upper small bowel where there is an acid environment. Solubility of these minerals decreases as pH increases, resulting in reduced absorption. Although some studies have not supported a role for acidity contributing to dietary calcium absorption, acidity clearly affects iron absorption.

The more effective a drug is in suppressing gastric acid production and the longer the duration of use, the greater the risk of drug nutrient interactions resulting in clinically depressed nutrient levels.

Examples

Drugs in this category include:

- Histamine H_2 antagonists: Cimetidine, famotidine, nizatidine, and ranitidine
- Proton pump inhibitors (PPIs): Esomeprazole, lansoprazole, omeprazole, pantoprazole, rabeprazole
- Prostaglandins: Misoprostol
- Protectants: Sucralfate (aluminum sucrose sulfate)

Interaction Notes

HISTAMINE H_2 ANTAGONISTS

- Agents in this category suppress gastric acid production. Drug-drug and drug-nutrient interactions reported for one drug in this class are likely to be similar for all the drugs when the interaction results from reduced gastric acidity. However, interactions resulting from hepatic microsomal enzyme activity differ substantially between agents.
- Cimetidine: Numerous drug interactions occur with cimetidine due to inhibition of hepatic microsomal CYP enzymes; however, few nutrient interactions are documented. Vitamin B-12 malabsorption from foods (protein-bound cobalamin) has been reported. Absorption of unbound cobalamin (vitamin B-12 supplement) does not seem to be altered (9–11). Folic acid absorption may be reduced by cimetidine, although the effect seems to be relatively small. The change in folic acid absorption was not significant with ranitidine; therefore, it is difficult to say whether the interaction occurs with other H_2 receptor antagonists (12). Zinc absorption is reduced after cimetidine administration, most likely as the result of reduced acidity. It is likely this interaction would occur with all H_2 receptor antagonists (13).
- Any (unspecified) histamine H_2 antagonists: Use of any histamine H_2 antagonists for 2 or more years increased the risk of vitamin B-12 deficiency in a large community-based population (odds ratio 1.25 [95% confidence interval 1.17–1.34]) (14).

PROTON PUMP INHIBITORS

- Agents in this category suppress gastric acid production. Drug-drug and drug-nutrient interactions reported for one PPI are likely to be similar for all PPIs when the interaction results from reduced gastric acidity. For example, use of any PPI for 2 or more years increased the risk of vitamin B-12 deficiency in a large community-based population. The effect of PPIs was greater than for histamine H_2 antagonists (odds ratio 1.65 vs 1.25), and higher doses were associated with vitamin B-12 deficiency to a greater extent than lower doses (14).
- Esomeprazole: Metabolism of drugs by CYP2C19 isoenzymes is inhibited by esomeprazole. No specific drug-nutrient interactions are reported.

- Omeprazole: Beta-carotene absorption seems to be reduced with omeprazole therapy. Based on a small study, significantly reduced beta-carotene absorption may occur with relatively short-term (7 days) use of omeprazole at standard doses (20 mg twice daily). All PPIs would likely have similar effects (15). Ginkgo increases metabolism of omeprazole based on a small, single-dose study in which omeprazole was administered after a 12-day course of standardized extract of ginkgo. The degree to which metabolism of omeprazole is altered varies with CYP2C19 genetic status (extensive metabolizer vs poor metabolizer). The mechanism of interaction is likely induction of CYP2C19, a hepatic isoenzyme involved in the metabolism of all PPIs (16). St. John's wort induces metabolism of omeprazole, likely through induction of hepatic microsomal isoenzymes CYP3A4 and CYP2C19. Efficacy of omeprazole therapy may reduce by this interaction, and the effect is likely to occur with all PPIs (17). Vitamin B-12 absorption may be reduced with PPI therapy. There are conflicting reports concerning serum concentrations of vitamin B-12 in those taking a PPI, although studies often fail to control for protein-bound (food sources) vs unbound (supplement) cobalamin. Absorption of protein-bound cobalamin does seem to be reduced (18–21).
- Rabeprazole: The metabolism of rabeprazole is much less dependent on CYP2C19 than is the metabolism of omeprazole. Therefore, the potential for interaction with St. John's wort may be lower with rabeprazole.

PROSTAGLANDINS

- Gastric acid secretion is reduced by synthetic analogs of prostaglandin E1.
- Misoprostol: Intestinal inflammation may be exacerbated in patients with inflammatory bowel disease, producing severe diarrhea.

PROTECTANTS

- Agents categorized as protectants form a barrier between gastric acid and tissue. In addition, pepsin is inhibited.
- Sucralfate (aluminum sucrose sulfate) (1): The aluminum content of sucralfate is expected to cause the same interaction with phosphorus and calcium as is noted with aluminum-containing antacids. Phosphate binding in the GI tract leads to increased bone loss and increased urinary calcium loss. Drugs known to bind divalent cations, such as ciprofloxacin, may be bound to sucralfate, resulting in significantly reduced bioavailability of the drug.

Recommendations

HISTAMINE H$_2$ ANTAGONISTS

- Administer drugs and nutrients requiring an acid environment for absorption, such as iron, at least 2 hours before or several hours after histamine H$_2$ antagonists. Calcium citrate solubility is less dependent on an acid environment than other calcium salts; therefore, calcium citrate may be a better choice for a calcium supplement when an H$_2$ receptor antagonist is used. Magnesium and iron may be better absorbed if taken with an acidic juice. Acid suppression by H$_2$ receptor antagonists can be reversed by food intake.
- Consider a vitamin B-12 supplement for anyone taking histamine H$_2$ antagonists; patients older than 50 years of age should routinely use a supplement (unbound source) of vitamin B-12.

Check the vitamin B-12 serum concentration in those using these medications long-term. The risk of interactions related to CYP enzymes is greatly reduced by use of histamine H_2 antagonists other than cimetidine.

PROTON PUMP INHIBITORS

- Administer drugs and nutrients requiring an acid environment for absorption, such as iron, at least 2 hours before or several hours after PPI administration. Calcium citrate solubility is less dependent on an acid environment than other calcium salts; therefore, calcium citrate may be a better choice for a calcium supplement when a PPI is used. Magnesium and iron may be better absorbed if taken with an acidic juice. Acid suppression by PPIs is not reversed by food intake.
- Consider a vitamin B-12 supplement for anyone taking a PPI; those older than 50 years of age should routinely use a supplement (unbound source) of vitamin B-12. Monitor vitamin B-12 status using either serum B-12 or methylmalonic acid levels.

PROSTAGLANDINS—MISOPROSTOL

- Misoprostol should be taken on an empty stomach because food decreases absorption.
- Avoid in patients with inflammatory bowel disease.

PROTECTANTS—SUCRALFATE (ALUMINUM SUCROSE SULFATE)

- Administer sucralfate 2 hours before or after drugs and mineral supplements known to bind to sucralfate.
- Consider patients receiving sucralfate for more than a few weeks to be at high risk for osteoporosis and monitor accordingly.

Prokinetic Agents

Agents classified as prokinetics can potentially alter absorption by increasing the rate of transit from the stomach and small bowel.

Examples

Drugs in this category include:

- Erythromycin
- Metoclopramide

Interaction Notes—Erythromycin

- The rate of gastric emptying is increased by erythromycin through effects on motilin, and a relatively small dose is required for this effect compared to the typical dose for effective antibiotic therapy.
- Despite the small dose, commensal GI flora, such as acidophilus and bifidobacteria, may be reduced when erythromycin is used as a prokinetic agent. The commensal GI flora produce significant quantities of several B vitamins and vitamin K (22–24).

Anti-Inflammatory Agents

Agents used to suppress inflammation in the GI tract are primarily aimed at control of inflammatory bowel disease. Mesalamine, sulfasalazine, and olsalazine all inhibit folate-dependent enzymes and are associated with a risk of folic acid depletion.

Examples

Drugs in this category include:

- Mesalamine
- Olsalazine
- Sulfasalazine

Interaction Notes

MESALAMINE
Folic acid depletion is a risk.

SULFASALAZINE

- Iron binds with sulfasalazine in the GI tract and may decrease absorption of both.
- Folic acid depletion may occur due to altered folic acid transport and competitive inhibition of the pathway for conversion to active folic acid (25).

Recommendations

- Anti-inflammatory agents should be taken after meals.
- Separate doses of iron by 2 hours before or after sulfasalazine, and consider the same for mesalamine and olsalazine.

Miscellaneous GI Drugs

Examples

Drugs in this category include:

- Alosetron
- Amoxicillin
- Clarithromycin
- Metronidazole
- Octreotide
- Orlistat
- Tegaserod
- Tetracycline

Interaction Notes

AMOXICILLIN
Commensal GI flora, such as acidophilus and bifidobacteria, may be reduced with antibiotic therapy. The commensal GI flora produce significant quantities of several B vitamins and vitamin K (22–24).

CLARITHROMYCIN
See comments under Amoxicillin pertaining to commensal GI flora.

METRONIDAZOLE

- *See* comments under Amoxicillin pertaining to commensal GI flora.
- Silymarin, the active constituent of milk thistle, reduces metronidazole levels by about 20% to 30% based on a small, short-term (7 to 10 days) study in healthy subjects. Metronidazole transport and metabolism are dependent upon CYP3A4 and P-glycoprotein, which seem to be induced by silymarin (26).

TETRACYCLINE

- *See* comments under Amoxicillin pertaining to commensal GI flora.
- Calcium, magnesium, and iron bind with tetracycline and reduce antibiotic efficacy.

ORLISTAT
The mechanism of action for orlistat-induced weight loss is fat malabsorption due to lipase inhibition. In addition to decreasing fat absorption, orlistat reduces absorption of fat-soluble vitamins, including A, D, E, K, and beta-carotene (27,28).

Recommendations

TETRACYCLINE

- Administer tetracycline on an empty stomach.
- Avoid milk, antacids, and supplements containing calcium, magnesium, or iron for 2 hours before or after a dose of tetracycline.

ORLISTAT

- Use a multivitamin containing the fat-soluble vitamins and separate vitamin administration by 2 hours from the orlistat dose.
- Nonprescription forms of orlistat are intended for short-term use and, as such, should carry minimal risk of clinically significant vitamin deficiencies unless there are other risk factors for deficiency.
- Consider monitoring fat-soluble vitamin status in anyone who is using orlistat routinely for more than a few weeks.

Lipid-Regulating Drugs

Drugs included in this category work within the GI tract to regulate lipid levels within the body.

Examples

Drugs in this category include:

- Cholestyramine
- Colesevelam
- Colestipol
- Ezetimibe

Interaction Notes

CHOLESTYRAMINE

- Cholestyramine is classified as a bile acid sequestrant. It is an anion-exchange resin that can bind to bile acids as well as a number of other compounds in the GI tract, and prevent their absorption. Enterohepatic recycling of bile acids is interrupted and absorption of fats is reduced. Interference with the absorption of vitamins, especially those that are fat-soluble, can occur due to bile acid binding and interference with fat absorption (29,30).
- Vitamins A, D, and K deficiencies have been reported with long-term therapy, although rarely.
- Lycopene and beta-carotene serum levels were reduced by about 30% and 40%, respectively, after 2 months of cholestyramine therapy in a study of 303 hypercholesterolemic subjects. This study used diet-derived lycopene and beta-carotene rather than supplements. Further reductions in lycopene and beta-carotene levels occurred with the addition of probucol, a drug no longer available in the United States (31).
- Folic acid absorption has been reported to be reduced. However, effects on water-soluble vitamins are not well studied.
- Chloride is released from cholestyramine resin and can be absorbed. Large doses of cholestyramine may result in hyperchloremic acidosis.
- Calcium excretion may be increased in the urine.
- Magnesium losses may increase slightly in the urine.
- Phosphorus, iron, zinc, and nitrogen absorption may be decreased.

COLESEVELAM

Like cholestyramine and colestipol, colesevelam is classified as a bile acid sequestrant. However, in recommended colesevelam doses, this drug does not seem to interfere with fat-soluble vitamin absorption.

COLESTIPOL

- Colestipol is classified as a bile acid sequestrant. Like cholestyramine, colestipol is an anion-exchange resin that can bind to bile acids, as well as a number of other compounds in the GI tract, and prevent their absorption. Enterohepatic recycling of bile acids is interrupted and absorption of fats is reduced. Interference with the absorption of vitamins, especially those that are fat-soluble, can occur due to bile acid binding and interference with fat absorption (32,33).

- Vitamins A, D, E, and K serum levels have been noted to decrease with colestipol therapy, although deficiencies are rare.
- Folic acid absorption may be reduced.

EZETIMIBE

- Ezetimibe is a cholesterol absorption inhibitor that localizes at the brush border of the small intestine and inhibits cholesterol absorption.
- Ezetimibe does not inhibit absorption of bile acid, triglycerides, or fatty acids; therefore, pharmacokinetic interactions with vitamins seem unlikely.

Recommendations

CHOLESTYRAMINE

- Monitor serum electrolytes periodically during cholestyramine therapy. There are no specific guidelines defining the period for monitoring; however, baseline values within the first couple weeks, followed by evaluation every few weeks to determine whether electrolyte concentrations are decreasing would be reasonable. Reduced dietary chloride intake may partially offset the effects of cholestyramine on serum electrolytes. Effects on electrolytes are most likely to be significant with high doses and prolonged periods of use.
- For children receiving cholestyramine therapy, routine supplementation of fat-soluble vitamins is not considered necessary. However, periodic monitoring of vitamin A and D levels and prothrombin time (PT) is suggested.
- Daily supplementation of vitamins A, D, and K in patients receiving high-dose cholestyramine should be considered. In addition, supplementation of fat-soluble vitamins would be reasonable in patients at risk of inadequate intake based on dietary assessment.
- Parenteral administration of vitamin K may be appropriate if bleeding associated with hypoprothrombinemia occurs.
- Monitor patients for folic acid deficiency and consider supplementation with 5 mg folic acid daily, especially for children and patients otherwise at risk of folic acid deficiency.
- Administer drugs and dietary supplements at least 1 hour before or 4 to 6 hours after cholestyramine to minimize the risk of interactions.

COLESEVELAM

Patients at risk of fat-soluble vitamin deficiency should be monitored for possible decline in vitamin status with long-term use of colesevelam.

COLESTIPOL

- For prolonged therapy, consider supplemental vitamins A and D.
- Serum folate and fat-soluble vitamin status should be monitored annually in children.
- Parenteral administration of vitamin K may be appropriate if bleeding associated with hypoprothrombinemia occurs.

Conclusion

Medications are clearly an integral part of the treatment of many conditions and diseases and the management of various adverse GI effects. However, clinicians need to recognize the potential for drug-nutrient interactions that could affect nutritional status and be prepared to make appropriate nutrition interventions to improve patient outcomes.

References

1. Spencer H, Lender M. Adverse effects of aluminum-containing antacids on mineral metabolism. *Gastroenterology*. 1979;76:603–606.
2. Khawaja IS, Marotta RF, Lippmann S. Herbal medicines as a factor in delirium. *Psychiatr Serv*. 1999;50:969–970.
3. Clark JH, Russell GJ, Fitzgerald JK, et al. Serum beta-carotene, retinol, and alpha-tocopherol levels during mineral oil therapy for constipation. *Am J Dis Child*. 1987;141:1210–1212.
4. Pelton R, laValle JB, Hawkins EB, Krinsky DL. *Drug-Induced Nutrient Depletion Handbook*. 2nd ed. Hudson, OH: Lexi-Comp and Cincinnati, OH: Natural Health Resources; 2001.
5. Pinto J, Huang YP, Pelliccione N, et al. Cardiac sensitivity to the inhibitory effects of chlorpromazine, imipramine and amitriptyline upon formation of flavins. *Biochem Pharmacol*. 1982;31:3495–3499.
6. Bell IR, Edman JS, Morrow FD, et al. Brief communication. Vitamin B1, B2, and B6 augmentation of tricyclic antidepressant treatment in geriatric depression with cognitive dysfunction. *J Am Coll Nutr*. 1992;11:159–163.
7. Vaddadi KS. The use of gamma-linolenic acid and linoleic acid to differentiate between temporal lobe epilepsy and schizophrenia. *Prostaglandins Med*. 1981;6:375–379.
8. Puri BK. The safety of evening primrose oil in epilepsy. *Prostaglandins Leukot Essent Fatty Acids*. 2007;77:101–103.
9. Streeter AM, Goulston KJ, Bathur FA, Hilmer RS, Crane GG, Pheils MT. Cimetidine and malabsorption of cobalamin. *Dig Dis Sci*. 1982; 27:13–16.
10. Steinberg WM, King CE, Toskes PP. Malabsorption of protein-bound cobalamin but not unbound cobalamin during cimetidine administration. *Dig Dis Sci*. 1980;25:188–191.
11. Salom IL, Silvis SE, Doscherholmen A. Effect of cimetidine on the absorption of vitamin B12. *Scand J Gastroenterol*. 1982; 17:129–131.
12. Russell RM, Golner BB, Krasinski SD, et al. Effect of antacid and H2 receptor antagonists on the intestinal absorption of folic acid. *J Lab Clin Med*. 1988;112:458–463.
13. Sturniolo GC, Montino MC, Rossetto L, et al. Inhibition of gastric acid secretion reduces zinc absorption in man. *Am J Coll Nutr*. 1991;10:372–375.
14. Lam JR, Schneider JL, Zhoa W, et al. Proton pump inhibitor and histamine 2 receptor antagonist use and vitamin B-12 deficiency. *JAMA*. 2013;310(22):2435–2442.
15. Tang G, Serfaty-Lacrosniere C, Camilo ME, Russell RM. Gastric acidity influences the blood response to a beta-carotene dose in humans. *Am J Clin Nutr*. 1996;64:622–626.
16. Yin OQ, Tomlinson B, Waye MM, Chow AH, Chow MS. Pharmacogenetics and herb-drug interactions: experience with Ginkgo biloba and omeprazole. *Pharmacogenetics*. 2004;14:841–850.
17. Wang LS, Zhou G, Zhu B, et al. St. John's wort induces both cytochrome P450 3A4-catalyzed sulfoxidation and 2C19-dependent hydroxylation of omeprazole. *Clin Pharmacol Ther*. 2004; 75:191–197.
18. Bradford GS, Taylor CT. Omeprazole and vitamin B12 deficiency. *Ann Pharmacother*. 1999;33:641–643.
19. Marcuard SP, Albernaz L, Khazanie PG. Omeprazole therapy causes malabsorption of cyanocobalamin (vitamin B12). *Ann Intern Med*. 1994;120:211–215.

20. King CE, Leibach J, Toskes PP. Clinically significant vitamin B12 deficiency secondary to malabsorption of protein-bound vitamin B12. *Dig Dis Sci.* 1979;24:397–402.

21. Schenk BE, Festen HP, Kuipers EJ, et al. Effect of short- and long-term treatment with omeprazole on the absorption and serum levels of cobalamine. *Aliment Pharmacol Ther.* 1996;10:541–545.

22. Cummings JH, Macfarlane G. Role of intestinal bacteria in nutrient metabolism. *JPEN J Parenter Enteral Nutr.* 1997;21:357–366.

23. Deguchi Y, et al. Comparative studies on synthesis of water-soluble vitamins among human species of bifidobacteria. *Agric Biol Chem.* 1985;19:13–19.

24. Hill MJ. Intestinal flora and endogenous vitamin synthesis. *Eur J Cancer Prev.* 1997;6(Suppl 1):S43–S45.

25. Sulfasalazine inhibits folate absorption. *Nutr Rev.* 1988;46:320–323.

26. Williamson E, Driver S, Baxter K. *Stockley's Herbal Medicines Interactions.* London, UK: Pharmaceutical Press; 2009:295.

27. Zhi J, Melia AT, Koss-Twardy SG, et al. The effect of orlistat, an inhibitor of dietary fat absorption, on the pharmacokinetics of beta-carotene in healthy volunteers. *J Clin Pharmacol.* 1996;36:152–159.

28. Finer N, James WP, Kopelman PG, et al. One-year treatment of obesity: a randomized, double-blind, placebo-controlled, multicenter study of orlistat, a gastrointestinal lipase inhibitor. *Int J Obes Relat Metab Disord.* 2000;24:306–313.

29. West RJ, Lloyd JK. The effect of cholestyramine on intestinal absorption. *Gut.* 1975;16:93–98.

30. Watkins DW, Khalafi R, Cassidy MM, et al. Alterations in calcium, magnesium, iron, and zinc metabolism by dietary cholestyramine. *Dig Dis Sci.* 1985;30:477–482.

31. Elinder LS, Hadell K, Johansson J, et al. Probucol treatment decreases serum concentrations of diet-derived antioxidants. *Arterioscler Thromb Vasc Biol.* 1995;15:1057–1063.

32. Schwartz KB, Goldstein PD, Witztum JL, et al. Fat-soluble vitamin concentrations in hypocholesterolemic children treated with colestipol. *Pediatrics.* 1980;65:243–250.

33. Tonstad S, Sivertsen M, Aksnes L, et al. Low dose colestipol in adolescents with familial hypercholesterolemia. *Arch Dis Child.* 1996;74:157–160.

CHAPTER 24

Nutraceutical Supplements

Gerard E. Mullin, MD, CNSP, FACN, AGAF

Nutraceutical supplement use in the patient population with gastrointestinal (GI) disorders is widespread and continues to grow. An estimated 50% of patients with digestive disorders use nutraceutical supplements, according to multiple studies on this topic (1–15). With more than 90 million Americans diagnosed with a GI condition—and with many of these patients seeking expert advice from a registered dietitian (RD) about which supplements have the most potential to effectively address their symptoms—it is imperative that dietetics practitioners familiarize themselves with the evidence supporting nutraceutical supplement use.

The vast majority of research for supplements used for GI and liver diseases has been conducted for only a small number of conditions, namely, irritable bowel syndrome (IBS), inflammatory bowel disease (IBD), and chronic liver disease (CLD). Further controlled clinical trials of the potential efficacy of natural supplementation in these and other GI and liver disorders are needed.

The most commonly used nutraceutical supplements seen in practice today are discussed in this chapter. The list of supplements covered here is by no means a comprehensive one.

Use of Supplements in Digestive Health and Disease

Although the nutraceutical supplement industry is growing in Europe, use of nutraceutical supplements for all digestive indications is seemingly more common in North America. The most popular form of alternative medicine for GI disorders is herbal therapy (16–19). Among all patients with digestive disorders, nutraceutical supplement use seems more common in the IBD and IBS patient populations (1,8,15), possibly because these disorders are chronic and refractory in nature (19,20); psychological factors may also play a role.

Considering the widespread nutraceutical supplement use among patients diagnosed with GI and liver disorders, physicians and RDs cannot ignore the potential benefits of these products. At the same time, health care providers must be aware of risks associated with supplement use. For example, many herbs have the potential for hepatotoxicity (see Table 24.1 for the most common hepatotoxic herbs).

TABLE 24.1 Hepatotoxic Herbal Preparations

Herb	Type of Liver Injury
Crotalaria, heliotropium, *Senecio longilobus*, *Symphytum officinale* (pyrrolizidine alkaloids)	Sinusoidal obstruction syndrome (veno-occlusive disease)
Chaparral leaf, germander	Zone 3 necrosis, cirrhosis, cholestasis, chronic hepatitis
Pennyroyal (squamit) oil	Zone 3 necrosis, microvesicular steatosis, fulminant liver failure
Jin bu huan	Acute and chronic cholestatic hepatitis, microvesicular steatosis, fibrosis
Mistletoe	Chronic hepatitis
Margosa oil	Microvesicular steatosis, Reye syndrome, hepatic necrosis
Usnic acid	Fulminant liver failure
Atractylis gummifera	Acute hepatitis, fulminant liver failure
Callilepis laureola	Acute hepatitis, fulminant liver failure
Impila	Acute hepatitis, fulminant liver failure
Camphor	Necrolytic hepatitis
Cascara sagrada	Cholestatic hepatitis
TJ-8, Dai saiko-toi	Autoimmune hepatitis
TJ-9, Sho-saiko-to	Acute and chronic hepatitis
Paeonia spp	Acute hepatitis, fulminant liver failure
Greater celandine	Chronic hepatitis, cholestasis, fibrosis
Germander	Acute and chronic hepatitis, fulminant liver failure
Isabgol	Giant cell hepatitis
Kava	Acute and chronic hepatitis, fulminant liver failure
Ma huang	Acute hepatitis, autoimmune hepatitis
Oil of cloves	Hepatic necrosis
Sassafras	Hepatocarcinogen
Saw palmetto	Mild hepatitis
Shou-wu-pian	Acute hepatitis
Valerian	Mild hepatitis

Herbal Therapies

Traditional Chinese Medicine (TCM)

The Chinese literature contains numerous reports concerning the treatment of digestive and liver disease with herbal remedies; however, only the abstracts for these articles are available in English.

In the treatment of IBD, all studies demonstrated that TCM was more effective than both placebo and conventional medical therapy for IBD (21–23).

For liver disease, several controlled studies using the TCM herbal preparation TJ9 for chronic hepatitis C establish that the preparation has impressive anti-inflammatory (24,25) and anti-fibrotic effects (26). (See Table 24.2 on page 314.)

TCM is popular among IBS patients; however, of the 75 randomized trials of TCM in IBS that were identified in one systematic review (27), only five double-blind, placebo-controlled trials were considered to be of high quality with mainly favorable results (28–32). Tong xie yao fang (TXYF), a TCM prepared from four herbs, has been shown to be effective for IBS in a meta-analysis of 1,125 subjects from

TABLE 24.2   Herbal Preparations Used in the Treatment of Chronic Liver Disease

Blended Herbal Preparations	Method of Action	Use
TJ-9	Anti-fibrotic; inhibits stellate cell activation; decreases hepatic lipid peroxidation; increases TNF-α and granulocyte colony stimulating factor (g-CSF)	Hepatitis B; prevention of hepatocellular carcinoma
TJ-108	Reduces HCV-RNA, hepatoprotective	Hepatitis C
Herbal medicine 861	Blocks cyclin/cyclin-dependent kinase, facilitates remodeling of fibrotic liver tissue	Hepatitis B
CH-100	No loss in HCV-RNA, however decreased ALT, hepatoprotective	Hepatitis C
Bing gan	Some improvement in HCV-RNA clearance	Hepatitis C
Liv 52	Inhibits lipid peroxidation; decreases TNF activity	Experimental liver injury; alcoholic liver disease

12 studies (33). Further studies to assess the efficacy of standard vs individualized herbal preparations for IBS would help practitioners appropriately advise patients.

Note: Some TCM products have been contaminated with heavy metals. Clinicians should warn patients to exercise caution when pursuing TCM therapies.

Aloe Vera

In patients with moderately active ulcerative colitis (UC), oral aloe vera gel given for 4 weeks proved to be more efficacious than placebo in a randomized, double-blind controlled study (34). Aloe has been shown to protect against dextran-induced colitis in animal models (35,36). Although aloe vera is used by many for peptic ulcers, Crohn's disease (CD), and gastroesophageal reflux disease (GERD), there are no controlled trials to demonstrate efficacy (37).

Glycyrrhizin (Licorice Root)

Glycyrrhiza glabra (licorice root) has been used for centuries in traditional medicine to treat cough, bronchitis, gastritis, and liver inflammation. In the United States, it is available over-the-counter in liquid, powder, and pill forms.

A large number of components have been isolated from licorice, including triterpene saponins, flavonoids, isoflavonoids, and chalcones, with glycyrrhizic acid (glycyrrhizin) normally being considered to be the main biologically active component. Glycyrrhizin has antioxidant, immunosuppressive and anti-inflammatory properties. It also enhances interferon production and stimulates natural killer cell activity (38–40).

Clinical trials using intravenous (IV) glycyrrhizin have mostly involved the treatment of hepatitis C, specifically, in patients who are refractory to, or intolerant of, interferon treatment (41). Very few studies have shown enhanced antiviral effects with glycyrrhizin.

Aly and associates found that oral licorice in combination with famotidine therapy could heal ulcers in rats as effectively as an H_2 blocker (42). Glycyrrhizinic acid has antiulcer properties and raises the local concentration of prostaglandins that promote mucous secretion and cell proliferation in the stomach, leading to healing of ulcers in experimental studies (43).

Several studies have confirmed that licorice root has activity against *Helicobacter pylori* (44–48). Despite the lack of evidence, many individuals with GERD use licorice root as first-line treatment.

The main side effects of glycyrrhizin treatment are fluid retention and hypokalemia due to its mineralocorticoid effect (49). Licorice root should be avoided in patients with cirrhosis and CLD.

Polyphenols

Polyphenols (phytochemicals in food substances) are nonessential nutrients, which means that the possibility of a person being polyphenol-deficient has not been identified in research. However, researchers have found polyphenols to be potentially immune-modulating and theorize that they may play a biologically active role (50). Polyphenols modify immunity and inflammation, downregulate inflammatory mediators, inhibit transcription of nuclear factor kappa beta (NFkB), and are prebiotic (ie, they help friendly bacteria thrive).

Among polyphenols studied for efficacy in treating colitis in animals, prophylactic and therapeutic effects were observed with resveratrol, epigallocatechin, curcumin, and quercetin, although quercetin was deemed the least effective (50). Clinical studies of polyphenol use in the treatment of IBD in humans have been limited to *Boswellia serrata* and *Curcuma longa*.

BOSWELLIA SERRATA

The immune-modulating properties of *B. serrata* (frankincense, a traditional Ayurvedic remedy and incense component) have been studied for their effect on IBD (51,52). A study in India comparing the efficacy of gum resin from *B. serrata* with sulfasalazine in moderately active UC found the remission rates in the Boswellia group (82%) comparable to those for patients given conventional therapy (75%) (53). In 2001, a similar study conducted by the same authors showed an improvement in the rate of remission among the Boswellia group, with a 70% remission rate in the 20 patients who took Boswellia for 6 weeks and a remission rate of 40% in the 10 patients who took sulfasalazine (54).

Another study compared the efficacy of the *B. serrata* extract with mesalamine in treating active CD. That randomized, double-blind controlled 8-week trial, which was powered to show noninferiority, included 102 patients (55). Similar to the results in previous trials with 5-ASA preparations, decreases in the mean CD Activity Index were measured in both groups, and H15 was well tolerated (56,57).

B. serrata is undergoing evaluation for its potential benefit for microscopic and collagenous colitis (58).

CURCUMA LONGA (TURMERIC)

In vitro studies have demonstrated multiple immunomodulatory and anti-inflammatory properties in curcumin, the yellow pigment of turmeric *(Curcuma longa)*, which is a key ingredient in curry powder (59–62). When taken orally, curcumin benefited four of five patients with Crohn's disease and five of five patients with ulcerative proctitis in an uncontrolled trial (63). The first study of curcumin's potential role in UC maintenance was a randomized, multicenter, double-blind placebo-controlled trial conducted in Japan by Hanai and colleagues (64). The results demonstrated that curcumin, when taken with mesalazine medication, maintained UC remission better than mesalazine alone. Thus, curcumin is emerging as a "rising star" in the digestive health supplement industry (65).

Peppermint Oil

Peppermint oil has been evaluated in patients with IBS and found to be beneficial in symptom relief (66). The presumed mechanism of action is via calcium-channel blockade-mediated smooth muscle relaxation.

Spanier et al reviewed five randomized, double-blind, placebo-controlled studies that have evaluated the supplement's efficacy (67). A meta-analysis showed an overall superiority of peppermint oil to placebo (68). The number of patients needed to be treated by peppermint oil to achieve benefit is only two (ie, NNT = 2), whereas the prescription-strength antispasmodic hyoscyamine has an NNT of 8 (69,70).

Iberogast is a German-derived multiherb combination for gut rescue from dyspepsia and IBS that features peppermint oil as a main ingredient. A study of 208 subjects demonstrated the efficacy in IBS of using the herbal preparations STW 5 (nine herbs: candytuft, chamomile, peppermint, caraway, licorice root, lemon balm, celandine, milk thistle, and angelica) and STW 5-II (six herbs: candytuft, chamomile, peppermint, caraway, licorice root, and lemon balm) (70,71). Both STW 5 formulations contain peppermint oil and chamomile, which act by relaxing intestinal smooth muscle.

Several studies have shown that Iberogast was superior to placebo for nonulcer dyspepsia (72–75). Clinicians are beginning to use Iberogast as an adjunctive treatment for gastroparesis since evidence is emerging for its use as a prokinetic (76,77).

Silymarin (Milk Thistle)

Silymarin is the active ingredient extracted from *Silybum marianum* (also known as *milk thistle*), which was used by ancient physicians and herbalists to treat a variety of liver and gallbladder diseases. The main effects of silymarin are the membrane-stabilizing and antioxidant effects. It is able to help with liver cell regeneration, and it can decrease the inflammatory reaction and inhibit the fibrogenesis in the liver. These results support the administration of silymarin preparations in the therapy of CLD.

A large number of animal studies have reported that silymarin offers hepatoprotection against a diverse range of toxins, including acetaminophen, carbon tetrachloride, mushroom poisoning (phalloidin), radiation, iron overload, phenylhydrazine, alcohol, cold ischemia, and thioacetamide (78). Silymarin works as an antioxidant by reducing free radical production, protecting against lipid peroxidation, stabilizing cell membranes, providing antifibrotic properties, and inhibiting NF-κB activation with favorable immunomodulatory effects (49,79–81).

In the United States, silymarin is one of the most commonly used complementary and alternative medicine agents in the treatment of liver disease, in part because of its good safety profile. A recent systematic review and meta-analysis by Saller et al concluded that the use of silymarin is reasonable as a supportive element in the therapy of *Amanita phalloides* poisoning, alcoholic liver disease (as an addition to abstinence), and Child's A cirrhosis (82). Large controlled trials of silymarin have evaluated its effects on liver function in CLD, with variable results, which may be attributed to low-quality clinical trials (49). Well-designed, multicenter randomized controlled trials of silymarin are required to prove its effectiveness in chronic liver disease, and trials sponsored by the National Institutes of Health are ongoing. (Other herbs used in the treatment of CLD are shown in Table 24.2, in the section on traditional Chinese medicine earlier in this chapter.)

Silymarin has been found to inhibit HCV replicon replication in cell culture (83), and a recent study using intravenous silymarin in combination with ribavirin demonstrated rapid suppression of hepatitis C viremia (84). Together, these and other data suggest that silymarin may be used for its antiviral effects in future clinical trials for hepatitis C.

Probiotics

See Chapter 25.

Prebiotics

Prebiotics are nondigestible fermentable food fibers that reportedly have demonstrated health benefits for the host because they encourage the growth and/or activity in the colon of one or a limited number of bacteria (85,86). Inulin, resistant maltodextrin, and oligosaccharides, including fructo-oligosaccharides (FOS) and galacto-oligosaccharides, are among the commonly consumed prebiotics.

Feeding prebiotics changes the composition of the intestinal microflora to favor more protective intestinal bacteria and alters systemic and mucosal immune responses of the host. Elevating endogenous numbers of bacterial strains with beneficial health effects (eg, lactobacillus and bifidobacterium) is the primary reason for consuming prebiotics (87,88). Prebiotics also increase short-chain fatty acid levels in the colon, which are important energy sources for the colonic enterocytes and have anti-inflammatory and antineoplastic properties.

In IBS, prebiotics may not be tolerated by all patients and can cause bloating and gas due to fermentation by resident bacteria in the small intestine. For patients with IBS, it is prudent to start with low doses of prebiotics (eg, 3 g FOS daily) and increase as tolerated.

Older as well as more recent studies show beneficial effects of prebiotics in experimental colitis, and later studies of human IBD, such as CD, UC, and chronic pouchitis, have also found benefits (89,90). For patients with left-sided UC that is resistant to medication, short-chain fatty acid rectal irrigation has been shown to be an effective alternative therapy (91–95). Probiotics have been studied more extensively than prebiotics in studies of therapeutic approaches to treating IBD. All four of the published studies on the effectiveness of prebiotic use in IBD support its application in treating active UC (91–94).

Fish Oils

A wide range of health benefits from consuming essential omega-3 fatty acids—namely, the prevention and treatment of a multitude of diseases—has been supported in the literature (96). The potent immunomodulatory effects of omega-3 fatty acids, which seem to be mediated via regulation of eicosanoid synthesis and through an eicosanoid-independent inhibitory effect on the proinflammatory cytokines, have been noted in cell culture and animal studies. Thus, the theory has advanced that relapse treatment or prevention for chronic inflammatory diseases could potentially benefit from omega-3 fatty acid supplementation.

In vivo and in vitro studies of omega-3 fatty acids in mice models have demonstrated effective prevention and treatment of colitis (97–102). A number of studies have shown the benefit of fish oils on the course of IBD (100,102–112).

Overall, fish oils have been shown to have efficacy for maintaining remission in UC. However, based on a Cochrane review, fish oils cannot be recommended as the only therapy for maintenance of UC (113).

In Crohn's disease, a Cochrane meta-analysis demonstrated that fish oils were efficacious for maintenance of remission (114). However, a more recent multicenter study failed to show a similar result, and, overall, fish oils cannot be relied upon as sole therapy for the maintenance of remission for CD (115,116).

Vitamin D

The highest prevalence of IBD is found in northern climates, including North America and northern Europe, where vitamin D from sunlight exposure is more limited than in southern regions (117,118). Vitamin D deficiency is common in patients with a number of digestive disorders characterized by intestinal malabsorption of fat-soluble vitamins and in patients with CLD (119).

Patients with IBD are deficient in vitamin D even when the disease is in remission (120). The mechanism that causes frequent deficiency of vitamin D in patients with both forms of IBD is unknown, although deficiency is likely the result of an aggregate of low vitamin D intake, malabsorption of vitamin D and other nutrients, and infrequent participation in outdoor activities because the climate for synthesizing vitamin D in the skin is suboptimal. Testing all individuals with IBD for 25-OH vitamin D_3 levels is essential, as risks for vitamin D deficiency and osteoporosis are elevated in this patient population (121). See Chapter 10 for more information on vitamin D supplementation in CLD.

Conclusion

Worldwide, approximately 50% of patients with digestive disease have tried nutraceutical supplements for better control of their illness. There is an abundance of clinical trials demonstrating efficacy of nutraceutical supplements in inflammatory bowel disease and irritable bowel syndrome. The mechanism of action of these nutraceutical supplements includes the downregulation of the inflammatory response, rebalancing the intestinal flora, and restoring proper gut immunity. Traditional Chinese medicine has been shown in limited trials to be effective, but study design and lack of reporting on toxicity are concerning. For IBD, probiotics, prebiotics, butyric acid enemas, *Curcumin longa*, *Boswellia serrata*, and fish oils have been shown to be superior to placebo and, in some cases, equal to standard medical therapy in well-designed randomized controlled trials. For IBS, peppermint oil has been shown in several studies and a meta-analysis to be superior to placebo. In chronic liver disease, use of silymarin may provide benefit and has no known adverse effects.

There is a need for clinical trials of the potential efficacy of natural approaches in combination with conventional therapy to achieve better outcomes in digestive disorders. Lastly, further education of physicians, RDs, and other health care professionals about the potential risks and benefits of nutraceutical supplements is essential if we are to give well-informed advice to patients who are considering or already using alternative therapies for GI and liver diseases.

References

1. Rawsthorne P, Shanahan F, Cronin NC, et al. An international survey of the use and attitudes regarding alternative medicine by patients with inflammatory bowel disease. *Am J Gastroenterol*. 1999;94(5):1298–1303.
2. Eisenberg DM, Davis RB, Ettner SL, et al. Trends in alternative medicine use in the United States, 1990–1997: results of a follow-up national survey. *JAMA*. 1998;280(18):1569–1575.
3. Garcia-Planella E, Marin L, Domènech E, et al. [Use of complementary and alternative medicine and drug abuse in patients with inflammatory bowel disease] [article in Spanish]. *Med Clin (Barc)*. 2007;128(2):45–48.
4. Joos S, Rosemann T, Szecsenyi J, et al. Use of complementary and alternative medicine in Germany—a survey of patients with inflammatory bowel disease. *BMC Complement Altern Med*. 2006;22(6):19.
5. Bensoussan M, Jovenin N, Garcia B, et al. Complementary and alternative medicine use by patients with inflammatory bowel disease: results from a postal survey. *Gastroenterol Clin Biol*. 2006;30(1):14–23.
6. McCann LJ, Newell SJ. Survey of paediatric complementary and alternative medicine use in health and chronic illness. *Arch Dis Child*. 2006;91(2):173–174.
7. Li FX, Verhoef MJ, Best A, Otley A, Hilsden RJ. Why patients with inflammatory bowel disease use or do not use complementary and alternative medicine: a Canadian national survey. *Can J Gastroenterol*. 2005;19(9):567–573.
8. Langhorst J, Anthonisen IB, Steder-Neukamm U, et al. Amount of systemic steroid medication is a strong predictor for the use of complementary and alternative medicine in patients with inflammatory bowel disease: results from a German national survey. *Inflamm Bowel Dis*. 2005;11(3):287–295.

9. Kong SC, Hurlstone DP, Pocock CY, et al. The incidence of self-prescribed oral complementary and alternative medicine use by patients with gastrointestinal diseases. *J Clin Gastroenterol*. 2005;39(2):138–141.

10. Day AS, Whitten KE, Bohane TD. Use of complementary and alternative medicines by children and adolescents with inflammatory bowel disease. *J Paediatr Child Health*. 2004;40(12):681–684.

11. Hilsden RJ, Verhoef MJ, Best A, Pocobelli G. Complementary and alternative medicine use by Canadian patients with inflammatory bowel disease: results from a national survey. *Am J Gastroenterol*. 2003;98(7):1563–1568.

12. Quattropani C, Ausfeld B, Straumann A, Heer P, Seibold F. Complementary alternative medicine in patients with inflammatory bowel disease: use and attitudes. *Scand J Gastroenterol*. 2003;38(3):277–282.

13. Langmead L, Chitnis M, Rampton DS. Use of complementary therapies by patients with IBD may indicate psychosocial distress. *Inflamm Bowel Dis*. 2002;8(3):174–179.

14. Hilsden RJ, Meddings JB, Verhoef MJ. Complementary and alternative medicine use by patients with inflammatory bowel disease: An Internet survey. *Can J Gastroenterol*. 1999;13(4):327–332.

15. Sutherland LR, Verhoef MJ. Why do patients seek a second opinion or alternative medicine? *J Clin Gastroenterol*. 1994;19(3):194–197.

16. Moody GA, Eaden JA, Bhakta P, Sher K, Mayberry JF. The role of complementary medicine in European and Asian patients with inflammatory bowel disease. *Public Health*. 1998;112(4):269–271.

17. Hilsden RJ, Scott CM, Verhoef MJ. Complementary medicine use by patients with inflammatory bowel disease. *Am J Gastroenterol*. 1998;93(5):697–701.

18. Hilsden RJ, Verhoef MJ. Complementary and alternative medicine: evaluating its effectiveness in inflammatory bowel disease. *Inflamm Bowel Dis*. 1998;4(4):318–323.

19. Verhoef MJ, Scott CM, Hilsden RJ. A multimethod research study on the use of complementary therapies among patients with inflammatory bowel disease. *Altern Ther Health Med*. 1998;4(4):68–71.

20. Moser G, Tillinger W, Sachs G, et al. Relationship between the use of unconventional therapies and disease-related concerns: a study of patients with inflammatory bowel disease. *J Psychosom Res*. 1996;40(5):503–509.

21. Chen ZS, Nie ZW, Sun QL. [Clinical study in treating intractable ulcerative colitis with traditional Chinese medicine]. *Zhongguo Zhong Xi Yi Jie He Za Zhi*. 1994;14(7):400–402.

22. Wang B, Ren S, Feng W, Zhong Z, Qin C. Kui jie qing in the treatment of chronic non-specific ulcerative colitis. *J Tradit Chin Med*. 1997;17(1):10–13.

23. Chen Q, Zhang H. Clinical study on 118 cases of ulcerative colitis treated by integration of traditional Chinese and Western medicine. *J Tradit Chin Med*. 1999;19(3):163–165.

24. Kusunose M, Qiu B, Cui T, et al. Effect of Sho-saiko-to extract on hepatic inflammation and fibrosis in dimethylnitrosamine induced liver injury rats. *Biol Pharm Bull*. 2002;25(11):1417–1421.

25. Stickel F, Brinkhaus B, Krahmer N, et al. Antifibrotic properties of botanicals in chronic liver disease. *Hepatogastroenterology*. 2002;49(46):1102–1108.

26. Sakaida I, Hironaka K, Kimura T, et al. Herbal medicine Sho-saiko-to (TJ-9) increases expression matrix metalloproteinases (MMPs) with reduced expression of tissue inhibitor of metalloproteinases (TIMPs) in rat stellate cell. *Life Sci*. 2004;74(18):2251–2263.

27. Bian Z, Wu T, Liu L, et al. Effectiveness of the Chinese herbal formula TongXieYaoFang for irritable bowel syndrome: a systematic review. *J Altern Complement Med*. 2006;12(4):401–407.

28. Bensoussan A, Talley NJ, Hing M, et al. Treatment of irritable bowel syndrome with Chinese herbal medicine: a randomized controlled trial. *JAMA*. 1998;280(18):1585–1589.

29. Leung WK, Wu JC, Liang FM, et al. Treatment of diarrhea-predominant irritable bowel syndrome with traditional Chinese herbal medicine: a randomized placebo-controlled trial. *Am J Gastroenterol*. 2006;101(7):1574–1580.

30. Wang ZJ, Li HX, Wang JH, Zhang F. Effect of Shugan Jianpi granule on gut mucosal serotonin-positive cells in patients with irritable bowel syndrome of stagnated Gan-qi attacking Pi syndrome type. *Chin J Integr Med*. 2008;14(3):185–189.

31. Sallon S, Ben-Arye E, Davidson R, et al. A novel treatment for constipation-predominant irritable bowel syndrome using Padma Lax, a Tibetan herbal formula. *Digestion.* 2002;65(3):161–171.

32. Wang G, Li TQ, Wang L, et al. Tong-xie-ning, a Chinese herbal formula, in treatment of diarrhea-predominant irritable bowel syndrome: a prospective, randomized, double-blind, placebo-controlled trial. *Chin Med J (Engl).* 2006;119(24):2114–2119.

33. Bian Z, Wu T, Liu L, et al. Effectiveness of the Chinese herbal formula TongXieYaoFang for irritable bowel syndrome: a systematic review. *J Altern Complement Med.* 2006;12(4):401–407.

34. Langmead L, Feakins RM, Goldthorpe S, et al. Randomized, double-blind, placebo-controlled trial of oral aloe vera gel for active ulcerative colitis. *Aliment Pharmacol Ther.* 2004;19(7):739–747.

35. Koetzner L, Grover G, Boulet J, Jacoby HI. Plant-derived polysaccharide supplements inhibit dextran sulfate sodium-induced colitis in the rat. *Dig Dis Sci.* 2010;55(5):1278–1285.

36. Korkina L, Suprun M, Petrova A, et al. The protective and healing effects of a natural antioxidant formulation based on ubiquinol and aloe vera against dextran sulfate-induced ulcerative colitis in rats. *Biofactors.* 2003;18(1–4):255–264.

37. Blitz JJ, Smith JW, Gerard JR. Aloe vera gel in peptic ulcer therapy: preliminary report. *J Am Osteopath Assoc.* 1963;62:731–735.

38. Yoshikawa M, Matsui Y, Kawamoto H, et al. Effects of glycyrrhizin on immune-mediated cytotoxicity. *J Gastroenterol Hepatol.* 1997;12(3):243–248.

39. Shiki Y, Ishikawa Y, Shirai K, Saito Y, Yoshida S. Effect of glycyrrhizin on lysosomes labilization by phospholipase A2. *Am J Chin Med.* 1986;14(3–4):131–137.

40. Shiki Y, Shirai K, Saito Y, et al. Effect of glycyrrhizin on lysis of hepatocyte membranes induced by anti-liver cell membrane antibody. *J Gastroenterol Hepatol.* 1992;7(1):12–16.

41. Suzuki H, Ohta T, Takino T, et al. Effects of glycyrrhizin on biochemical tests in patients with chronic hepatitis: double blind trial. *Asian Med J.* 1983;26:423–438.

42. Aly AM, Al-Alousi L, Salem HA. Licorice: a possible anti-inflammatory and anti-ulcer drug. *AAPS Pharm Sci Tech.* 2005;6(1):E74–E82.

43. Baker ME. Licorice and enzymes other than 11 beta-hydroxysteroid dehydrogenase: an evolutionary perspective. *Steroids.* 1994;59(2):136–141.

44. Wittschier N, Faller G, Hensel A. Aqueous extracts and polysaccharides from liquorice roots (Glycyrrhiza glabra L.) inhibit adhesion of Helicobacter pylori to human gastric mucosa. *J Ethnopharmacol.* 2009;125(2):218–223.

45. Fukai T, Marumo A, Kaitou K, et al. Anti-Helicobacter pylori flavonoids from licorice extract. *Life Sci.* 2002;71(12):1449–1463.

46. Krausse R, Bielenberg J, Blaschek W, Ullmann U. In vitro anti-Helicobacter pylori activity of Extractum liquiritiae, glycyrrhizin and its metabolites. *J Antimicrob Chemother.* 2004;54(1):243–246.

47. Nariman F, Eftekhar F, Habibi Z, Falsafi T. Anti-Helicobacter pylori activities of six Iranian plants. *Helicobacter.* 2004;9(2):146–151.

48. O'Mahony R, Al-Khtheeri H, Weerasekera D, et al. Bactericidal and anti-adhesive properties of culinary and medicinal plants against Helicobacter pylori. *World J Gastroenterol.* 2005;11(47):7499–7507.

49. Hanje AJ, Fortune B, Song M, Hill D, McClain C. The use of selected nutrition supplements and complementary and alternative medicine in liver disease. *Nutr Clin Pract.* 2006;21(3):255–272.

50. Shapiro H, Singer P, Halpern Z, Bruck R. Polyphenols in the treatment of inflammatory bowel disease and acute pancreatitis. *Gut.* 2007;56(3):426–435.

51. Ammon HP. Modulation of the immune system by Boswellia serrata extracts and boswellic acids. *Phytomedicine.* 2010;17(11):862–867.

52. Ammon HP. Boswellic acids in chronic inflammatory diseases. *Planta Med.* 2006;72(12):1100–1116.

53. Gupta I, Parihar A, Malhotra P, et al. Effects of Boswellia serrata gum resin in patients with ulcerative colitis. *Eur J Med Res.* 1997;2(1):37–43.

54. Gupta I, Parihar A, Malhotra P, et al. Effects of gum resin of Boswellia serrata in patients with chronic colitis. *Planta Med.* 2001;67(5):391–395.

55. Gerhardt H, Seifert F, Buvari P, Vogelsang H, Repges R. [Therapy of active Crohn disease with Boswellia serrata extract H 15] [article in German]. *Z Gastroenterol*. 2001;39(1):11–17.

56. Hanauer SB. The case for using 5-aminosalicyclates in Crohn's disease: pro. *Inflamm Bowel Dis*. 2005;11(6):609–612.

57. Hanauer SB. Supplemental evidence. *Nat Clin Pract Gastroenterol Hepatol*. 2005;2(9):375.

58. Chande N, MacDonald JK, McDonald JW. Interventions for treating microscopic colitis: a Cochrane Inflammatory Bowel Disease and Functional Bowel Disorders Review Group systematic review of randomized trials. *Am J Gastroenterol*. 2009;104(1):235–241.

59. Gautam SC, Gao X, Dulchavsky S. Immunomodulation by curcumin. *Adv Exp Med Biol*. 2007;595:321–341.

60. Camacho-Barquero L, Villegas I, Sánchez-Calvo JM, et al. Curcumin, a Curcuma longa constituent, acts on MAPK p38 pathway modulating COX-2 and iNOS expression in chronic experimental colitis. *Int Immunopharmacol*. 2007;7(3):333–342.

61. Kurup VP, Barrios CS, Raju R, et al. Immune response modulation by curcumin in a latex allergy model. *Clin Mol Allergy*. 2007;5:1.

62. Sharma S, Chopra K, Kulkarni SK, Agrewala JN. Resveratrol and curcumin suppress immune response through CD28/CTLA-4 and CD80 co-stimulatory pathway. *Clin Exp Immunol*. 2007;147(1):155–163.

63. Holt PR, Katz S, Kirshoff R. Curcumin therapy in inflammatory bowel disease: a pilot study. *Dig Dis Sci*. 2005;50(11):2191–2193.

64. Hanai H, Iida T, Takeuchi K, et al. Curcumin maintenance therapy for ulcerative colitis: randomized, multicenter, double-blind, placebo-controlled trial. *Clin Gastroenterol Hepatol*. 2006;4(12):1502–1506.

65. Hanai H, Sugimoto K. Curcumin has bright prospects for the treatment of inflammatory bowel disease. *Curr Pharm Des*. 2009;15(18):2087–2094.

66. Pittler MH, Ernst E. Peppermint oil for irritable bowel syndrome: a critical review and meta-analysis. *Am J Gastroenterol*. 1998;93(7):1131–1135.

67. Spanier JA, Howden CW, Jones MP. A systematic review of alternative therapies in the irritable bowel syndrome. *Arch Intern Med*. 2003;163(3):265–274.

68. Pittler MH, Ernst E. Peppermint oil for irritable bowel syndrome: a critical review and meta-analysis. *Am J Gastroenterol*. 1998;93(7):1131–1135.

69. Ford AC, Talley NJ, Spiegel BM, et al. Effect of fibre, antispasmodics, and peppermint oil in the treatment of irritable bowel syndrome: systematic review and meta-analysis. *BMJ*. 2008;337:a2313.

70. Madisch A, Holtmann G, Plein K, Hotz J. Treatment of irritable bowel syndrome with herbal preparations: results of a double-blind, randomized, placebo-controlled, multi-centre trial. *Aliment Pharmacol Ther*. 2004;19(3):271–279.

71. Madisch A, Holtmann G, Plein K, Hotz J. Treatment of irritable bowel syndrome with herbal preparations: results of a double-blind, randomized, placebo-controlled, multi-centre trial. *Aliment Pharmacol Ther*. 2004;19(3):271–279.

72. Raedsch R, Hanisch J, Bock P, et al. [Assessment of the efficacy and safety of the phytopharmacon STW 5 versus metoclopramide in functional dyspepsia—a retrolective cohort study] [article in German]. *Z Gastroenterol*. 2007;45(10):1041–1048.

73. Allescher HD, Wagner H. [STW 5/Iberogast: multi-target-action for treatment of functional dyspepsia and irritable bowel syndrome]. *Wien Med Wochenschr*. 2007;157(13–14):301–307.

74. von Arnim, U, Peitz U, Vinson B, Gundermann KJ, Malfertheiner P. STW 5, a phytopharmacon for patients with functional dyspepsia: results of a multicenter, placebo-controlled double-blind study. *Am J Gastroenterol*. 2007;102(6):1268–1275.

75. Rosch W, Liebregts T, Gundermann KJ, Vinson B, Holtmann G. Phytotherapy for functional dyspepsia: a review of the clinical evidence for the herbal preparation STW 5. *Phytomedicine*. 2006;13(Suppl 5):114–121.

76. Braden B, Caspary W, Börner N, Vinson B, Schneider AR. Clinical effects of STW 5 (Iberogast) are not based on acceleration of gastric emptying in patients with functional dyspepsia and gastroparesis. *Neurogastroenterol Motil*. 2009;21(6):632–638.

77. Rosch W, Vinson B, Sassin I. A randomised clinical trial comparing the efficacy of a herbal preparation STW 5 with the prokinetic drug cisapride in patients with dysmotility type of functional dyspepsia. *Z Gastroenterol.* 2002;40(6):401–408.

78. Jacobs BP, Dennehy C, Ramirez G, Sapp J, Lawrence VA. Milk thistle for the treatment of liver disease: a systematic review and meta-analysis. *Am J Med.* 2002;113(6):506–515.

79. Dehmlow C, Erhard J, de Groot H. Inhibition of Kupffer cell functions as an explanation for the hepatoprotective properties of silibinin. *Hepatology.* 1996;23(4):749–754.

80. Saliou C, Rihn B, Cillard J, Okamoto T, Packer L. Selective inhibition of NF-kappaB activation by the flavonoid hepatoprotector silymarin in HepG2. Evidence for different activating pathways. *FEBS Lett.* 1998;440(1–2):8–12.

81. Manna SK, Mukhopadhyay A, Van NT, Aggarwal BB. Silymarin suppresses TNF-induced activation of NF-kappa B, c-Jun N-terminal kinase, and apoptosis. *J Immunol.* 1999;163(12):6800–6809.

82. Saller R, Brignoli R, Melzer J, Meier R. An updated systematic review with meta-analysis for the clinical evidence of silymarin. *Forsch Komplementmed.* 2008;15(1):9–20.

83. Ahmed-Belkacem A, Ahnou N, Barbotte L, et al. Silibinin and related compounds are direct inhibitors of hepatitis C virus RNA-dependent RNA polymerase. *Gastroenterology.* 2010;138(3):1112–1122.

84. Biermer M, Berg T. Rapid suppression of hepatitis C viremia induced by intravenous silibinin plus ribavirin. *Gastroenterology.* 2009;137(1):390–391.

85. Bengmark S, Martindale R. Prebiotics and synbiotics in clinical medicine. *Nutr Clin Pract.* 2005;20(2):244–261.

86. Lim CC, Ferguson LR, Tannock GW. Dietary fibres as "prebiotics": implications for colorectal cancer. *Mol Nutr Food Res.* 2005;49(6):609–619.

87. Roberfroid MB. Prebiotics and synbiotics: concepts and nutritional properties. *Br J Nutr.* 1998;80(4 Suppl):S197–S202.

88. Salminen S, Bouley C, Boutron-Ruault MC, et al. Functional food science and gastrointestinal physiology and function. *Br J Nutr.* 1998;80(Suppl 1):S147–S171.

89. Steed H, Macfarlane GT, Macfarlane S. Prebiotics, synbiotics and inflammatory bowel disease. *Mol Nutr Food Res.* 2008;52(8):898–905.

90. Macfarlane S, Macfarlane GT, Cummings JH. Review article: prebiotics in the gastrointestinal tract. *Aliment Pharmacol Ther.* 2006;24(5):701–714.

91. Hallert C, Björck I, Nyman M. Increasing fecal butyrate in ulcerative colitis patients by diet: controlled pilot study. *Inflamm Bowel Dis.* 2003;9(2):116–121.

92. Sartor RB. Therapeutic manipulation of the enteric microflora in inflammatory bowel diseases: antibiotics, probiotics, and prebiotics. *Gastroenterology.* 2004;126(6):1620–1633.

93. Fernandez-Banares F, Hinojosa J, Sánchez-Lombraña JL, et al. Randomized clinical trial of Plantago ovata seeds (dietary fiber) as compared with mesalamine in maintaining remission in ulcerative colitis. Spanish Group for the Study of Crohn's Disease and Ulcerative Colitis (GETECCU). *Am J Gastroenterol.* 1999;94(2):427–433.

94. Kanauchi O, Serizawa I, Araki Y, et al. Germinated barley foodstuff, a prebiotic product, ameliorates inflammation of colitis through modulation of the enteric environment. *J Gastroenterol.* 2003;38(2):134–141.

95. Welters CF, Heineman E, Thunnissen FB, et al. Effect of dietary inulin supplementation on inflammation of pouch mucosa in patients with an ileal pouch-anal anastomosis. *Dis Colon Rectum.* 2002;45(5):621–627.

96. Ruxton CH, Reed S, Simpson M, Millington K. The health benefits of omega-3 polyunsaturated fatty acids: a review of the evidence. *J Hum Nutr Diet.* 2007;20(3):275–285.

97. Bassaganya-Riera J, Hontecillas R. CLA and n-3 PUFA differentially modulate clinical activity and colonic PPAR-responsive gene expression in a pig model of experimental IBD. *Clin Nutr.* 2006;25(3):454–465.

98. Hudert CA, Weylandt KH, Lu Y, et al. Transgenic mice rich in endogenous omega-3 fatty acids are protected from colitis. *Proc Natl Acad Sci U S A.* 2006;103(30):11276–11281.

99. Whiting CV, Bland PW, Tarlton JF. Dietary n-3 polyunsaturated fatty acids reduce disease and colonic pro-inflammatory cytokines in a mouse model of colitis. *Inflamm Bowel Dis.* 2005;11(4):340–349.

100. Meister D, Ghosh S. Effect of fish oil enriched enteral diet on inflammatory bowel disease tissues in organ culture: differential effects on ulcerative colitis and Crohn's disease. *World J Gastroenterol.* 2005;11(47):7466–7472.

101. Arita M, Yoshida M, Hong S, et al. Resolvin E1, an endogenous lipid mediator derived from omega-3 eicosapentaenoic acid, protects against 2,4,6-trinitrobenzene sulfonic acid-induced colitis. *Proc Natl Acad Sci U S A.* 2005;102(21):7671–7676.

102. Shoda R, Matsueda K, Yamato S, Umeda N. Therapeutic efficacy of N-3 polyunsaturated fatty acid in experimental Crohn's disease. *J Gastroenterol.* 1995;30(Suppl 8):98–101.

103. Arslan G, Brunborg LA, Frøyland L, et al. Effects of duodenal seal oil administration in patients with inflammatory bowel disease. *Lipids.* 2002;37(10):935–940.

104. Belluzzi A, Boschi S, Brignola C, et al. Polyunsaturated fatty acids and inflammatory bowel disease. *Am J Clin Nutr.* 2000;71(1 Suppl):339S–342S.

105. Hawkey CJ, Mahida YR, Hawthorne AB. Therapeutic interventions in gastrointestinal disease based on an understanding of inflammatory mediators. *Agents Actions.* 1992;Spec No:C22–C26.

106. Hillier K, Jewell R, Dorrell L, Smith CL. Incorporation of fatty acids from fish oil and olive oil into colonic mucosal lipids and effects upon eicosanoid synthesis in inflammatory bowel disease. *Gut.* 1991;32(10):1151–1155.

107. Jorquera Plaza F, Espinel Diez J, Olcoz Goni JL. [Inflammatory bowel disease: importance of nutrition today]. *Nutr Hosp.* 1997;12(6):289–298.

108. Lorenz R, Weber PC, Szimnau P, et al. Supplementation with n-3 fatty acids from fish oil in chronic inflammatory bowel disease—a randomized, placebo-controlled, double-blind cross-over trial. *J Intern Med Suppl.* 1989;731:225–232.

109. O'Morain C, Tobin A, Suzuki Y, O'Riordan T. Risk factors in inflammatory bowel disease. *Scand J Gastroenterol Suppl.* 1989;170:58–68.

110. Razack R, Seidner DL. Nutrition in inflammatory bowel disease. *Curr Opin Gastroenterol.* 2007;23(4):400–405.

111. Simopoulos AP. Omega-3 fatty acids in inflammation and autoimmune diseases. *J Am Coll Nutr.* 2002;21(6):495–505.

112. Vilaseca J, Salas A, Guarner F, et al. Dietary fish oil reduces progression of chronic inflammatory lesions in a rat model of granulomatous colitis. *Gut.* 1990;31(5):539–544.

113. De Ley M, de Vos R, Hommes DW, Stokkers P. Fish oil for induction of remission in ulcerative colitis. *Cochrane Database Syst Rev.* 2007(4):CD005986.

114. Turner D, Zlotkin SH, Shah PS, Griffiths AM. Omega 3 fatty acids (fish oil) for maintenance of remission in Crohn's disease. *Cochrane Database Syst Rev.* 2009(1):CD006320.

115. von Roon AC, Reese GE, Orchard TR, Tekkis PP. Crohn's disease. *Clin Evid (Online).* 2007. www.ncbi.nlm.nih.gov/pmc/articles/PMC2943777. Accessed April 9, 2014.

116. Turner D, Shah PS, Steinhart AH, Zlotkin S, Griffiths AM. Maintenance of remission in inflammatory bowel disease using omega-3 fatty acids (fish oil): a systematic review and meta-analyses. *Inflamm Bowel Dis.* 2011;17(1):336–345.

117. Podolsky DK. Inflammatory bowel disease (2). *N Engl J Med.* 1991;325(14):1008–1016.

118. Podolsky DK. Inflammatory bowel disease (1). *N Engl J Med.* 1991;325(13):928–937.

119. Rode A, Fourlanos S, Nicoll A. Oral vitamin D replacement is effective in chronic liver disease. *Gastroenterol Clin Biol.* 2010;34(11):618–620.

120. Pappa HM, Gordon CM, Saslowsky TM, et al. Vitamin D status in children and young adults with inflammatory bowel disease. *Pediatrics.* 2006;118(5):1950–1961.

121. Lichtenstein GR, Sands BE, Pazianas M. Prevention and treatment of osteoporosis in inflammatory bowel disease. *Inflamm Bowel Dis.* 2006;12(8):797–813.

CHAPTER 25

Probiotics

Gerard E. Mullin, MD, CNSP, FACN, AGAF

The theory that there are therapeutic benefits to administering probiotics when treating a range of gastrointestinal (GI) and systemic conditions is supported by abundant data. The gut microbiota support host nutrition and homeostasis maintenance. Clinical trials of probiotics for GI and systemic disorders are reviewed in this chapter. The beneficial effects of probiotics are presented in Figure 25.1.

The Gut Microbiome

There are approximately 100 trillion microbial organisms—microbiota—in the intestinal tract of an adult human (1). Only 60% of the more than 500 species of gut microbes have been cultured. The upper digestive tract contains 10^3 to 10^5 species (predominated by aerobes) per gram of luminal contents, whereas the colon contains 10^{10} to 10^{11} organisms (mostly anaerobic bacteria) per gram of luminal content (2).

Facilitation of metabolic functions (eg, conversion of malabsorbed carbohydrates to energy via fermentation) is among the multitude of host benefits yielded by probiotic administration. Additional benefits include the production of short-chain fatty acids, which adds to trophic action on the epithelium; improved intestinal barrier function, which yields greater mucous production, stimulates tight cellular junctions, and boosts intestinal motility; and production of B vitamins and vitamin K. By producing bateriocin, probiotics prevent both pathologic bacteria invasion and pathologic organism adhesion while increasing resistance to bacteria colonization and decreasing luminal pH via organic acid formation (3). Probiotics are a fundamental component in immune system development and maintenance.

What Are Probiotics?

Probiotics are "live microbial feed supplements that beneficially affect the host animal by improving its intestinal microbial balance" (4). The World Health Organization (WHO) has established criteria for probiotic classification, and a number of organisms meet those standards (see Box 25.1).

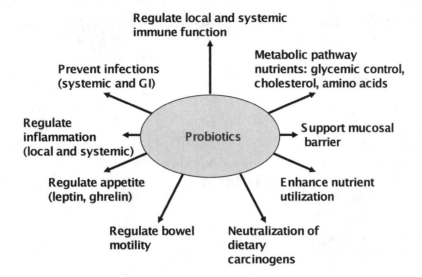

FIGURE 25.1 **The beneficial effects of probiotics and their substrates in the human host.** Probiotics have a substantial effect on the adaptive and innate immunity of the gut. The demonstrated benefits of probiotic administration include interference in clonal expansion and mucosal binding of enteric pathogens; facilitation in destroying *Helicobacter pylori, Clostridium difficile,* and a variety of other pathogens that develop in the colon; and prevention of the development of systemic infections. Gut immune function is positively affected via induction of T regulatory cells, secretory IgA production, and regulation of Th1 and Th2 cytokine production. Because a range of metabolic pathways (eg, carbohydrate, cholesterol, and protein metabolism in the liver) has been supported by probiotic administration, probiotics have been used to treat hepatic encephalopathy, decrease serum cholesterol levels, and regulate blood glucose. Mineral absorption increases while lactose intolerance decreases with probiotic administration because B vitamin and vitamin K synthesis is facilitated by the effects of probiotics in nutrient utilization and metabolism. Gut movement regulation in patients with bowel motility disorders (eg, irritable bowel syndrome) is supported by probiotics. Recent studies of leptin and ghrelin, which play a role in energy balance and appetite, have demonstrated the effect of probiotics in balancing these hormone levels and thus regulating appetite. Maintenance of the production of short-chain fatty acids for the colonocyte as its primary energy source is facilitated by probiotics, and in the gastrointestinal tract, probiotics induce anti-inflammatory and anti-neoplastic effects. Probiotics should be considered colonic foods because of how they interact with gut microflora, which is newly considered a vital organ for nourishing the body, regulating development of epithelial cells, and facilitating the functions of inborn immunity.

Clinical Uses for Probiotics

Lactose Intolerance

Diarrhea, abdominal pain, and flatulence that follow consumption of milk or milk products comprise the clinical symptoms of lactose intolerance. It is a global health problem, with prevalence ranging from 7% to 20% among whites, 50% among Hispanics, 75% among Africans and African-Americans, and more than 90% in Asian populations.

Lactose intolerance may be effectively managed with probiotic use. In individuals with lactose intolerance, the glycocalyx of the proximal small bowel has a lesser amount of lactase enzymes, and lactose therefore cannot hydrolyze to glucose and galactose. Diarrhea, abdominal pain, and flatulence result from the short-chain fatty acids and excesses of hydrogen, methane, and carbon dioxide gases produced when malabsorbed lactose is metabolized by colonic microbiota in the colon.

BOX 25.1   Selected Organisms That Are Used As Probiotic Agents

Yeast
- *Saccharomyces boulardii*

Gram-negative bacteria
- *Bifidobacterium bifidum*
- *Bifidobacterium infantis*
- *Lactococcus lactis* (engineered to produce IL-10 or trefoil factors)
- *Lactobacillus rhamnosus GG* (used with lactoferrin)
- *Lactobacillus plantarum* 299v
- *Lactobacillus acidophilus*
- *Lactobacillus casei*
- *Bacillus polyfermenticus*

Multi-strain agents
- *Lactobacillus rhamnosus GG* combined with *Bifidobacterium lactis*
- VSL#3 *(Lactobacillus casei, Lactobacillus plantarum, Lactobacillus acidophilus, Lactobacillus bulgaricus, Bifidobacterium longum, Bifidobacterium breve, Bifidobacterium infantis,* and *Streptococcus thermophilus)*

Reduction in lactose intake and/or administration of enzyme substitutes (eg, lactase supplements) or probiotics encompass typical management of lactose intolerance (5,6). However, despite six crossover trials and one parallel-group randomized trial that investigated how probiotics might improve lactose intolerance symptoms, there has not yet been sufficient evidence to support any claim that yogurt and probiotics ameliorate these GI manifestations (7–12).

Necrotizing Enterocolitis

Necrotizing enterocolitis—a severe form of enterocolitis that leads to serious morbidity (intestinal perforation, intestinal stricture, and sepsis) and has a high incidence of mortality—is a GI emergency most frequently seen in neonates, particularly those who are born prematurely. Males and black infants are at highest risk. Systematic reviews of randomized controlled trials indicate that probiotics can lower mortality from necrotizing enterocolitis and shorten time to full feeds in preterm (<34 weeks' gestation) very-low-birth weight (birth weight <1,500 g) neonates (13). In 2010, the advantages of probiotic supplementation in preterm neonates as a means to reduce incidence of death and disease was confirmed in a Cochrane meta-analysis (14).

Irritable Bowel Syndrome

Lactobacillus, Bifidobacteria, and *Saccharomyces boulardii* are the probiotic species most commonly studied and used as treatment for irritable bowel syndrome (IBS) (15–17). With the exception of stool frequency and consistency, administration of *Bifidobacterium infantis* 35624 (*B. infantis*) has been linked to IBS symptom improvement (18,19). In one study, when compared with placebo, *Lactobacillus* GG had a greater likelihood of successful treatment outcomes and reduced frequency of pain symptoms (20). Total IBS symptom scores improved with administration of a probiotic mixture of *Lactobacillus rhamnosus* GG, *L. rhamnosus* LC705, *Bifidobacterium breve* Bb99, *Propionibacterium freudenreichii* ssp, and *Propionibacterium shermanii* JS in a few studies (21,22). In another trial, bloating and flatulence improved in IBS patients taking the probiotic preparation VSL#3 compared with placebo (23). See Box 25.1 as well as the section on ulcerative colitis (later in this chapter) for more information about VSL#3. When fermented milk comprising *Bifidobacterium animalis*, *S. thermophilus*, and *L. bulgaricus* was administered to IBS patients with predominant constipation, it yielded better results than placebo in alleviating symptoms (24). In a smaller study that researched the impact of multispecies probiotic formulation on composite IBS scores, compared with placebo, the probiotic formulation effectively improved symptoms (abdominal distension and pain in particular) (25). In the pediatric IBS population, VSL#3 has been shown to be significantly more effective than placebo (26). See Chapter 9 for more information on IBS.

Traveler's Diarrhea

The most common causative bacterial organism of traveler's diarrhea (ie, diarrhea experienced by many individuals who travel from developed countries to developing countries, which can be disruptive to work and vacation plans) is enterotoxigenic *Escherichia coli*. Antibiotic administration was once the suggested prophylactic treatment for traveler's diarrhea, but probiotics recently have been included in the recommendations. McFarland's meta-analysis determined that traveler's diarrhea was significantly reduced as a result of probiotic administration (27). There is no standard recommended probiotic dosage for preventing traveler's diarrhea. However, it is generally suggested that travelers begin dosing for several days in advance of travel to attain adequate colonization and maximize protection for the first days of the trip, when risk is greatest.

Clostridium difficile infection

Accounting for 15% to 25% of antibiotic-associated diarrhea (AAD) in hospital cases, the prevalence and severity of *Clostridium difficile* (a nosocomial, toxin-mediated infection) has been increasing. Marked by characteristic clinical and pathologic features (28), toxin A and B assays confirm *C. difficile* diagnosis.

Dosages of 250 mg *Saccharomyces boulardii* twice a day for preventing *C. difficile* and four times daily for preventing recurrent *C. difficile* colitis have been proven as effective adjunctive therapy in conjunction with either metronidazole or vancomycin (29). In a meta-analysis that studied probiotics in *C. difficile*–infected patients, it was determined that the frequency of acute diarrhea decreased with probiotic administration (30). For treating recurrent *C. difficile* infections, *S. boulardii* have demonstrated effectiveness (31,32).

Antibiotic-Associated Diarrhea

AAD occurs in 5% to 25% of patients receiving antibiotics, with increased risk in elderly and immunosuppressed patients and in patients who have had GI surgery. Extensive studies of acute diarrhea in pediatric patients have shown that twice-daily dosage of one capsule of *Lactobacillus* GG is an effective treatment (33). Compared with a control group that received a placebo, AAD patients administered a daily dose of *L. plantarum*, strain 299v, had reduced severity in GI symptoms (34). Additionally, oral *L. rhamnosus* has been shown to prevent AAD onset in a pediatric population (35), whereas a 2008 meta-analysis demonstrated the therapeutic efficacy of *S. boulardii* in preventing AAD in adult patients (30).

Infectious Diarrhea

After a person ingests contaminated food or water, a common result is acute enteritis and enterocolitis. In a multicenter trial, compared with unsupplemented yogurt, yogurt supplemented with *L. casei*, strain DN-114 001, demonstrated beneficial effects in decreasing diarrhea frequency and duration in healthy children (36). Probiotic treatment in children was also shown to reduce risk and decrease duration of diarrhea in children in five meta-analyses (three studied a variety of probiotics whereas the other two focused on single organisms) (37).

Inflammatory Bowel Disease

ULCERATIVE COLITIS

In studies of the treatment of ulcerative colitis (UC), probiotic use has shown some promising results. The probiotic preparation VSL#3, which has 450 billion live bacteria per packet in each dose, has been extensively studied for this purpose. The bacteria in this preparation (which is available in the United States) include *Bifidobacterium breve, B. longum, B. infantis, L. acidophilus, L. plantarum, L. paracasei, L. bulgaricus,* and *Streptococcus thermophilus*. A number of well-designed clinical trials have shown that VSL#3 can facilitate both the induction and maintenance of remission in UC better than when medication is used alone (38–41). In a 2010 meta-analysis of the effects of administering probiotics in the treatment of UC, UC maintenance was generally improved with the probiotic compared with placebo, though the same was not true for induction of remission (42). Refer to Chapter 7 for additional information on UC.

CROHN'S DISEASE

Several published trials have evaluated the efficacy of using probiotics in the maintenance of Crohn's disease remission. A recent meta-analysis (43) that evaluated the efficacy of bacterial-derived probiotics indicated that only seven of these studies (44–50) merited consideration. Probiotics generally failed to provide an advantage for the maintenance of remission for Crohn's disease ($P = .71$; risk ratio = 1.09); thus, the use of probiotics as an adjunctive treatment for Crohn's disease is not warranted (43).

Trials using *Saccharomyces boulardii* seem to have yielded mixed results, and it has been demonstrated that *S. boulardii* does not prevent relapse of Crohn's disease (51,52). However, McFarland et al (51) conducted a systematic review for the potential efficacy of *S. boulardii* in the treatment of a number of GI conditions, including the maintenance of remission of Crohn's disease. In McFarland and colleagues' report of two randomized, double-blind placebo-controlled clinical trials (53,54), results showed that *S. boulardii* prevented relapse in patients in remission with Crohn's disease. Plein et al randomly assigned 20 patients with quiescent Crohn's disease to *S. boulardii* treatment with either 750 mg *S. boulardii* or placebo for 7 weeks, and the *S. boulardii* group had an improvement in daily stool output compared with controls (3/3 ± 1.2 vs 4.6 ± 1.9; $P<.05$) (53). In a randomized, double-blind, placebo-controlled trial to evaluate the combination of 1,000 mg *S. boulardii* with 3 g mesalamine per day compared with 3 g mesalamine per day alone in 32 patients with Crohn's disease in remission for a 6-month period, Guslandi et al determined that the *S. boulardii*–mesalamine group had a 6% relapse rate (1 of 16) compared with a rate of 38% in the mesalamine-only group (6 of 16) (54).

In a much larger prospective study of 165 patients who experienced remission after treatment with steroids or salicylates, patients were randomly assigned to groups given *S. boulardii* (1 g/d) or placebo for 52 weeks (52). There were no significant differences between groups in mean Crohn's disease activity index scores, erythrocyte sedimentation rates, or median levels of C-reactive protein.

Additional well-designed trials are needed before probiotics can be recommended for the therapy of Crohn's disease. Refer to Chapter 7 for additional information on Crohn's disease.

POUCHITIS

A nonspecific inflammation of the ileal reservoir, pouchitis occurs in approximately half of all patients after receiving ileal pouch-anal anastomosis for UC. Probiotic use has demonstrated therapeutic benefits in addressing the diminished amounts of lactobacilli and bifidobacteria in the pouch contents (55–57). For preventing pouchitis or maintaining inflammatory disease remission, VSL#3 generally has had promising results.

Safety Issues

Lactobacillus and *S. boulardii* have been associated with clinical infection in immunosuppressed, severely debilitated patients (58,59). Probiotics are not indicated in the following patient populations: those who are severely immunocompromised, those with synthetic valves, and those with indwelling central venous catheters (60,61).

Breaking capsules to add probiotics to enteral tube feedings is an unsafe practice that should never be used. Furthermore, administering probiotic preparations to patients with acute, severe (necrotizing) pancreatitis via intraduodenal delivery significantly increases the risk of death (62,63). A carefully conducted clinical research protocol is probably the only setting where probiotics should be administered to intensive care unit patients and patients with severe immune deficiencies.

Conclusion

Probiotics play a role in the amelioration of illnesses such as lactose intolerance, infantile necrotizing enterocolitis, AAD and *C. difficile* colitis, IBS, traveler's diarrhea, infantile diarrhea, *Helicobacter* IBD, and pouchitis. Ongoing and future research into the use of probiotics to maximize health will yield more evidence about their efficaciousness and benefits in preventing and treating illness and disease.

References

1. Backhed F, Ley RE, Sonnenburg JL, Peterson DA, Gordon JI. Host-bacterial mutualism in the human intestine. *Science.* 2005;307(5717):1915–1920.
2. Berg RD. The indigenous gastrointestinal microflora. *Trends Microbiol.* 1996;4(11):430–435.
3. Fedorak RN, Madsen KL. Probiotics and the management of inflammatory bowel disease. *Inflamm Bowel Dis.* 2004;10(3):286–299.
4. Fuller R. Probiotics in man and animals. *J Appl Bacteriol.* 1989;66(5):365–378.
5. Zhong Y, Huang CY, He T, Harmsen HM. Effect of probiotics and yogurt on colonic microflora in subjects with lactose intolerance. *Wei Sheng Yan Jiu.* 2006;35(5):587–591.
6. He T, Priebe MG, Zhong Y, et al. Effects of yogurt and bifidobacteria supplementation on the colonic microbiota in lactose-intolerant subjects. *J Appl Microbiol.* 2008;104(2):595–604.
7. Adhikari K, Mustapha A, Grün IU, Fernando L. Viability of microencapsulated bifidobacteria in set yogurt during refrigerated storage. *J Dairy Sci.* 2000;83(9):1946–1951.
8. Shaukat A, Levitt MD, Taylor BC, et al. Systematic review: effective management strategies for lactose intolerance. *Ann Intern Med.* 2010;152(12):797–803.
9. Liu Z, Jiang Z, Zhou K, et al. Screening of bifidobacteria with acquired tolerance to human gastrointestinal tract. *Anaerobe.* 2007;13(5–6):215–219.

10. Lin MY, Yen CL, Chen SH. Management of lactose maldigestion by consuming milk containing lactobacilli. *Dig Dis Sci.* 1998;43(1):133–137.

11. Mustapha A, Jiang T, Savaiano DA. Improvement of lactose digestion by humans following ingestion of unfermented acidophilus milk: influence of bile sensitivity, lactose transport, and acid tolerance of Lactobacillus acidophilus. *J Dairy Sci.* 1997;80(8):1537–1545.

12. Martini MC, Kukielka D, Savaiano DA. Lactose digestion from yogurt: influence of a meal and additional lactose. *Am J Clin Nutr.* 1991;53(5):1253–1258.

13. Deshpande G, Rao S, Patole S. Probiotics for prevention of necrotising enterocolitis in preterm neonates with very low birthweight: a systematic review of randomised controlled trials. *Lancet.* 2007;369(9573):1614–1620.

14. Deshpande G, Rao S, Patole S, Bulsara M. Updated meta-analysis of probiotics for preventing necrotizing enterocolitis in preterm neonates. *Pediatrics.* 2010;125(5):921–930.

15. Quigley EM. Bacterial flora in irritable bowel syndrome: role in pathophysiology, implications for management. *J Dig Dis.* 2007;8(1):2–7.

16. Quigley EM, Bytzer P, Jones R, Mearin F. Irritable bowel syndrome: the burden and unmet needs in Europe. *Dig Liver Dis.* 2006;38(10):717–723.

17. Quigley EM, Flourie B. Probiotics and irritable bowel syndrome: a rationale for their use and an assessment of the evidence to date. *Neurogastroenterol Motil.* 2007;19(3):166–172.

18. O'Mahony L, McCarthy J, Kelly P, et al. Lactobacillus and bifidobacterium in irritable bowel syndrome: symptom responses and relationship to cytokine profiles. *Gastroenterology.* 2005;128(3):541–551.

19. Whorwell PJ, Altringer L, Morel J, et al. Efficacy of an encapsulated probiotic Bifidobacterium infantis 35624 in women with irritable bowel syndrome. *Am J Gastroenterol.* 2006;101(7):1581–1590.

20. Gawronska A, Dziechciarz P, Horvath A, Szajewska H. A randomized double-blind placebo-controlled trial of Lactobacillus GG for abdominal pain disorders in children. *Aliment Pharmacol Ther,* 2007;25(2):177–184.

21. Kajander K, Hatakka K, Poussa T, Färkkilä M, Korpela R. A probiotic mixture alleviates symptoms in irritable bowel syndrome patients: a controlled 6-month intervention. *Aliment Pharmacol Ther.* 2005;22(5):387–394.

22. Guslandi M, Mezzi G, Sorghi M, Testoni PA. Saccharomyces boulardii in maintenance treatment of Crohn's disease. *Dig Dis Sci.* 2000;45(7):1462–1464.

23. Kim HJ, Vazquez Roque MI, Camilleri M, et al. A randomized controlled trial of a probiotic combination VSL#3 and placebo in irritable bowel syndrome with bloating. *Neurogastroenterol Motil.* 2005;17(5):687–696.

24. Guyonnet D, Chassany O, Ducrotte P, et al. Effect of a fermented milk containing Bifidobacterium animalis DN-173 010 on the health-related quality of life and symptoms in irritable bowel syndrome in adults in primary care: a multicentre, randomized, double-blind, controlled trial. *Aliment Pharmacol Ther.* 2007;26(3):475–486.

25. Kajander K, Krogius-Kurikka L, Rinttilä T, et al. Effects of multispecies probiotic supplementation on intestinal microbiota in irritable bowel syndrome. *Aliment Pharmacol Ther.* 2007;26(3):463–473.

26. Ghoshal UC, Park H, Gwee KA. Bugs and irritable bowel syndrome: the good, the bad and the ugly. *J Gastroenterol Hepatol.* 2010;25(2):244–251.

27. McFarland LV. Meta-analysis of probiotics for the prevention of traveler's diarrhea. *Travel Med Infect Dis.* 2007;5(2):97–105.

28. Bartlett JG. Clostridium difficile-associated enteric disease. *Curr Infect Dis Rep.* 2002;4(6):477–483.

29. McFarland LV. Meta-analysis of probiotics for the prevention of antibiotic associated diarrhea and the treatment of Clostridium difficile disease. *Am J Gastroenterol.* 2006;101(4):812–822.

30. McFarland LV, Dublin S. Meta-analysis of probiotics for the treatment of irritable bowel syndrome. *World J Gastroenterol.* 2008;14(17):2650–2661.

31. Tung JM, Dolovich LR, Lee CH. Prevention of Clostridium difficile infection with Saccharomyces boulardii: a systematic review. *Can J Gastroenterol.* 2009;23(12):817–821.

32. Pillai A, Nelson R. Probiotics for treatment of Clostridium difficile-associated colitis in adults. *Cochrane Database Syst Rev.* 2008(1):CD004611.

33. Doron S, Snydman DR, Gorbach SL. Lactobacillus GG: bacteriology and clinical applications. *Gastroenterol Clin North Am.* 2005;34(3):483–498.

34. Lonnermark E, Friman V, Lappas G, et al. Intake of Lactobacillus plantarum reduces certain gastrointestinal symptoms during treatment with antibiotics. *J Clin Gastroenterol.* 2010;44(2):106–112.

35. Ruszczynski M, Radzikowski A, Szajewska H. Clinical trial: effectiveness of Lactobacillus rhamnosus (strains E/N, Oxy and Pen) in the prevention of antibiotic-associated diarrhoea in children. *Aliment Pharmacol Ther.* 2008;28(1):154–161.

36. Parassol N, Freitas M, Thoreux K, et al. Lactobacillus casei DN-114 001 inhibits the increase in paracellular permeability of enteropathogenic Escherichia coli-infected T84 cells. *Res Microbiol.* 2005;156(2):256–262.

37. Szajewska H, Skórka A, Ruszczyński M, Gieruszczak-Białek D. Meta-analysis: Lactobacillus GG for treating acute diarrhoea in children. *Aliment Pharmacol Ther.* 2007;25(8):871–881.

38. Bibiloni R, Fedorak RN, Tannock GW, et al. VSL#3 probiotic-mixture induces remission in patients with active ulcerative colitis. *Am J Gastroenterol.* 2005;100(7):1539–1546.

39. Miele E, Pascarella F, Giannetti E, et al. Effect of a probiotic preparation (VSL#3) on induction and maintenance of remission in children with ulcerative colitis. *Am J Gastroenterol.* 2009;104(2):437–443.

40. Sood A, Midha V, Makharia GK, et al. The probiotic preparation, VSL#3 induces remission in patients with mild-to-moderately active ulcerative colitis. *Clin Gastroenterol Hepatol.* 2009;7(11):1202–1209.

41. Tursi A. Balsalazide plus high-potency probiotic preparation (VSL#3) in the treatment of acute mild-to-moderate ulcerative colitis and uncomplicated diverticulitis of the colon. *J Clin Gastroenterol.* 2008;42(Suppl 3 Pt 1):S119–S122.

42. Sang LX, Chang B, Zhang WL, et al. Remission induction and maintenance effect of probiotics on ulcerative colitis: a meta-analysis. *World J Gastroenterol.* 2010;16(15):1908–1915.

43. Shen J, Zuo ZX, Mao AP. Effect of probiotics on inducing remission and maintaining therapy in ulcerative colitis, Crohn's disease, and pouchitis: meta-analysis of randomized controlled trials. *Inflamm Bowel Dis.* 2014;20(1):21–23.

44. Malchow HA. Crohn's disease and Escherichia coli. A new approach in therapy to maintain remission of colonic Crohn's disease? *J Clin Gastroenterol.* 1997;25:653–658.

45. Prantera C, Scribano ML, Falasco G, et al. Ineffectiveness of probiotics in preventing recurrence after curative resection for Crohn's disease: a randomised controlled trial with Lactobacillus GG. *Gut.* 2002;51:405–409.

46. Schultz M, Timmer A, Herfarth HH, et al. Lactobacillus GG in inducing and maintaining remission of Crohn's disease. *BMC Gastroenterol.* 2004;4:5.

47. Bousvaros A, Guandalini S, Baldassano RN, et al. A randomized, double-blind trial of Lactobacillus GG versus placebo in addition to standard maintenance therapy for children with Crohn's disease. *Inflamm Bowel Dis.* 2005;11:833–839.

48. Marteau P, Lémann M, Seksik P. Ineffectiveness of Lactobacillus johnsonii LA1 for prophylaxis of post-operative recurrence in Crohn's disease: a randomised, double blind, placebo controlled GETAID trial. *Gut.* 2006;55:842–847.

49. Van Gossum A, Dewit O, Louis E, et al. Multicenter randomized-controlled clinical trial of probiotics (Lactobacillus johnsonii, LA1) on early endoscopic recurrence of Crohn's disease after Ileo-caecal resection. *Inflamm Bowel Dis.* 2007;13(2):135–142.

50. Steed H, Macfarlane GT, Blackett KL, et al. Clinical trial: the microbiological and immunological effects of synbiotic consumption: a randomized double-blind placebo-controlled study in active Crohn's disease. *Aliment Pharmacol Ther.* 2010;32:872–883.

51. McFarland LV. Systematic review and meta-analysis of Saccharomyces boulardii in adult patients. *World J Gastroenterol.* 2010;16(18):2202–2222.

52. Bourreille A, Cadiot G, Le Dreau G, et al. Saccharomyces boulardii does not prevent relapse of Crohn's disease. *Clin Gastroenterol Hepatol.* 2013;11(8):982–987.

53. Plein K, Hotz J. Therapeutic effects of Saccharomyces boulardii on mild residual symptoms in a stable phase of Crohn's disease with special respect to chronic diarrhea: a pilot study. *Z Gastroenterol*. 1993;31:129–134.

54. Guslandi M, Mezzi G, Sorghi M, Testoni PA. Saccharomyces boulardii in maintenance treatment of Crohn's disease. *Dig Dis Sci*. 2000;45:1462–1464.

55. Gionchetti P, Rizzello F, Venturi A, et al. Oral bacteriotherapy as maintenance treatment in patients with chronic pouchitis: a double-blind, placebo-controlled trial. *Gastroenterology*. 2000;119(2):305–309.

56. Mimura T, Rizzello F, Helwig U, et al. Once daily high dose probiotic therapy (VSL#3) for maintaining remission in recurrent or refractory pouchitis. *Gut*. 2004;53(1):108–114.

57. Elahi B, Nikfar S, Derakhshani S, Vafaie M, Abdollahi M. On the benefit of probiotics in the management of pouchitis in patients who underwent ileal pouch anal anastomosis: a meta-analysis of controlled clinical trials. *Dig Dis Sci*. 2008;53(5):1278–1284.

58. Gasser F. Safety of lactic acid bacteria and their occurrence in human clinical infection. *Bull Inst Pasteur*. 1994;92:45–67.

59. Schlegel L, Lemerel S, Geslin P. Lactobacillus species as opportunistic pathogens in immune-compromised patients. *Clin Microbiol Infect*. 1998;17:87–88.

60. Hennequin C, Kauffmann-Lacroix C, Jobert A, et al. Possible role of catheters in Saccharomyces boulardii fungemia. *Eur J Clin Microbiol Infect Dis*. 2000;19(1):16–20.

61. Land MH, Rouster-Stevens K, Woods CR, et al. Lactobacillus sepsis associated with probiotic therapy. *Pediatrics*. 2005;115(1):178–181.

62. Besselink MG, van Santvoort HC, Renooij W, et al. Intestinal barrier dysfunction in a randomized trial of a specific probiotic composition in acute pancreatitis. *Ann Surg*. 2009;250(5):712–719.

63. McClave SA, Heyland DK, Wischmeyer PE. Comment on: probiotic prophylaxis in predicted severe acute pancreatitis: a randomized, double-blind, placebo-controlled trial. *JPEN J Parenter Enteral Nutr*. 2009;33(4):444–446.

CHAPTER 26

Ethical and Legal Issues in Gastrointestinal Nutrition Interventions

Denise Baird Schwartz, MS, RD, CNSC, FADA, FAND, FASPEN

Gastrointestinal (GI) nutrition can involve ethical and legal issues for health care professionals, patients, and the families of patients. In particular, the provision of nutrients through tubes into the GI tract or through intravenous lines is a form of medical therapy, and decisions about the initiation, continued use, or discontinuation of this treatment have important ethical and legal dimensions, such as:

- Who is empowered (legally and ethically) to make these decisions?
- On what basis should these decisions be made? (eg, quality of life or likely clinical outcomes; the patient's or family's desires; cultural and religious values)
- What types of institutional policies and procedures will help clinicians and patients make timely and ethical choices for care?

This chapter explores these sorts of questions regarding the ethics and legality of GI nutrition and hydration and offers general guidance for clinicians navigating this challenging aspect of patient care. Readers unfamiliar with terminology used when dealing with ethical and legal aspects of GI nutrition care will find a list of definitions in the appendix to this book. The appendix also includes a list of useful resources for additional exploration of this topic.

The Law and End-of-Life Decisions

The legal history related to the discontinuation of GI nutrition through tubes spans several decades. Box 26.1 summarizes three of the landmark court cases that have shaped current legal opinion (1,2). A more in-depth discussion of this area of law is beyond the scope of this chapter. Legal positions on end-of-life care are continually evolving, and state and local laws and regulations can vary. Therefore, health care providers should seek appropriate legal counsel to guide their own practice.

BOX 26.1   Notable Legal Cases Related to the Ethics of Tube Feeding

Karen Ann Quinlan (1954–1985)

In 1975 Quinlan had a brain injury that left her in a PVS. In 1976 the New Jersey Supreme Court ruled that the ventilator, a life-sustaining measure, could be removed if the prognosis was "no reasonable possibility of a patient returning to a cognitive, sapient state" and a hospital ethics committee could confirm such a conclusion. Quinlan was removed from ventilator. Tube feeding continued. The following are implications of this case for ethical decision-making:

- It introduced the "substitutional judgment" or "subjective test," which allows a proxy to decide what the individual would have wanted.
- It provided for criminal and civil legal protection for all involved parties in the decision-making process.
- It helped establish hospital ethics committees and enactment of "living will" legislation at the state level.

Nancy Beth Cruzan (1957–1990)

In 1983 Cruzan sustained injuries in a car accident that resulted in a PVS. In 1990 the Missouri Supreme Court determined that her feeding tube could lawfully be removed only if there were "clear and convincing evidence" that removal was in accordance with her wishes. In 1990 the US Supreme Court acknowledged a constitutional right that grants a competent person a right to refuse life-saving hydration and nutrition, ruled that a surrogate may act for the patient in electing to withdraw treatment, and indicated that clear and convincing evidence of an incompetent person's wishes to withdraw treatment to be an appropriate standard of proof. The US Supreme Court thus rejected the coguardians' contentions that the state must accept the substituted judgment of close family members and established ANH as life-sustaining medical treatment, no different than ventilators and hemodialysis. The court recommended use of DPAHC and living wills as valuable safeguards to a patient's interest in directing medical care. Cruzan's tube feeding was stopped. This case stimulated increased use of health care proxies or DPAHC, and it was the reason for the enactment of the Patient Self Determination Act of 1990.

Theresa Marie (Terri) Schiavo (1963–2005)

In 1990 Schiavo went into cardiac arrest, which resulted in a PVS. In 1998 her husband filed a Florida petition to have the feeding tube removed on grounds that Schiavo would not wish to be maintained in a PVS. Her parents argued the opposite position. Their legal debate led to two feeding tube removals and reinsertions, four rejected appeals to the Supreme Court, and intervention by the Florida legislature and governor, Congress, and the president. In 2005 the federal district court refused to order the reinsertion of the feeding tube, and Schiavo's tube feeding was permanently stopped. The political reaction to this case resulted in refinement of living will legislation with regards to ANH in several states.

Abbreviations: ANH, artificial nutrition and hydration; DPAHC, durable power of attorney for health care; GI, gastrointestinal; PVS, persistent vegetative state, TF, tube feeding.
Source: Data are from references 1 and 2.

Recommendations from Professional Societies

In clinical practice, the inclusion of an interprofessional perspective is essential to achieve the best outcomes for the patient. For this reason, it is important for clinicians to understand the positions and recommendations of leading national organizations involved in health and nutrition care (3–15). Common themes in these documents include the following:

- Autonomy
- Use of informed surrogate decision-makers when individuals are unable to speak for themselves
- Artificial nutrition as medical therapy
- The burden vs benefit of the life-sustaining therapies based on the individual's quality-of-life goals
- The importance of advance care planning in the process

For registered dietitians, the positions of the Academy of Nutrition and Dietetics (3,4) and American Society for Parenteral and Enteral Nutrition (A.S.P.E.N.) (5) on ethics in feeding and hydration are of particular relevance, and these perspectives are therefore presented here. See references 6 through 15 for the positions and recommendations of other leading organizations.

Academy of Nutrition and Dietetics Position and Practice Papers

In 2013 the Academy of Nutrition and Dietetics published position and practice papers regarding ethical and legal issues of feeding and hydration (3,4). The two papers should be used together, as the practice paper provides a proactive, integrated systematic process to implement the Academy's position. Box 26.2 (page 336) presents the Academy position and summary guidelines for feeding (3). Box 26.3 (pages 336–338) draws from the associated practice paper to outline an ethical deliberative process that can align clinical decision-making with the Academy's position (4).

American Society for Parenteral and Enteral Nutrition Ethics Position

The A.S.P.E.N. 2010 position paper on ethics (5) provides a critical summary of the major ethical and legal issues related to the provision of artificial nutrition and hydration (ANH), offers guidance for practitioners confronted with these dilemmas, and directs readers to additional references for further study. See Box 26.4 (pages 338–339) for key points from this paper (5).

Religious, Cultural, and Ethnic Considerations

Religious, cultural, and ethnic factors may shape an individual's views on end-of-life care and the use of life-sustaining therapies, such as GI tube feedings. Box 26.5 on page 340 (16,17) identifies differences among religious perspectives on end-of-life decisions. However, it is important to keep in mind that each individual is unique, and one person's decision-making process will not necessarily be the same as the process for another person who practices the same religion or comes from a similar cultural or ethnic background.

BOX 26.2 Academy of Nutrition and Dietetics Position on Ethical and Legal Issues in Feeding and Hydration and Summary Guidelines for Feeding

Position

It is the position of the Academy of Nutrition and Dietetics that individuals have the right to request or refuse nutrition and hydration as medical treatment. Registered dietitians should work collaboratively as part of an interprofessional team to make recommendations on providing, withdrawing, or withholding nutrition and hydration in individual cases and serve as active members of institutional ethics committees.

Summary Guidelines for Feeding

The nutritional concept of "when in doubt, feed" is applicable to most individuals. Feeding should start immediately upon being medically stable and continue until treatment is futile. During feeding, the goals are to provide adequate nutrients to maintain or achieve reasonable weight and muscle mass, and achieve hydration when possible. Feeding may be discontinued if authorized by the individual or surrogate, if it is clinically contraindicated, or after the individual is diagnosed as permanently unconscious, with evidence of the individual's wish to stop feeding. In cases where evidence strongly suggests that feeding or hydration does not provide benefit, it is the responsibility of the interprofessional health care team to explain this to the individual or authorized surrogate, but it is the individual or authorized surrogate that decides.

Source: Reprinted with permission from reference 3: O'Sullivan Maillet J, Schwartz DB, Posthauer ME. Position of the Academy of Nutrition and Dietetics: ethical and legal issues of feeding and hydration. *J Acad Nutr Diet.* 2013;113;828–833.

BOX 26.3 Suggested Ethical Deliberations about Nutrition and Hydration

1. The individual's expressed desire for extent of medical care is a primary guide for determining the level of nutrition intervention.
2. The decision to forgo hydration or nutrition should be weighed carefully, because such a decision may result in nutrient deficits that are difficult or impossible to reverse.
3. The expected benefits, in contrast to the potential burdens, of non-oral feeding must be evaluated by the health care team and discussed with the person. The focus of care should include the individual's physical and psychological comfort.
4. Artificial nutrition and hydration are considered medical interventions.
5. Consider whether or not nutrition, either oral or through a tube, will improve the individual's preferred quality of life during the end-of-life period.
6. Consider whether or not nutrition, either oral or through a tube, can be expected to provide the person with emotional comfort, decreased anxiety about disease cachexia, improved self-esteem with cosmetic benefits, improved interpersonal relationships, or relief of fear or abandonment.
7. If death is imminent and feeding will not alter the condition, consider whether or not artificial nutrition through tubes will be burdensome, creating discomfort for the individual.
8. When oral intake is appropriate:
   a. Oral feeding should be advocated whenever possible, based on an individual's desire. Food and control of food intake may give comfort, pleasure and a sense of autonomy

Continues

BOX 26.3 Suggested Ethical Deliberations about Nutrition and Hydration *(Continued)*

and dignity. The most important priority is to provide food according to the individual's wishes.

b. Efforts should be made to enhance the person's physical and emotional enjoyment of food by encouraging staff and family assistance in feeding the individual, as needed.

c. Nutrition supplements, including commercial products and other alternatives, may be used to encourage intake and ameliorate symptoms associated with hunger, thirst, or malnutrition, if these occur.

d. Dietary restrictions should be individualized and/or liberalized. Coordination of medication or medication schedules with the diet should be discussed with the physician, with the objective of maximizing food choices and intake by the person.

e. The person's right to self-determination must be considered in determining whether to allow the individual to consume foods that are not generally permitted within the diet prescription.

f. Suboptimal oral feedings may be more appropriate than burdensome enteral tube feedings or parenteral feedings.

9. When enteral tube feeding or parenteral feeding is being considered:

a. The informed individual's preference for the level of nutrition intervention is primary. The person or designated surrogate decisionmaker should be advised on how to accomplish whatever feeding is desired.

b. When palliative care is the agreed goal, consideration of use or discontinuation of artificial nutrition should be part of the discernment process, based on the informed person's wishes, including benefit and risk burden.

c. Feeding may not be desirable if death is expected within hours or a few days and the effects of partial dehydration or the withdrawal of nutrition support (enteral tube feeding or parenteral nutrition) will not adversely alter the individual's comfort.

d. Health care facilities and/or agencies should provide and distribute written protocols for the provision of and termination of enteral tube feedings and parenteral feedings. The protocols should be reviewed periodically, and revised if necessary, by the interprofessional health care team. Legal and ethical counsel, as needed, should be routinely sought during the development and interpretation of the guidelines. The health care facilities' ethics committee, if available, should assist in establishing and implementing defined, written guidelines for a nutrition support policy. The registered dietitian should be a contributing member of the committee.

e. Conflict within the family or among stakeholders can be resolved by referring to an ethics committee or consultant if available within the institution.

f. The potential benefits versus burdens of enteral tube feeding or parenteral feeding should be weighed on the basis of specific facts concerning the individual's medical and mental status, as well as on the facility's options and limitations.

g. Health care facilities limitations that should be considered:

   (1) Lack of staffing, limiting ability to manage and monitor feeding

   (2) Financial limitations

   (3) If a feeding strategy is started in one site, it may have to be stopped when the individual is transferred to another site within the same facility or to another facility. This can lead to a sense of abandonment for the person.

Continues

**BOX 26.3   Suggested Ethical Deliberations about Nutrition and Hydration
*(Continued)***

10. Either short- or long-term parenteral nutrition should be considered only when other routes are impossible or inadequate to meet the comfort needs of the person.
11. When the physician's diet order in medical record documents the decision to forgo nutrition support:
    a. The registered dietitian (RD) should participate in the decision process.
    b. If a decision is made that the RD does not agree with, the RD should first contact the ordering physician to discuss; then the RD would discuss with the primary physician if the ordering physician was a consultant. The RD should discuss with individual's nurse and document in the medical record, indicating persons contacted and the outcome. If the RD felt this was not resolved, contacting the facility's ethics mechanism (committee or consultant) is appropriate and document in the medical record.
    c. If the court has ordered feeding or no feeding and there is disagreement with the court's decision, appeal to the facility's ethics mechanism is appropriate.

Source: Reprinted with permission from reference 4: Schwartz DB, Posthauer ME, O'Sullivan Maillet J. Practice paper of Academy of Nutrition and Dietetics: ethical and legal issues of feeding and hydration. Abstract: *J Acad Nutr Diet.* 2013;113(7):981. Full paper: www.eatright.org/Members/content.aspx?id=6442476744. Accessed October 9, 2013.

**BOX 26.4   American Society for Parenteral and Enteral Nutrition Ethics Position
Paper Summary**

1. To the extent possible, decisions regarding ANH [artificial nutrition and hydration] should be based on EBM [evidence-based medicine], best practices, and clinical experience and judgment in discussion with the patient, family, or significant others.
2. From a scientific, ethical, and legal perspective there should be no differentiation between withholding and withdrawing of ANH, thus this paper employs the term "forgoing" for both, recognizing that withdrawing is more emotionally laden than withholding, especially within specific cultures.
3. Decisions regarding forgoing ANH should incorporate a benefit-risk-burden analysis based on EBM and best practice in discussion with the patient, family, or significant others.
4. Limited time trials are an acceptable alternative when the benefits of ANH are questionable and the trial nature of ANH is communicated and consented to by the patient and family prior to its initiation.
5. Scientific evidence on the physiology of patients with brain death, in a coma, or in a persistent vegetative state (PVS), indicates these patients do not experience thirst or hunger, and therefore are not likely to suffer.
6. ANH may not provide any benefit and may have associated risks in patients with severe dementia or in a PVS.
7. Artificial hydration of terminally ill patients can lead to discomfort due to fluid overload, pulmonary and generalized edema, shortness of breath, etc. and may be discontinued on clinical and ethical grounds provided such discontinuation is not in conflict with existing laws, institutional policies and consent/consensus of decision-makers.

Continues

BOX 26.4   American Society for Parenteral and Enteral Nutrition Ethics Position Paper Summary *(Continued)*

8. Forgoing ANH in infants and children at the end-of-life may be ethically acceptable when competent parents and the medical team concur that the intervention no longer confers a benefit to the child or creates a burden that cannot be justified.

9. The religious, cultural and ethnic background of patients and families needs to be respected to the extent it is consistent with other ethical principles and duties.

10. Consent, respect, and preservation of dignity should be paramount during ethical and legal deliberations regarding ANH.

11. Many states in the U.S. require "clear and convincing evidence" to forgo ANH in decisionally incapacitated patients without documented ANH preferences.

12. Patients with decisional-making capacity and authority should be the appropriate moral agents to make choices regarding ANH based on evidence-based information qualified practitioners present to them.

13. For patients lacking decision-making capacity, the health care professional has an ethical and legal obligation to reference an advance directive or discussion with the authorized surrogate decision-maker, whether appointed through mechanisms of a durable power of attorney for health care directive, court or statutory process.

14. Surrogate decision-makers (including but not limited to family members and/or significant others) should be given the same considerations as individual patients with decision-making capacity.

15. Health care professionals should not be ethically obligated to offer ANH if in their clinical judgment there is not adequate evidence for the therapy, or the burden or risk of the intervention far outweighs its benefit.

16. The establishment of interdisciplinary teams and conferences with the patient and family is highly encouraged. Interdisciplinary ethics committees or panels should be consulted when the involved parties cannot resolve the ethical dilemma.

17. Care should continue until the conflict regarding ANH is resolved. If unable to resolve conflicts, even with an ethics consultation, orderly transfer of care assuring continuity of care is recommended to an equally qualified and willing practitioner and/or institution. At no time should patients or family feel abandoned.

Source: Reprinted from reference 5: Barrocas A, Geppert G, Durfee SM, O'Sullivan Maillet J, Monturo C, Mueller C, Stratton K, Valentine C, A.S.P.E.N. Board of Directors. A.S.P.E.N. Ethics Position Paper. *Nutr Clin Pract.* 2010;25:672–679. Copyright © 2010 *Nutrition in Clinical Practice.* Reprinted by permission of SAGE Publications.

Creating Institution-Specific Policies and Procedures

Despite the availability of legal precedents, position and practice papers, and sociocultural information, there remains a practice gap in the ethical decision-making process related to GI nutrition as a life-sustaining medical therapy. To improve in this area, health care facilities should establish a proactive, integrated, systematic process and encourage increased communication of health care wishes and advance care planning. A sample quality improvement project for ethics and artificial nutrition is presented in Box 26.6 (page 341). Box 26.7 (page 342) offers an example of an intensive care unit (ICU) artificial nutrition health care choices communication policy and procedure. Development of this type of policy and

BOX 26.5   Religious Perspectives on Health Care and End-of-Life Decisions

Catholicism (16)
- Person has a moral obligation to use ordinary or proportionate means of preserving his or her life.
- Person may forgo extraordinary or disproportionate means of life.
- Medically assisted nutrition and hydration become morally optional when they cannot reasonably be expected to prolong life or when they would be excessively burdensome for individual or would cause significant physical discomfort, for example resulting from complications in use of means employed.
- Free and informed judgment made by a competent adult individual concerning use or withdrawal of life-sustaining procedures should always be respected and normally complied with, unless it is contrary to Catholic moral teaching.

Greek Orthodoxy (17)
- Withholding or withdrawing of artificial nutrition is not allowable even if there is no prospect of recovery.

Hinduism and Sikh (17)
- Duty-based rather than rights-based faiths, with belief in karma (a casual law where all acts and human thoughts have consequences).
- Death is viewed as a passage to a new life; way you die is important.
- A do not attempt resuscitation order is usually accepted or desired because death should be peaceful.

Islam (17)
- Premature death should be prevented, but treatments can be withheld or withdrawn in terminally ill individuals when physicians are certain about inevitability of death, and that treatment in no way will improve condition or quality of life.
- Intention must never be to hasten death, only to abstain from overzealous treatment.

Judaism (17)
- Withdrawal of continuous life-sustaining therapy is not allowed, but withholding further treatment is allowed as part of dying process if it is an intermittent life-sustaining treatment, and if it was a clear wish of patient.
- Food and fluid are regarded as basic needs and not treatment.
- It is permissible to withhold food and fluid if this is individual's expressed wishes, when individual approaches final days of life, when food and even fluids may cause suffering and complications.

Protestantism (17)
- Most Protestants will, if there is little hope of recovery, accept and understand withholding or withdrawal of therapy.

BOX 26.6 Sample Quality Improvement Project for Ethics and Artificial Nutrition

1. Determine the number patients in the intensive care unit (ICU) on artificial nutrition (gastrointestinal tube feedings and intravenous nutrition) and the percentage of these patients that have an advance directive on chart, family care conference, palliative care and bioethics consults.
2. Collect patient data of all individuals receiving artificial nutrition and analyze with inter-professional health care team.
3. Compare results with current benchmarked data in literature.
4. Develop an institution policy and procedure for communication and ethical decision-making for artificial nutrition collaboratively with health care team; obtain approval of the policy and procedure through medical committees.
5. Educate the interprofessional health care team on the policy and procedure process and implement it.
6. Remeasure the patients in the ICU on artificial nutrition to determine the effects of the change in practice and assess its sustainability.
7. Share best practices for ethics and artificial nutrition among health care institutions and organizations.

---

procedure should involve an interprofessional health care team. The components of the policy and procedure should be derived from a review of the position and practice papers, statements, and/or guidelines of relevant national organizations (3–16) and also modified as appropriate for the patient population of the facility. Box 26.8 (page 343) lists selected resources that can be used in the policy and procedures team's discussion of quality-of-life goals for the facility.

Health care facilities that develop a proactive, integrated, systematic process for artificial nutrition decision-making will improve the communication process for patients, their families, and health care professionals. Written documentation in the medical record is important, but verbal communication between the patient, his or her family, and the health care team about wishes for medical therapies, including GI nutrition, is also beneficial. For example, discussion between the health care team and the hospitalized patient and the patient's family about the uses and potential benefits and risks of nutrition support therapy through tubes may provide an opening for a broader conversation about the goals of care (18).

Ideally, the decision-making process should start early, before a patient is ill and hospitalized, with individuals engaging and becoming empowered by advance care planning (19–21). The appendix to this book lists numerous resources for both the health care professional and the public related to advance care planning.

Conclusion

Ethical and legal issues related to the use and discontinuation of GI nutrition through tubes have been addressed for decades. Several national health care organizations, including the Academy of Nutrition and Dietetics and A.S.P.E.N., have provided recommendations on this topic. Common themes in these recommendations are autonomy, use of informed surrogate decision-makers when individuals are unable to speak for themselves, the need for an interdisciplinary approach, consideration of the burden vs benefit of the life-sustaining therapies based on the individual's quality-of-life goals, and the importance of advance care planning.

BOX 26.7   Sample Artificial Nutrition Health Care Choices Communication Policy and Procedure for Intensive Care Units

Policy: Policy is to provide ethically and medically appropriate artificial nutrition in the intensive care unit (ICU), based on evidence-based guidelines and recommendations of national organizations.

Purpose: Purpose is to promote health literacy and written documentation in the medical record concerning health care decisions for artificial nutrition. The intent is to promote early communication between health care professionals, patients, and families/surrogate decision-makers, with attention to spiritual/faith and cultural diversity.

Important considerations: Include components from the following organizations and other organizations as appropriate for the institution population, culture, and religious affiliation:
  a. Academy Nutrition and Dietetics Position Paper and Practice Paper on Ethical and Legal Issues in Feeding and Hydration
  b. American Society for Parenteral and Enteral Nutrition (A.S.P.E.N.) Ethics Position Paper

Procedure:
1. Health care clinicians would be involved in training sessions dealing with communication, spiritual and cultural diversity, difficult subjects, role playing, and teach-back method.
2. An evaluation tool would be completed after the discussion with the patient/family. This tool would incorporate both health care professional and patient/family evaluation. The results would be evaluated for revisions and re-evaluated periodically.
3. Information obtained about patient's health care choices for artificial nutrition would be communicated verbally with health care team and in medical record.
4. Patients in ICU ≥3 days should be screened for palliative care needs based on defined screening criteria, as developed by the palliative care team. Patients would be identified during ICU rounds at high risk for palliative care team need to help with health care choices for quality-of-life goals, including use of artificial nutrition.
5. Family care conferences are recommended for patients in ICU 5 to 7 days or less, incorporating a discussion on artificial nutrition, as appropriate. Include documentation in progress notes and family care conference outcome/recommended plan.

References: [Add citations of relevance to the facility.]

Approval: [Signed and dated by the Medical Committee.]

An individual's views on end-of-life care and use of life-sustaining therapies, such as GI nutrition through tubes, may be shaped by his or her religious convictions and ethnic and cultural background. Health care providers should always respect the values and uniqueness of every individual in their care. To this end, health care facilities need institutional policies and procedures to assist clinicians in ethical and legal areas and empower patients in planning for their own care.

BOX 26.8   Sources for Quality-of-Life Goals for Artificial Nutrition Decision-Making

- Advance directives
- Durable power of attorney for health care (DPAHC)
- Physician orders for life-sustaining treatment (POLST)
- Interprofessional unit rounds
- Discussion with health care professionals, including physicians, registered dietitians, nurses, social workers, chaplains, case managers, and palliative care team members
- Comments made during discussion by individuals and their family, when assessing nutritional status and during nutrition support education
- Futility of treatment based on an individual's overall clinical status, as assessed by the physician and documented in medical record

---

Source: Data are from reference 2.

References

1. Geppert CMA, Barrocas A, Schwartz DB. Ethics and law. In: Mueller C, Kovacevich D, McClave S, Miller S, Schwartz DB, eds. *The A.S.P.E.N. Adult Nutrition Support Core Curriculum.* 2nd ed. Springfield, MD: American Society for Parenteral and Enteral Nutrition. 2012:656–676.

2. Schwartz DB. Ethical considerations in the critically ill patient. In: Cresci G, ed. *Nutritional Therapy for the Critically Ill Patient: A Guide to Practice.* 2nd ed. Boca Raton, FL: Taylor & Francis; 2014 (in press).

3. O'Sullivan Maillet J, Schwartz DB, Posthauer ME. Position of the Academy of Nutrition and Dietetics: ethical and legal issues of feeding and hydration. *J Acad Nutr Diet.* 2013;113;828–833.

4. Schwartz DB, Posthauer ME, O'Sullivan Maillet J. Practice Paper of Academy of Nutrition and Dietetics: ethical and legal issues of feeding and hydration. Abstract: *J Acad Nutr Diet.* 2013;113(7):981. Full paper: www.eatright.org/Members/content.aspx?id=6442476744. Accessed October 9, 2013.

5. Barrocas A, Geppert G, Durfee SM, O'Sullivan Maillet J, Monturo C, Mueller C, Stratton K, Valentine C, A.S.P.E.N. Board of Directors. A.S.P.E.N. Ethics Position Paper. *Nutr Clin Pract.* 2010;25:672–679.

6. Alzheimer's Association. Assisted Oral Feeding and Tube Feeding. 2011. www.alz.org/documents_custom /statements/assisted_oral_tube_feeding.pdf. Accessed July 4, 2013.

7. American Academy of Hospice and Palliative Medicine. Five Things Physicians and Patients Should Question. www.choosingwisely.org/doctor-patient-lists/american-academy-of-hospice-palliative-medicine. Accessed October 9, 2013.

8. Snyder L. American College of Physicians Ethics Manual 6th ed. *Ann Intern Med.* 2012;156:73–104.

9. American Geriatric Society (AGS). Feeding Tubes in Advanced Dementia Position Statement. May 2013. www.americangeriatrics.org/files/documents/feeding.tubes.advanced.dementia.pdf. Accessed June 28, 2013.

10. American Medical Association. AMA Policy on Provision of Life-Sustaining Medical Treatment. www.ama-assn.org/ama/pub/physician-resources/medical-ethics/about-ethics-group/ethics-resource-center /end-of-life-care/ama-policy-provision-life-sustaining-medical.page? Accessed June 25, 2013.

11. American Medical Association. AMA Statement on End-of-Life Care. www.ama-assn.org/ama/pub/physician -resources/medical-ethics/about-ethics-group/ethics-resource-center/end-of-life-care/ama-statement-end-of -life-care.page?#. Accessed June 25, 2013.

12. American Nurses Association Board of Directors. Position Statement: Forgoing Nutrition and Hydration. 2011. www.nursingworld.org/MainMenuCategories/Policy-Advocacy/Positions-and-Resolutions/ANA PositionStatements/Position-Statements-Alphabetically/prtetnutr14451.pdf. Accessed June 23, 2013.

13. CMS Center for Clinical Standards and Quality/ Survey & Certification Group. F322 Feeding Tubes. Centers for Medicare & Medicaid Services. September 27, 2012. www.cms.gov/Medicare/Provider -Enrollment-and-Certification/SurveyCertificationGenInfo/Downloads/Survey-and-Cert-Letter-12-46.pdf. Accessed October 9, 2013.

14. Hospice and Palliative Nurses Association. HPNA Position Statement Artificial Nutrition and Hydration in Advanced Illness 2011. www.hpna.org/pdf/Artifical_Nutrition_and_Hydration_PDF.pdf. Accessed June 27, 2013.

15. NASW Standards for Social Work Practice in Palliative and End of Life Care 2013. www.socialworkers.org /practice/bereavement/standards. Accessed June 27, 2013.

16. Ethical and Religious Directives Issued by the United States Conference of Catholic Bishops. November 17, 2009. 5th ed. www.usccb.org/issues-and-action/human-life-and-dignity/health-care/upload/Ethical-Religious -Directives-Catholic-Health-Care-Services-fifth-edition-2009.pdf. Accessed December 11, 2013.

17. Preedy VR, ed. *Diet and Nutrition in Palliative Care*. Boca Raton, FL:CRC Press, 2011.

18. Schwartz DB. RD role in ethical decision-making for enteral and parenteral nutrition. *Today's Dietitian*. 2013;15(1):28.

19. Schwartz DB. Three Steps for Improving End-of-Life Nutrition Care. *Clin Nutr Insight*. 2012;38:4–5.

20. Schwartz DB. Clinical ethics and nutrition support. *J Nutr Therapeutics*. 2012;1:86–90. www.lifescience global.com/journals/journal-of-nutritional-therapeutics/current-issue.

21. Schwartz DB. Integrating patient-centered care and clinical ethics into nutrition practice. *Nutr Clin Pract*. October 2013;28:543–555.

APPENDIX

Resources on
Artificial Nutrition

Denise Baird Schwartz, MS, RD, CNSC, FADA, FAND, FASPEN

Definitions of Ethical and Legal Terms

- **Artificial nutrition and hydration**: Nutrition received in any form other than taking food and fluid through mouth (orally). This can be achieved through a nasogastric tube (NG), a gastrostomy tube (G tube) or percutaneous endoscopic gastrostomy (PEG) tube, a jejunostomy tube (J tube), a nasojejunal tube (NJ tube), or intravenous (IV) tube (peripheral) or central total parenteral nutrition (TPN).
- **Autonomy**: A multidimensional ethical concept. The ability and right of a capable person to decide his or her own course of action. Self-determination is a legal right.
- **Decisional capacity**: The ability of a person to make decisions. Adults are presumed capable unless declared incompetent by a court of law or judge. Some states require two physicians to determine decisional capacity of a particular person. Decisional capacity is specific to a point in time and a specific decision. A clinical evaluation of capacity centers on a person's ability to (a) take in information; (b) understand relevant information and apply it to his/her own condition; (c) have insight into condition and consequences of treatment options; (d) be able to communicate decision and reasoning for choices.
- **Evidence-based medicine**: A practice that is based on research, clinical expertise, and patient preferences that guides decision about health care of individual patients. Evidence-based clinical practice stresses use of research findings, quality improvement data (as appropriate), other operational and evaluation data, consensus of recognized experts, and affirmed experience to substantiate practice.
- **Forgoing life-sustaining treatment**: To do without a medical intervention that would be expected to extend a patient's life. Forgoing includes withholding (noninitiation) and withdrawing (stopping).
- **Health care agent or proxy**: A person appointed by the patient to make health care decisions if the patient becomes incapable of making her or his own decisions. The proxy has a responsibility

to act in accordance with the known preferences of patient; if preferences are not specifically known, the responsibility is to act on similar known preferences of the patient. Decisions made by the agent or proxy carry the same legal weight as if made by the patient.

- **Interdisciplinary team**: A group of health care professionals from diverse fields who work in a coordinated fashion toward a common goal for a patient.
- **Life-sustaining therapies**: Life-sustaining therapies include but are not limited to cardio-pulmonary resuscitation (CPR); cardiac support devices (pacemakers, internal cardioverters/defibrillators, intra-aortic balloon pumps) and cardiac medications; respiratory support devices (invasive and noninvasive mechanical ventilation), oxygen, and respiratory medications; renal support devices (dialysis in any form) and renal medications; blood products; parenteral and enteral nutrition and hydration; cancer treatments; and surgery.
- **Palliative care**: Care that aims to prevent and relieve suffering and to support best possible quality of life for patients and their families, regardless of stage of disease or needs for other therapies. A philosophy of care and an organized, highly structured system for delivering care. Expands the traditional disease-model medical treatments to include goals of enhancing the quality of life for patients and their families, optimizing function, helping with decision-making, and providing opportunities for personal growth. Can be delivered concurrently with life-prolonging care or be the main focus of care.
- **Proxy decision-making**: A type of decision-making allowed if a person lacks the capacity to make an informed choice. Such surrogate decisions are guided by written advanced directives or substituted judgments based on either the subjective knowledge of a person's values, views on quality of life, or goals, or the "best interest" of a person whose wishes and values are unknown based on the benefits-burden weighing of recommended actions.
- **Surrogate decision-maker**: Someone authorized to make decisions, usually medical or legal, for another person. The role of surrogate decision-maker is to make decisions for a patient that he or she thinks the patient would have made for himself or herself based on knowing the patient's values and previously expressed wishes.

Advanced Care Planning Resources for Health Care Professionals and the Public

- *Breathe* by Anne Bland (www.breathe-annebland.com): A health care professional tells her personal story to help individuals begin dialogue with family about end-of-life health care decisions. Focus is on dealing with family relationships, religion, and values that impact health care decisions. The book is intended for the public and health care professionals.
- **Consider the Conversation** (www.considertheconversation.org): Consider the Conversation uses film to inspire person-centered care. The goal is to inspire cultural change that results in end-of-life care that is more person-centered and less system-centered.
- **The Conversation Project** (www.theconversationproject.org): Developed in collaboration with Institute for Healthcare Improvement, this project aims to have every person's end-of-life preferences expressed and respected. The project provides a starter kit to help gather one's thoughts and then have conversations with a loved one on wishes for end-of-life care.
- **Five Wishes—Aging With Dignity** (www.agingwithdignity.org/five-wishes.php): Five Wishes is a useful guide and documentation tool of individuals' wishes, written in everyday language. It helps start and structure important conversations about care in times of serious illness.

- **National Healthcare Decisions Day** (www.nhdd.org): National Healthcare Decisions Day is a collaborative effort of national, state, and community organizations in the United States with the goal of inspiring, educating, and empowering the public and providers about importance of advance care planning. The site provides specific resources for activities to promote National Healthcare Decisions Day (held annually on April 16). These resources are provided as templates and can be adapted to include local contacts and other information as needed.
- **Physician Orders for Life-Sustaining Treatment** (www.polst.org): This is a paradigm program designed to improve quality of care people receive at the end of life. Emphasis is on effective communication of patient wishes. Materials include documentation of medical orders on a brightly colored form and a promise by health care professionals to honor these wishes.
- **PREPARE** (www.prepareforyourcare.org): An online program that can help individuals make medical decisions for themselves and others, talk with their doctors, and get medical care that is right for them. Written at a fifth-grade reading level; features large type, voice-overs, and how-to videos.
- **Speak Up Campaign** (www.advancecareplanning.ca): This campaign promotes advance care planning in Canada and raises awareness of issues related to an aging population, a strained health care system, and end-of-life care. Speak Up Campaign Kit contains material to promote advance care planning.

Index

Page number followed by *b* indicates a box; *f* indicates a figure; *t* indicates a table.